Genitourinary Emergencies

Guest Editor

JONATHAN E. DAVIS, MD, FACEP, FAAEM

EMERGENCY MEDICINE CLINICS OF NORTH AMERICA

www.emed.theclinics.com

Consulting Editor

AMAL MATTU, MD

August 2011 • Volume 29 • Number 3

SAUNDERS an imprint of ELSEVIER, Inc.

W.B. SAUNDERS COMPANY

A Division of Elsevier Inc.

1600 John F. Kennedy Boulevard • Suite 1800 • Philadelphia, Pennsylvania 19103-2899

http://www.theclinics.com

EMERGENCY MEDICINE CLINICS OF NORTH AMERICA Volume 29, Number 3
August 2011 ISSN 0733-8627, ISBN-13: 978-1-4557-1036-2

Editor: Patrick Manley
Developmental Editor: Donald Mumford

Emergency Medicine Clinics of North America (ISSN 0733-8627) is published quarterly by Elsevier Inc., 360 Park Avenue South, New York, NY, 10010-1710. Months of issue are February, May, August, and November. Business and Editorial Offices: 1600 John F. Kennedy Boulevard, Suite 1800, Philadelphia, PA 19103-2899. Customer Service Office: 6277 Sea Harbor Drive, Orlando, FL 32887-4800. Periodicals postage paid at New York, NY, and additional mailing offices. Subscription prices are $133.00 per year (US students), $264.00 per year (US individuals), $455.00 per year (US institutions), $189.00 per year (international students), $379.00 per year (international individuals), $549.00 per year (international institutions), $189.00 per year (Canadian students), $326.00 per year (Canadian individuals), and $549.00 per year (Canadian institutions). International air speed delivery is included in all *Clinics'* subscription prices. All prices are subject to change without notice. **POSTMASTER:** Send address changes to *Emergency Medicine Clinics of North America*, Elsevier Periodicals Customer Service, 11830 Westline Industrial Drive, St. Louis, MO 63146. Customer Service (orders, claims, online, change of address): Elsevier Periodicals Customer Service, 11830 Westline Industrial Drive, St. Louis, MO 63146. Tel: 1-800-654-2452 (U.S. and Canada); 314-453-7041 (outside U.S. and Canada). Fax: 314-453-5170. E-mail: journalscustomerservice-usa@elsevier.com (for print support); journalsonline support-usa@elsevier.com (for online support).

Reprints. For copies of 100 or more of articles in this publication, please contact the Commercial Reprints Department, Elsevier Inc., 360 Park Avenue South, New York, NY 10010-1710. Tel.: 212-633-3812; Fax: 212-462-1935; E-mail: reprints@elsevier.com.

Emergency Medicine Clinics of North America is covered in *MEDLINE/PubMed (Index Medicus), Current Contents/Clinical Medicine, EMBASE/Excerpta Medica, BIOSIS, SciSearch, CINAHL, ISI/BIOMED,* and *Research Alert.*

Printed and bound by CPI Group (UK) Ltd, Croydon, CR0 4YY

Transferred to Digital Print 2011

Contributors

CONSULTING EDITOR

AMAL MATTU, MD, FAAEM, FACEP
Program Director, Emergency Medicine Residency; Professor, Department of Emergency Medicine, University of Maryland School of Medicine, Baltimore, Maryland

GUEST EDITOR

JONATHAN E. DAVIS, MD, FACEP, FAAEM
Associate Program Director, Georgetown University Hospital and Washington Hospital Center; Associate Professor of Emergency Medicine, Georgetown University School of Medicine, Washington, DC

AUTHORS

MICHAEL S. ANTONIS, DO, RDMS, FACEP
Assistant Professor of Clinical Emergency Medicine, Georgetown University School of Medicine; Director, Emergency Medicine Ultrasound, and Emergency Medicine Ultrasound Fellowship, Department of Emergency Medicine, MedStar Health: Washington Hospital Center and Georgetown University, Washington, DC

RAHUL G. BHAT, MD, FACEP
Assistant Professor of Clinical Emergency Medicine, Department of Emergency Medicine, Georgetown University Hospital; Washington Hospital Center, Washington, DC

DIANE M. BIRNBAUMER, MD
Professor of Medicine; Associate Program Director, Department of Emergency Medicine, Harbor University of California, Los Angeles Medical Center, David Geffen School of Medicine at University of California, Los Angeles, Torrance, California

MICHAEL BLAIVAS, MD, RDMS, FACEP
Professor of Emergency Medicine; Associate Professor of Internal Medicine, Department of Emergency Medicine, Northside Hospital Forsyth, Atlanta, Georgia

JOELLE BORHART, MD
Attending Physician, Department of Emergency Medicine, Georgetown University/ Washington Hospital Center, Washington, DC

JONATHAN E. DAVIS, MD, FACEP, FAAEM
Associate Program Director, Georgetown University Hospital and Washington Hospital Center; Associate Professor of Emergency Medicine, Georgetown University School of Medicine, Washington, DC

HEATHER K. DEVORE, MD
Clinical Instructor, Department of Emergency Medicine, Washington Hospital Center and Georgetown University; Medical Director, District of Columbia Sexual Assault Nurse Examiner Program, Washington, DC

JEFFREY DUBIN, MD, MBA
Vice Chairman, Department of Emergency Medicine, Washington Hospital Center; Assistant Professor of Clinical Emergency Medicine, Georgetown University School of Medicine, Washington, DC

AUTUMN GRAHAM, MD
Assistant Residency Director of Education, Department of Emergency Medicine, Washington Hospital Center, Georgetown University, Washington, DC

JOHN M. HOWELL, MD
Department of Emergency Medicine, Inova Fairfax Hospital/Inova Fairfax Hospital for Children, Falls Church, Virginia

KORIN B. HUDSON, MD, FACEP
Assistant Professor, Department of Emergency Medicine, Georgetown University Hospital and Washington Hospital Center, Washington, DC

TAMARA A. KATY, MD, FAAP
Assistant Professor of Clinical Pediatrics and Emergency Medicine, Georgetown University Hospital, Washington, DC

DAVID R. LANE, MD
Assistant Professor and Clerkship Director, Department of Emergency Medicine, Georgetown University Hospital & Washington Hospital Center, Georgetown University School of Medicine, Washington, DC

SAMUEL LUBER, MD, MPH
Assistant Professor, Program Director Emergency Medicine Residency, Department of Emergency Medicine, University of Texas Health Sciences Center at Houston, Houston, Texas

NORINE A. MCGRATH, MD
Attending Physician, Department of Emergency Medicine, Georgetown University Hospital, Washington Hospital Center, Washington, DC

CAROLYN A. PHILLIPS, MD, RDMS, FACEP
Associate Director, Emergency Medicine Ultrasound, and Emergency Medicine Ultrasound Fellowship, Department of Emergency Medicine, MedStar Health: Washington Hospital Center, Washington, DC

FREDERICK C. PLACE, MD
Clinical Assistant Professor of Pediatrics, INOVA Fairfax Hospital, Virginia Commonwealth University, Falls Church, Virginia

KEVIN C. REED, MD
Assistant Professor, Department of Emergency Medicine, Georgetown University Hospital, Washington, DC

CAROLYN J. SACHS, MD, MPH
Associate Professor of Medicine, Departments of Emergency Medicine and Medicine, University of California, Los Angeles, Los Angeles; Medical Director, Forensic Nurse Specialists, Orange County, Los Alamitos, California

GILLIAN SCHMITZ, MD
Assistant Professor, Department of Emergency Medicine, Georgetown University, Washington Hospital Center, Washington, DC

SANJAY SHEWAKRAMANI, MD
Assistant Professor, Department of Emergency Medicine, Georgetown University Hospital, Washington, DC

MICHAEL SILVERMAN, MD
Chairman, Department of Emergency Medicine, Virginia Hospital Center, Arlington, Virginia; Instructor of Emergency Medicine, The Johns Hopkins University School of Medicine, Baltimore, Maryland

RICHARD SINERT, DO
Associate Professor of Emergency Medicine, Department of Emergency Medicine, State University of New York Downstate Medical Center, Brooklyn, New York

SUKHJIT S. TAKHAR, MD
Attending Physician, Department of Emergency Medicine, Brigham and Women's Hospital; Harvard Medical School, Boston, Massachusetts

CARRIE TIBBLES, MD
Associate Director, Department of Graduate Medical Education; Attending Physician, Harvard Affiliated Emergency Medicine Residency, Beth Israel Deaconess Medical Center, Boston, Massachusetts

ALLAN B. WOLFSON, MD
Professor of Emergency Medicine; Program Director Emergency Medicine Residency, Department of Emergency Medicine, University of Pittsburgh, Pittsburgh, Pennsylvania

Contents

Foreword: Genitourinary Emergencies in Emergency Medicine xiii

Amal Mattu

Preface xv

Jonathan E. Davis

Scrotal Emergencies 469

Jonathan E. Davis and Michael Silverman

An acute scrotum is defined as an acute painful swelling of the scrotum or its contents, accompanied by local signs or general symptoms. Early identification and skillful management of testicular torsion is critical, as it may threaten testicular viability and future fertility if not managed expediently and appropriately. The cremasteric reflex and testicular sonography are frequently used, yet imperfect, diagnostic tools in assessing for testicular torsion. Other emergent conditions include incarcerated inguinal hernia, Fournier's gangrene, and any form of genitourinary trauma until proven otherwise. This article reviews the evaluation and management of the acute scrotum in the emergency department.

Penile Emergencies 485

Jeffrey Dubin and Jonathan E. Davis

The penis is a very sensitive organ and even minor injury or discomfort may cause a patient to seek emergency evaluation. Emergency practitioners must be most concerned with the entities that, if left untreated, can result in ischemia and necrosis of the penis, namely ischemic priapism, paraphimosis, and entrapment injury. Any penile trauma should be considered an emergency until proven otherwise. This article discusses emergent penile complaints in adults, with emphasis on the most serious and common conditions.

Genitourinary Trauma 501

Sanjay Showakramani and Kevin C. Reed

Injury to the genitourinary (GU) tract occurs in up to 10% of all traumas, with the kidneys being the most frequently affected. Trauma to different areas of the GU tract can be caused in a variety of ways, and the diagnostics and management of the injuries vary widely depending on the mechanism and location. Overall, fatalities from GU trauma are not common. However, significant morbidity can occur without prompt recognition and appropriate intervention. A basic understanding of urologic trauma is necessary for all emergency practitioners when caring for trauma patients.

Urolithiasis in the Emergency Department 519

Autumn Graham, Samuel Luber, and Allan B. Wolfson

Urolithiasis commonly presents to the emergency department with acute, severe, unilateral flank pain. Patients with a suspected first-time stone or atypical presentation should be evaluated with a noncontrast computed tomography scan to confirm the diagnosis and rule out alternative diagnoses. Narcotics remain the mainstay of pain management but in select patients, nonsteroidal anti-inflammatories alone or in combination with narcotics provide safe and effective analgesia in the emergency department. Whereas most kidney stones can be managed with pain control and expectant management, obstructing kidney stones with a suspected proximal urinary tract infection are urological emergencies requiring emergent decompression, antibiotics, and resuscitation.

Diagnosis and Management of Urinary Tract Infection and Pyelonephritis **539**

David R. Lane and Sukhjit S. Takhar

Urinary tract infections (UTIs) are the most common bacterial infections treated in the outpatient setting and range in severity from minimally symptomatic cystitis to severe septic shock in a wide array of patients. Diagnosis of uncomplicated cystitis can be inferred from history and physical, and confirmed by urinalysis. Appropriate antimicrobial therapy should rapidly improve symptoms in all UTIs. Treatment can be further tailored according to severity of illness, analysis of individualized risk factors, and antimicrobial resistance patterns. This article discusses treatment options in light of bacterial resistance in the twenty-first century.

Genitourinary Imaging in the Emergency Department **553**

Michael S. Antonis, Carolyn A. Phillips, and Michael Blaivas

The emergency medicine (EM) specialist has a wide-ranging armamentarium of imaging modalities available for use in the patient with genitourinary complaints. This article covers the various imaging options, with a discussion of the advantages and disadvantages of each of these different modalities. Special emphasis is placed on point-of-care EM ultrasound performed by the EM specialist at the patient bedside.

Renal Failure: Emergency Evaluation and Management **569**

Korin B. Hudson and Richard Sinert

Patients with altered renal function are frequently encountered in the emergency department (ED) and emergency physicians often play an important role in the evaluation and management of renal disease. Early recognition, diagnosis, prevention of further iatrogenic injury, and management of renal disease have important implications for long-term morbidity and mortality. This article reviews basic renal physiology, discusses the differential diagnosis and approach to therapy, as well as strategies to prevent further renal injury, for adult patients who present to the ED with renal injury or failure.

Emergency Department Management of Sexually Transmitted Infections **587**

Joelle Borhart and Diane M. Birnbaumer

Patients seeking treatment for sexually transmitted infections (STIs) account for a large number of emergency department (ED) visits per year.

Despite the large volume of patients, STIs are often missed or treated inappropriately. Due to the high prevalence and incidence of STIs in the United States, it is important that emergency practitioners recognize symptoms consistent with STIs, and treat presumptively. This practice leads to overtreatment of STIs; however, when weighed against the public health risk and complications of untreated disease, empiric treatment is recommended. This article provides an overview of STIs encountered in the ED and recommendations for their treatment.

Sexual Assault **605**

Heather K. DeVore and Carolyn J. Sachs

Sexual assault is a problem that permeates all socioeconomic classes and impacts hundreds of thousands in the United States and millions worldwide. Most victims do not report the assault; those that do often present to an emergency department. Care must encompass the patients' physical and emotional needs. Providers must be cognizant regarding handling of evidence and possible legal ramifications. This article discusses the emergency medicine approach to history taking, physical examination, evidence collection, chain of custody, psychological and medical treatment, and appropriate follow-up. Special circumstances discussed include intimate partner violence, male examinations, pediatric examinations, suspect examinations, and drug-facilitated assaults.

Genitourinary Emergencies in the Nonpregnant Woman **621**

Gillian Schmitz and Carrie Tibbles

Lower abdominal and pelvic pains are common symptoms in women who present to the emergency department (ED). Once pregnancy has been ruled out, attention should focus on other potential life or fertility threats. Ultrasound remains the most helpful initial diagnostic modality. Time-sensitive and serious conditions, such as large ovarian masses or abnormal vaginal bleeding, need gynecologic consultation. Because many patients do not have access to primary care, ED physicians should be familiar with the treatment of sexually transmitted diseases. However, most nonpregnant women with pelvic complaints can safely be managed in the outpatient setting after ED evaluation.

Pediatric Urinary Tract Infections **637**

Rahul G. Bhat, Tamara A. Katy, and Frederick C. Place

Urinary tract infections (UTIs) in children are commonly seen in the emergency department and pose several challenges to establishing the proper diagnosis and determining management. This article reviews pediatric UTI and addresses epidemiology, diagnosis, treatment, and imaging, and their importance to the practicing emergency medicine provider. Accurate and timely diagnosis of pediatric UTI can prevent short-term complications, such as severe pyelonephritis or sepsis, and long-term sequelae including scarring of the kidneys, hypertension, and ultimately chronic renal insufficiency and need for transplant.

Pediatric Genitourinary Emergencies **655**

Norine A. McGrath, John M. Howell, and Jonathan E. Davis

Pediatric medical complaints and differential diagnoses often vary from adults, requiring a specialized knowledge base and behavioral skill set. This article addresses a variety of congenital and acquired pediatric genitourinary disorders. Genitourinary emergencies include paraphismosis, priapism, serious infection, significant traumatic injury and gonadal torsion.

Index **667**

FORTHCOMING ISSUES

November 2011

Cardiovascular Emergencies

J. Stephen Bohan, MD, and
Joshua M. Kosowsky, MD,
Guest Editors

February 2012

Cardiac Arrest

William Brady, MD,
Nathan Charlton, MD,
Ben Lavner, MD, and
Sara Sutherland, MD, *Guest Editors*

May 2012

Thoracic Emergencies

Joel Turner, MD, *Guest Editor*

RECENT ISSUES

May 2011

Gastrointestinal Emergencies

Angela M. Mills, MD, and
Anthony J. Dean, MD, *Guest Editors*

February 2011

Seizures

Andy Jagoda, MD, and
Edward P. Sloan, MD, MPH,
Guest Editors

November 2010

Orthopedic Emergencies

Michael C. Bond, MD, *Guest Editor*

RELATED INTEREST

Ultrasound Clinics, January 2008, Vol. 3, No. 1 (pages 1–178)
Emergency Ultrasound
Vikram S. Dogra, MD, and Shweta Bhatt, MD, *Guest Editors*

GOAL STATEMENT

The goal of *Emergency Medicine Clinics of North America* is to keep practicing physicians up to date with current clinical practice in emergency medicine by providing timely articles reviewing the state of the art in patient care.

ACCREDITATION

The *Emergency Medical Clinics of North America* is planned and implemented in accordance with the Essential Areas and Policies of the Accreditation Council for Continuing Medical Education (ACCME) through the joint sponsorship of the University of Virginia School of Medicine and Elsevier. The University of Virginia School of Medicine is accredited by the ACCME to provide continuing medical education for physicians.

The University of Virginia School of Medicine designates this educational activity for a maximum of 15 *AMA PRA Category 1 Credits*™ for each issue, 60 credits per year. Physicians should only claim credit commensurate with the extent of their participation in the activity.

The American Medical Association has determined that physicians not licensed in the US who participate in this CME activity are eligible for a maximum of 15 *AMA PRA Category 1 Credits*™ for each issue, 60 credits per year.

The Emergency Medicine Clinics of North America CME program is approved by the American College of Emergency Physicians for 60 hours of ACEP Category I Credit per year.

Credit can be earned by reading the text material, taking the CME examination online at http://www.theclinics.com/home/cme, and completing the evaluation. After taking the test, you will be required to review any and all incorrect answers. Following completion of the test and evaluation, your credit will be awarded and you may print your certificate.

FACULTY DISCLOSURE/CONFLICT OF INTEREST

The University of Virginia School of Medicine, as an ACCME accredited provider, endorses and strives to comply with the Accreditation Council for Continuing Medical Education (ACCME) Standards of Commercial Support, Commonwealth of Virginia statutes, University of Virginia policies and procedures, and associated federal and private regulations and guidelines on the need for disclosure and monitoring of proprietary and financial interests that may affect the scientific integrity and balance of content delivered in continuing medical education activities under our auspices.

The University of Virginia School of Medicine requires that all CME activities accredited through this institution be developed independently and be scientifically rigorous, balanced and objective in the presentation/discussion of its content, theories and practices.

All authors/editors participating in an accredited CME activity are expected to disclose to the readers relevant financial relationships with commercial entities occurring within the past 12 months (such as grants or research support, employee, consultant, stock holder, member of speakers bureau, etc.). The University of Virginia School of Medicine will employ appropriate mechanisms to resolve potential conflicts of interest to maintain the standards of fair and balanced education to the reader. Questions about specific strategies can be directed to the Office of Continuing Medical Education, University of Virginia School of Medicine, Charlottesville, Virginia.

The faculty and staff of the University of Virginia Office of Continuing Medical Education have no financial affiliations to disclose.

The authors/editors listed below have identified no professional or financial affiliations for themselves or their spouse/partner:

Michael S. Antonis, DO, RDMS; Rahul G. Bhat, MD; Diane M. Birnbaumer, MD; Michael Blaivas, MD, RDMS; Joelle Borhart, MD; Jonathan E. Davis, MD (Guest Editor); Heather K. DeVore, MD; Jeffrey Dubin, MD, MBA; Autumn Graham, MD; John M. Howell, MD; Korin B. Hudson, MD; Tamara A. Katy, MD; David R. Lane, MD; Samuel Luber, MD, MPH; Patrick Manley, (Acquisitions Editor); Amal Mattu, MD (Consulting Editor); Norine A. McGrath, MD; Carolyn A. Phillips, MD, RDMS; Frederick C. Place, MD; Kevin C. Reed, MD; Carolyn J. Sachs, MD, MPH; Gillian Schmitz, MD; Sanjay Shewakramani, MD; Michael Silverman, MD; Richard Sinert, DO; Sukhjit S. Takhar, MD; Carrie Tibbles, MD; Allan B. Wolfson, MD; and Bill Woods, MD (Test Author).

Disclosure of Discussion of Non-FDA Approved Uses for Pharmaceutical Products and/or Medical Devices

The University of Virginia School of Medicine, as an ACCME provider, requires that all faculty presenters identify and disclose any off-label uses for pharmaceutical and medical device products. The University of Virginia School of Medicine recommends that each physician fully review all the available data on new products or procedures prior to clinical use.

TO ENROLL

To enroll in the Emergency Medicine Clinics of North America Continuing Medical Education program, call customer service at 1-800-654-2452 or visit us online at www.theclinics.com/home/cme. The CME program is available to subscribers for an additional fee of $190.00.

Foreword

Genitourinary Emergencies in Emergency Medicine

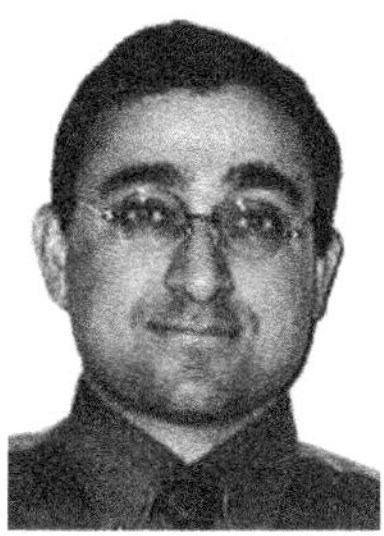

Amal Mattu, MD
Consulting Editor

One of my former medical school professors once referred to the genitourinary (GU) system as *the* most important system of the human body. He went on to describe the GU system as the reason that we all *can* live as well as the reason that we all *want* to live. Without a properly functioning GU system, waste products would build up and cause us to die within days. The GU system also is responsible for mankind's ability to reproduce and carry on the species. His point was well-taken.

Maladies of the GU system, especially sexual transmitted infections, have affected historical figures such as Hitler, Beethoven, Van Gogh, Al Capone, Napoleon, the Tsar of Russia, Churchill, and King Henry VII. Urinary system diseases, including kidney failure, have affected other well-known figures such as Mozart, James Michener, Emily Dickenson, Erma Bombeck, Art Buchwald, Barry White, and even the beloved fictional character Tiny Tim from the Charles Dickens classic *A Christmas Carol*. But for every celebrity and historical figure afflicted with a disease of the GU system are countless tens of thousands of others whose lives have been changed or lost. Although cardiovascular, neurological, and gastrointestinal diseases receive far more attention in emergency medicine, there's no question that GU diseases are common and associated with significant morbidity and even mortality in our patients.

In this issue of *Emergency Medicine Clinics of North America*, Guest Editor Dr Jonathan Davis has assembled an outstanding group of authors to educate us on this vital aspect of our specialty. Articles discuss core topics such as kidney disease, urinary tract infections, and sexually transmitted infections. Special focus is placed throughout also on conditions that may affect reproductive viability such as testicular torsion and acute ovarian pathologies. Special articles are added focusing on GU tract trauma, specific pediatric disorders, sexual assault, and special imaging techniques. The contributors have also added articles focusing on less common but critically important topics such as Fournier's gangrene, paraphimosis, and entrapment injuries.

Emerg Med Clin N Am 29 (2011) xiii–xiv
doi:10.1016/j.emc.2011.06.002 emed.theclinics.com
0733-8627/11/$ – see front matter

This issue of *Clinics* represents an important addition to the emergency medicine literature. It is perhaps one of the only resources ever published that focuses on the spectrum of GU emergencies encountered in emergency medicine practice. It will certainly bring greater knowledge to an important but often neglected area of the emergency medicine core curriculum. Whether or not one considers the GU system the most important body system, there's no doubt that this issue of *Clinics* will serve as one of your most important resources to keep on hand during routine emergency medicine practice. Kudos to Dr Davis and the authors for this outstanding work!

Amal Mattu, MD
Department of Emergency Medicine
University of Maryland School of Medicine
110 S. Paca Street, 6th Floor, Suite 200
Baltimore, MD 21201, USA

E-mail address:
amattu@smail.umaryland.edu

Preface

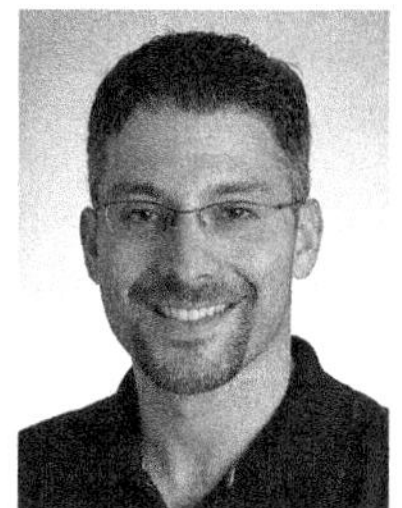

Jonathan E. Davis, MD
Guest Editor

Genitourinary (GU) complaints can be quite distressing for the patient, parent, or caretaker (and even, at times, for the health care provider!). Presentations may be delayed as a result of embarrassment or apprehension. The emergency care provider must remain particularly sensitive to both the emotional and the physical needs of the patient. Furthermore, certain GU conditions such as testicular torsion are particularly high risk from a medicolegal perspective.[1,2]

The goal of this issue of *Emergency Clinics* is to provide an evidence-based, best practice approach to the patient presenting to the emergency department (ED) with a complaint involving the GU system. Useful pearls for daily practice, as well as areas of treachery and avoidable pitfalls, are highlighted throughout.

This issue will tackle a wide spectrum of GU diagnoses in adult and pediatric patients, both male and female, including medical and surgical disorders. Updates in the classification and management of kidney disease, sexually transmitted infections, imaging of the GU system, and in the approach to sexual assault will be presented. Special considerations for GU conditions in the pediatric patient will also be covered.

The challenge in emergency practice is often to differentiate conditions requiring prompt evaluation and action from less urgent conditions. Missed or delayed diagnosis of testicular or ovarian torsion threatens gonadal viability and future fertility. Infectious conditions such as Fournier's gangrene, obstructing/infected ureteral calculus, or ascending urinary tract infection may lead to rapid deterioration and septic shock. Emergent penile conditions include priapism, paraphimosis, and entrapment injury. Traumatic injury to the GU tract should be presumed an emergency in all but the most minor cases until proven otherwise.

Contributors to this issue include emergency medicine specialists with additional training and expertise in nephrology, urology, and infectious disease. Senior authors with extensive experience and background in their respective content areas have been kind enough to contribute their collective wisdom from the trenches.

A project of this scope is not possible without the contributions of many dedicated individuals. I would like to thank the faculty of the Georgetown University/Washington Hospital Center Emergency Medicine Residency Program for their dedication, our departmental leadership for their support, and our residents for their constant inspiration.

Emerg Med Clin N Am 29 (2011) xv–xvi
doi:10.1016/j.emc.2011.06.001 **emed.theclinics.com**
0733-8627/11/$ – see front matter

I would also like to thank my wife and children—you are a source of perpetual strength, grounding, and encouragement that forever reminds me of the really important things in life.

It is my hope that you will find this issue to be both practical and useful in providing the best possible care for your patients in the ED each and every day.

Jonathan E. Davis, MD
Georgetown University Hospital
and Washington Hospital Center
Georgetown University School of Medicine
3800 Reservoir Road, NW, Washington, DC 20007, USA

E-mail address:
jdthere@yahoo.com

REFERENCES

1. Matteson JR, Stock JA, Hanna MK, et al. Medicolegal aspects of testicular torsion. Urology 2001;57(4):783–7.
2. Selbst SM, Friedman MJ, Singh SB. Epidemiology and etiology of malpractice lawsuits involving children in US emergency departments and urgent care centers. Pediatr Emerg Care 2005;21(3):165–9.

Scrotal Emergencies

Jonathan E. Davis, MD[a,*], Michael Silverman, MD[b,c]

KEYWORDS

• Male • Genital • Emergency • Scrotum • Testicle • Torsion

Although acute scrotal pain comprises fewer than 1% of overall emergency department (ED) visits, this presentation may provoke great anxiety for the patient or caretaker given its highly sensitive nature.[1] An acute scrotum is defined as an acute painful swelling of the scrotum or its contents, accompanied by local signs or general symptoms.[2] Although the list of diagnostic possibilities for a patient with an undifferentiated acute scrotum is extensive, early identification and skillful management of testicular torsion is critical, as it may threaten testicular viability and future fertility if not managed expediently and appropriately. Differentiating this genitourinary (GU) emergency from alternative conditions takes precedence over definitive diagnosis. The cremasteric reflex and testicular sonography are frequently used, yet imperfect, diagnostic tools in assessing for testicular torsion. Other emergent conditions include necrotizing fasciitis of the perineum (Fournier's disease), incarcerated or strangulated inguinal hernia, and any form of GU trauma until proven otherwise. This article reviews the evaluation and management of the acute scrotum in the ED setting.

DIFFERENTIAL DIAGNOSIS

A diligent and focused history and physical examination of the male complaining of acute scrotal symptoms is the cornerstone of formulating an appropriate plan of action. One of the most challenging aspects of scrotal complaints is that a wide variety of clinical conditions may present in a similar fashion: a male patient complaining of an acute, painful, swollen, and tender hemiscrotum. Indeed, the differential diagnosis of the acute scrotum is extensive (**Table 1**).

For patients presenting with an acute scrotum, several life-threatening or fertility-threatening conditions should always be considered and ruled out: testicular torsion, Fournier's disease, or incarcerated/strangulated inguinal hernia. When scrotal pain is associated with systemic symptoms, such as nausea or vomiting, additional vigilance is prudent in searching for these dangerous conditions. The 3 aforementioned conditions can occur at any age. With this said, Fournier's disease tends to occur in adult

[a] Department of Emergency Medicine, Georgetown University Hospital & Washington Hospital Center, 3800 Reservoir Road, NW, Washington, DC, 20007, USA
[b] Department of Emergency Medicine, Virginia Hospital Center, 1701 North George Mason Drive, Arlington, VA 22205, USA
[c] The Johns Hopkins University School of Medicine, Baltimore, MD, USA
* Corresponding author.
E-mail address: jed27@georgetown.edu

Emerg Med Clin N Am 29 (2011) 469–484
doi:10.1016/j.emc.2011.04.011
emed.theclinics.com

Table 1
Differential diagnosis of scrotal pain

Diagnosis	Symptoms	Signs	Evaluation
Appendage torsion	Typically a more indolent onset of symptoms compared with testicular torsion; less likely to present with nausea or vomiting	Tender nodule typically at head of testicle or epididymis; blue dot sign pathognomonic	US examination may demonstrate infarcted appendage
Epididymitis	Typically a more indolent onset of symptoms compared with testicular torsion; less likely to present with nausea or vomiting	*Early*: firmness and nodularity isolated to epididymis. *Late*: with progression, inflammation may become contiguous with testicle (termed epididymo-orchitis)	US examination may reveal increased intratesticular blood flow, although this is a nonspecific finding
Epididymo-orchitis	More likely to present with systemic findings, including nausea, vomiting, fever	Large, swollen scrotal mass typically with indistinct border between testicle and epididymis	US examination may reveal increased intratesticular blood flow, although this is a nonspecific finding
Fournier's disease	Perineal pain, swelling, redness; fever, vomiting, lethargy	May present with an absence of visible local findings on skin inspection in early stages (pain out of proportion to examination); ecchymosis, crepitus, necrotic eschar may be present in more advanced disease	Emergent surgical consultation for debridement, broad-spectrum antimicrobials
Hematocele	Large, painful scrotal mass; often antecedent history of trauma	Ecchymoses of scrotal skin; testicular tenderness or firmness	US examination may reveal fluid-filled tunica vaginalis
Hernia	Unilateral inguinal or scrotal swelling and pain	Reducible, incarcerated and strangulated forms; incarcerated/strangulated hernia may be particularly tender on examination	Emergent surgical consultation when incarcerated or strangulated; outpatient surgical referral reasonable if readily reducible
Hydrocele	Typically a gradual progression of swelling	Scrotal transillumination may be helpful	US examination may reveal fluid-filled tunica vaginalis
Idiopathic scrotal edema	Typically unilateral scrotal swelling and edema; primarily seen in children younger than 10 years	Scrotal, perineal, inguinal erythema and edema; may be difficult to distinguish from an acute skin-soft tissue infection	US examination
Orchitis	Typically gradual onset of unilateral (or bilateral) testicular swelling and pain	Swelling and tenderness isolated to testis/testes without epididymal involvement	US examination; often seen in conjunction with other systemic diseases (viral, other); treatment is disease specific

(*continued on next page*)

Table 1
(continued)

Diagnosis	Symptoms	Signs	Evaluation
Scrotal skin infection	Variable depending on cause	Must distinguish between lesions localized to scrotal wall and those contiguous with deeper scrotal structures	US or CT imaging may be helpful in determining the depth and extent of involvement if invasive process suspected
Testicular torsion	Typically a sudden and severe onset of pain; more likely to be associated with nausea or emesis	Classic findings include an elevated testis with a transverse lie	Emergent surgery consultation in high-probability cases
Trauma	History of blunt or penetrating mechanism of injury	Variable depending on mechanism	US examination; low threshold for surgical consultation in all but the most minor injuries
Tumor	Typically a gradually progressive testicular mass; may be painless or painful	May palpate testicular mass, firmness, or induration	US examination
Varicocele	Typically a gradual onset of unilateral swelling, often painless	Abnormally enlarged spermatic cord (pampiniform) venous plexus (often described as a "bag of worms")	US examination
Vasculitis (eg, HSP)	Testicular swelling and pain	Associated vasculitis findings (such as buttock/lower extremity purpura and renal involvement in HSP)	US examination, other diagnostic testing guided by suspected cause (eg, complete blood count, serum electrolytes with renal function in HSP)

Abbreviations: CT, computed tomography; HSP, Henoch-Schönlein purpura; US, ultrasonography.

patients, whereas incarcerated inguinal hernia is most common at the extremes of age, particularly in the first year of life.[3]

Although the differential is extensive and includes relatively rare life threats such as strangulated inguinal hernia and Fournier's gangrene, the acute scrotum can frequently be distilled to 3 principal diagnostic possibilities: testicular torsion, epididymitis, and appendage torsion[4]; this serves to better focus the ED evaluation. Testicular torsion is the fertility threat that needs to be ruled out. There is, however, significant overlap in the clinical signs and symptoms of these 3 conditions (**Table 2**).[5] Appendage torsion results from twisting of an appendage, which are embryologic remnants without known physiologic function (**Fig. 1**). Testicular torsion and epididymitis are the principal diagnostic considerations in the adult.[4]

The vast majority of series reported in the medical literature addressing the diagnosis and management of the acute scrotum are limited to pediatric cohorts, although testicular torsion in adults does occur.[6] The frequency of testicular torsion, appendage torsion, and epididymitis in children varies significantly from study to study. Differences in factors such as the age distribution and study setting make it difficult to draw definitive conclusions from the available data.[7,8] With this said, each of these

Table 2
Differentiating characteristics of testicular torsion, epididymitis, and appendage torsion

	Testicular Torsion	Epididymitis	Appendage Torsion
Historical Features			
Age	Incidence peaks in neonatal and adolescent groups, but may occur at any age	Primarily adolescents and adults, but may occur at any age	Typically prepubertal males
Risk factors	Undescended testicle (neonate), rapid increase in testicular size (adolescent), failure of prior orchiopexy	Sexual activity/ promiscuity, genitourinary anomalies, genitourinary instrumentation	Presence of appendages
Pain onset	Sudden	Gradual	Gradual or sudden
Prior episodes of similar pain	Possible (spontaneous detorsion)	Unlikely	Occasional
History of trauma	Possible	Possible	Possible
Nausea/vomiting	More likely	Less likely	Less likely
Dysuria	Less likely	More likely	Less likely
Physical Findings			
Fever	Less likely	More likely, particularly in advanced disease (epididymo-orchitis)	Less likely
Location of swelling/ tenderness	Testicle, progressing to diffuse hemiscrotal involvement	Epididymis, progressing to diffuse hemiscrotal involvement	Localized to head of affected testicle or epididymis
Cremasteric reflex	Testicular torsion less likely if present	May be present or absent	May be present or absent
Testicle position	High riding testicle, transverse alignment	Normal position, vertical alignment	Normal position, vertical alignment
Pyuria	Less likely	More likely	Less likely

diagnoses contributes to roughly one-third of pediatric acute scrotum cases in series from surgery or urology services.[9] However, this probably does not reflect the patient mixture seen in the ED setting. In fact, a recent large retrospective series from a pediatric ED (patients aged 0–18 years) showed a testicular torsion rate of only 3.3% in 523 patient visits reviewed.[5] The incidence was even lower than the 12% to 16% incidence of testicular torsion found in other ED-based studies.[1,10–12] In this same series, epididymitis and appendage torsion accounted for 32% and 8%, respectively. Of importance, scrotal pain of unknown etiology was the most frequent (34%) final diagnosis.

In another review of consecutive cases presenting to a children's hospital ED, the most common diagnosis varied by age group: testicular torsion in the first year of life, appendage torsion in the toddler to prepubertal (3- to 13-year-old) age range, and epididymitis after 13 years of age.[1] Specifically, bimodal peaks in the incidence of testicular torsion were noted in newborns and peripubertal males, which are concordant with other investigations (**Fig. 2**).[13,14] Up to 20% of acute scrotum cases, however, may result from other causes entirely, including incarcerated inguinal hernia

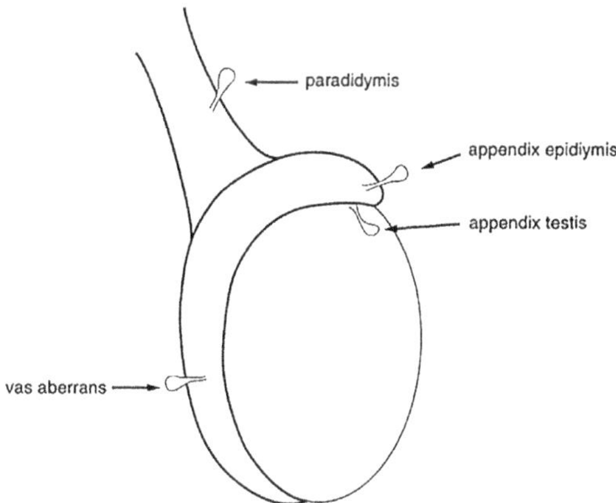

Fig. 1. Position of appendages. (*From* Sidhu PS. Clinical and imaging features of testicular torsion: role of ultrasound. Clin Radiol 1999;54:346; Courtesy of Royal College of Radiologists; with permission.)

or idiopathic scrotal edema, among others.[14,15] In addition, as previously noted, reaching a final diagnosis of scrotal pain of unclear etiology is not uncommon, particularly when evaluating all-comers in the ED setting.

EVALUATION IN THE EMERGENCY DEPARTMENT

History

The presence of systemic symptoms may provide additional diagnostic clues in the patient presenting with an acute scrotum. As noted, the vast majority of studies

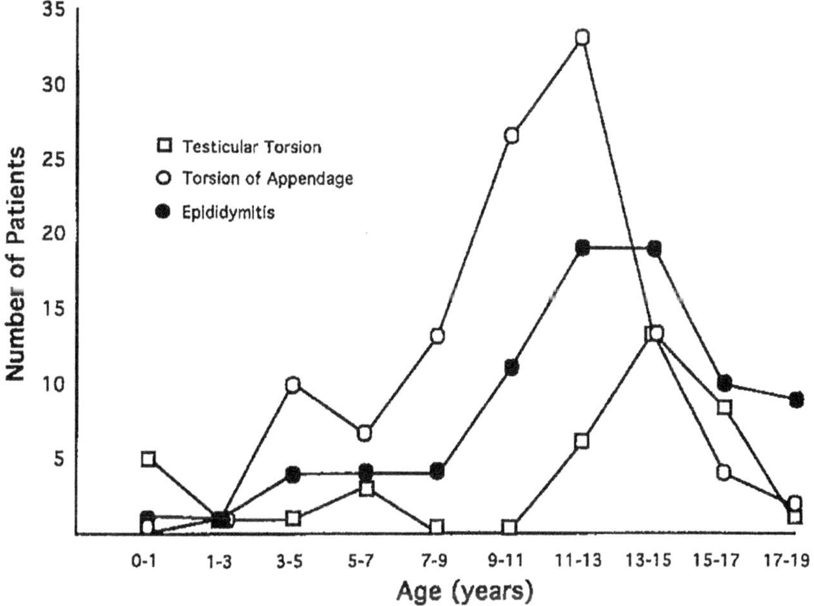

Fig. 2. Relative incidence of torsion, appendage torsion, and epididymitis as a function of age. (*From* Lewis AG, Bukoswki TP, Jarvis PD, et al. Evaluation of the acute scrotum in the emergency department. J Pediatr Surg 1995;30(2):278; with permission.)

addressing the evaluation and management of the acute scrotum are derived from pediatric cohorts. Therefore, the information that follows is based on analysis of pediatric cases unless noted otherwise.

As a general rule, patients with testicular torsion are more likely to have associated systemic symptoms such as nausea and vomiting when compared with patients with the other commonest causes of acute scrotal pain, such as uncomplicated epididymitis or appendage torsion.[16,17] Beni-Israel and colleagues[5] reported an odds ratio of 8.9 (95% confidence interval 2.6–30.1) for the association between the presence of nausea or vomiting and the diagnosis of testicular torsion. Another variable associated with testicular torsion in this study was duration of symptoms for less than 24 hours (odds ratio 6.7, 95% confidence interval 1.5–33.3). A second study confirmed a shorter symptom duration (<12 hours) for testicular torsion when compared with epididymitis.[10] Although these features have been associated with testicular torsion, their absence should certainly not preclude the diagnosis.[16]

Whereas patients with epididymitis may present with nausea, malaise, or low-grade fever, it is typically those with more advanced degrees of infection (epididymo-orchitis) who exhibit more systemic involvement.[18,19] It must be noted that patients with Fournier's disease or an incarcerated/strangulated inguinal hernia typically present with systemic symptoms as well.[20]

The distinction between constant/progressive and intermittent/colicky pain can be useful in the diagnosis of acute scrotal pain. Scrotal pain that begins abruptly and severely should be considered testicular torsion until proven otherwise.[16] Although urinary symptoms may accompany many causes of acute scrotal pain, epididymitis in particular may present with accompanying urinary complaints such as dysuria and urgency.[16]

Other important historical features include inquiring about prior similar episodes, which may occur in intermittent torsion-detorsion.[21] Eliciting a history of minor trauma is also important, as trauma-induced testicular torsion has been reported.[22]

Examination

Differentiating among the causes of acute scrotal pain by physical examination is challenging. Often confounding the problem is the exquisite pain and discomfort elicited by the examination itself. There are several examination findings which, if present, may facilitate a more accurate diagnosis.[10] High position of the testis was associated with an odds ratio of 58.8 (95% confidence interval 19.2–166.6) for testicular torsion in one study,[5] and when absent had a negative predictive value of 95% in a second study.[16] Other examination findings that have been associated with testicular torsion include transverse location of the testis (sensitivity 83%, specificity 94%, negative predictive value 95%) and anterior rotation of the epididymis from its typical posterolateral position (sensitivity 69%, specificity 98%, negative predictive value 92%).[16] Along these lines, Kadish and Bolte[10] found a statistically significant association between the following variables and the diagnosis of epididymitis: normal testicular position, presence of a tender epididymis, and the absence of testicular tenderness. Furthermore, they found a strong association between the presence of isolated tenderness at the superior pole of the testis and the diagnosis of appendage torsion.

A congenital anomaly of fixation of the testis, termed the bell-clapper deformity, is associated with the development of testicular torsion.[23] This condition occurs when the intrascrotal portion of the spermatic cord lacks firm posterior adhesion to the scrotal wall and remains surrounded by the tunica vaginalis (**Fig. 3**). As a result of the abnormal attachment, the testis may be suspended horizontally.[24] These anatomic features predispose the affected testis to rotation.

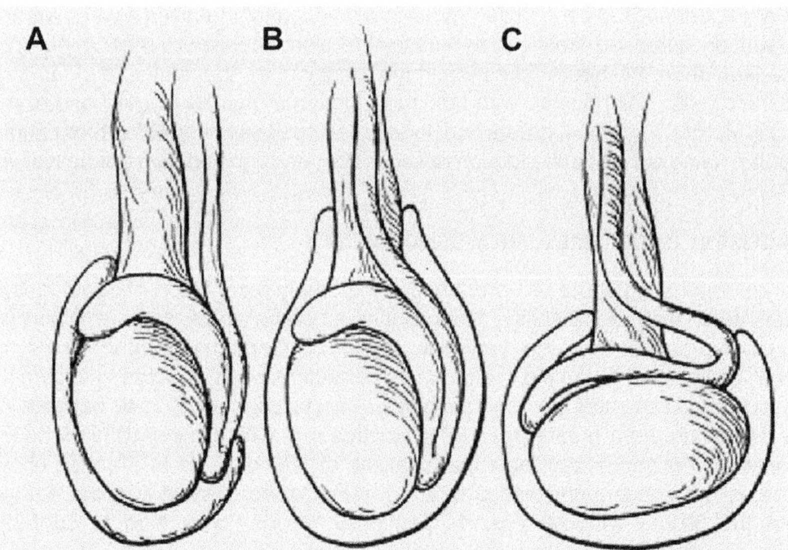

Fig. 3. Testis position within the tunica vaginalis. (*A*) Normal anatomy. (*B*) Bell-clapper deformity. (*C*) Bell-clapper deformity with horizontal testis. (*From* Testis torsion. In: Oldham KT, Colombani PM, Foglia RP, editors. Surgery of infants and children: scientific principles and practice. Philadelphia: Lippincott-Raven; 1997. p. 1552–3; with permission.)

The cremasteric reflex is elicited by stroking the inner thigh, resulting in reflexive elevation of the ipsilateral testicle through contraction of the cremaster muscle. The absence of the reflex is nonspecific. Some healthy individuals lack the reflex altogether (particularly males in their first few years of life), and inflammation or swelling from any cause may blunt or otherwise limit the ability to appreciate the reflex.[25]

It has been suggested that the presence of an intact ipsilateral cremasteric reflex can be helpful in excluding the diagnosis of testicular torsion.[13,26,27] However, there have been several published reports of testicular torsion presenting with an intact cremasteric reflex.[28–30] Beni-Israel and colleagues[5] reported that 5 of the 17 patients (29%) included in their study who were ultimately diagnosed with testicular torsion had a normal cremasteric reflex noted on initial examination. This finding is concordant with those of other studies suggesting that the presence of a normal cremasteric reflex does not necessarily rule out testicular torsion. Specifically, Karmazyn and colleagues[31] noted the presence of a normal cremasteric reflex in 3 of 31 patients (10%) with testicular torsion, whereas Van Glabeke and colleagues[32] noted the lack of an absence of the cremasteric reflex in 10 of 25 patients (40%) with testicular torsion. The bottom line is that, like many diagnostic adjuncts, the cremasteric reflex needs to be cautiously interpreted in the context of the overall clinical picture. Even though it has been suggested that the presence of an ipsilateral cremasteric reflex makes testicular torsion less likely, it is not powerful enough to exclude this fertility-threatening diagnosis.

Prehn's sign, or relief of pain with scrotal elevation, was historically taught as a method to aid in differentiating epididymitis (pain relief with scrotal elevation) from testicular torsion.[33] However, this sign is entirely unreliable in distinguishing these two disorders.[34] Therefore, its use should be abandoned. The blue dot sign is pathognomonic for appendage torsion.[35] This finding is very specific, yet insensitive.[10,13,14]

In a large pediatric ED cohort, Ben-Israel and coleagues[5] identified 4 variables associated with an increased likelihood of testicular torsion: nausea or vomiting, pain duration of less than 24 hours' duration, high position of the testis, and abnormal cremasteric reflex. All patients with testicular torsion in their study had one or more of the risk factors. The investigators concluded that the absence of all 4 of these findings is helpful in ruling out testicular torsion based on its very high negative predictive value.

MANAGEMENT IN THE EMERGENCY DEPARTMENT

The key to managing acute GU problems is the timely recognition of conditions that threaten life or testicular viability. Most routine laboratory aids, such as blood work or urinalysis, cannot exclude testicular torsion.[36] Certain laboratory tests may, however, be important in ruling in alternative conditions such as acute epididymitis.[37]

Testicular salvage rates are time sensitive. A meta-analysis of 1140 patients in 22 series demonstrated a greater than 90% salvage rate with surgery within 6 hours of pain onset.[38] An accompanying meta-analysis of 535 patients in 8 series showed that the risk of subsequent testicular atrophy increased despite surgical detorsion beyond the 6-hour window (**Fig. 4**). Testicular atrophy may lead to subfertility.

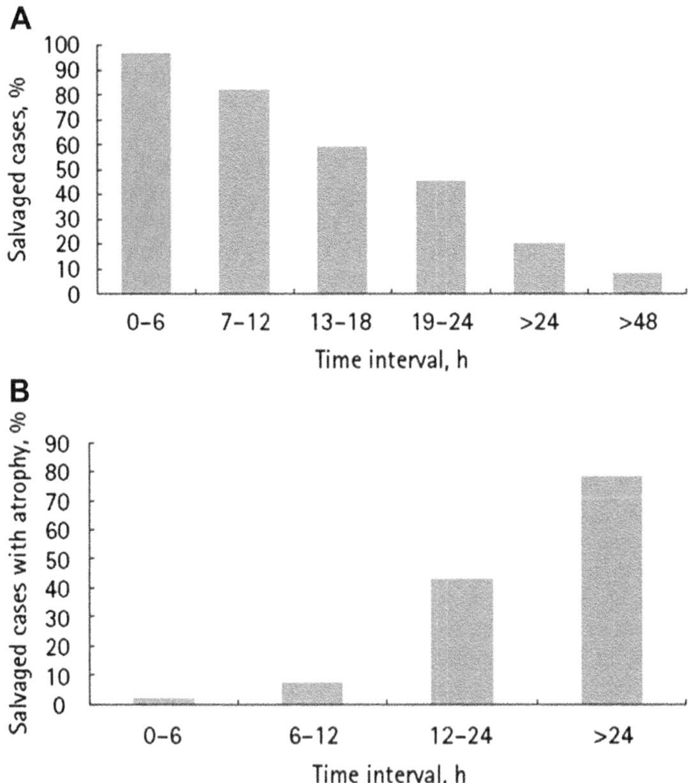

Fig. 4. Testicular salvage and atrophy rates over time in testicular torsion. (*A*) Immediate (early) surgical salvage after torsion. (*B*) Subsequent atrophy of surgically salvaged testes after torsion of various time intervals. (*Reprinted from* Visser AJ, Heyns CF. Testicular function after torsion of the spermatic cord. BJU Int 2003;92:201; with permission.)

Furthermore, testicular loss may lead to contralateral testis dysfunction through immune-mediated or other mechanisms.[38]

A retrospective review of 162 cases of testicular torsion demonstrated a median of 360° of torsion in cases of testicular salvage, and a median of 540° of torsion in nonviable cases.[39] There was overlap between the categories, however, with a range of 180° to 1080° of torsion found in both categories. Of importance, testicular infarction can occur with as little as 180° of torsion.

Diagnostic Imaging

If the history and examination suggests the diagnosis of testicular torsion, surgical consultation and plans for immediate exploration should be initiated without delay. A patient with compelling historical and examination findings of testicular torsion does not require any diagnostic tests. In other cases, a confirmatory diagnostic study such as color flow Doppler ultrasonography (CDUS) is indicated.[40] Surgical exploration is the initial treatment of choice with a strong clinical suspicion for testicular torsion, although guidelines published by the American College of Radiology recommend that confirmatory imaging can be performed if readily available and obtained within 30 to 60 minutes of the request to *simultaneously* prepare the operating room.[41] At present, however, there are no such guidelines specific to emergency medicine.

When used in the appropriate clinical setting, sonography remains the most useful diagnostic modality in the evaluation of GU complaints. A patient with compelling historical and examination findings of testicular torsion does not require any preoperative diagnostic tests. CDUS may be very helpful in all other cases. The classic sonographic finding suggestive of testicular torsion is diminished intratesticular blood flow. In addition, examination of the spermatic cord with high-resolution gray-scale ultrasonography (HRUS) may reveal "coiling" or "kinking" of the cord at the site of torsion.[42–44] Sonography is used not only to exclude testicular torsion but also to search for alternative causes of acute scrotal pain.[45] In epididymitis, perfusion may be normal (or increased) because of the effects of inflammatory mediators on local vascular beds, although this is a nonspecific finding.[46,47] An infarcted appendage may be visualized on ultrasonography as well.[48] Ultrasonography may also identify hydroceles, hematoceles, varicoceles, hernias, tumors, abscesses, and gonadal vasculitis, among others. It has been suggested that emergency physicians may be able to accurately assess for intratesticular blood flow in patients presenting with acute scrotal pain using bedside sonography.[49]

CDUS has long been regarded as the diagnostic modality of choice in assessing for testicular torsion. However, reports of false-negative ultrasound results have been reported.[50–56] Many of these studies are case reports or case series, limited by small numbers and retrospective design. Two larger series reported documented intratesticular blood flow with CDUS in 6 of 23 (26%) and 50 of 208 cases (24%), respectively, of confirmed testicular torsion.[42,57] Doppler ultrasonography may reveal seemingly adequate intratesticular blood flow in partial torsion, which can be very misleading to the practitioner.[58]

Radionuclide scintigraphy and CDUS show similar sensitivity, as well as false-negative rates, for the diagnosis of testicular torsion.[59] However, given the widespread availability and expertise with ultrasound technology, combined with the risks of isotope radiation exposure, radionuclide procedures have fallen out of favor. The use of magnetic resonance imaging has been explored, but limitations include speed of imaging and availability.[60,61]

Ultrasound evaluation of the acute scrotum has its limitations. Ultrasonography may be helpful in identifying an alternate diagnosis. However, surgical scrotal exploration remains the only definitive diagnostic modality in assessing for testicular torsion, but this needs to be balanced with the potential for unnecessary operations. The real question is: when is the risk low enough to safely send a patient home following a "normal" ultrasound imaging study? Whereas some series have found ultrasonography to be unreliable, other larger series have reported a negative predictive value approaching 97%.[62] Overall, it is wise for the emergency practitioner to approach the acute scrotum with a "play not to lose" rather than a "play to win" mentality. If the ultrasonogram is nondiagnostic for testicular torsion, and the clinical story is still concerning, emergent surgical consultation is prudent.

Manual Detorsion

The pain of testicular torsion may be relieved following a trial of manual detorsion. A study of 162 cases of testicular torsion revealed that anticipated lateral to medial rotation occurred in 67% of cases, with medial to lateral rotation in the remaining 33%.[39] This result challenges the standard dogma of medial to lateral rotation, or "opening the book," as the standard method for detorsion. The end-point of manual detorsion is relief of pain, or the return of intratesticular blood flow as seen on ultrasound imaging.[63] Although manual detorsion may allow for reperfusion of the testis, a lesser degree of residual torsion may remain. Given that infarction can occur with as little as 180° of torsion, immediate surgical exploration after what is thought to be a successful manual detorsion is still advocated.[39] If attempted in the ED, preprocedure local anesthesia or systemic analgesia is prudent. The bottom line is that specialty consultation and plans for possible immediate surgical exploration need to occur regardless of outcome of the detorsion procedure.

EPIDIDYMITIS

Antibiotics are the mainstay of therapy for epididymitis. Antimicrobial selection is guided by patient demographics: younger (<35 years of age), sexually active males are treated with agents to cover *Neisseria gonorrhoeae* and *Chlamydia trachomatis*, such as single-dose intramuscular (IM) ceftriaxone with a 10-day course of oral doxycycline.[37] Fluoroquinolones are no longer recommended for the treatment of gonococcal infections.[64] Antimicrobials covering common urinary pathogens are recommended for males older than 35 years with epididymitis. This age distinction, however, is arbitrary, and variability exists.

Epididymitis may also occur in prepubescent males[65]; this is thought to be caused by reflux of sterile urine into the epididymis, although the precise mechanisms remain unclear.[66,67] Reflux may result from congenital GU anomalies that require diagnostic evaluation. Recommendations regarding treatment of the resulting inflammation vary from treating all boys to limiting antimicrobial use to patients with documented urinary findings such as pyuria or a positive urine culture.[11,66] If used, prophylactic antibiotics should cover the common urinary pathogens.

APPENDAGE TORSION

Appendage torsion occurs most frequently in the prepubertal age group, likely resulting from the increased size of the pedunculated structures as a result of hormonal stimulation.[68] Appendage torsion is self-limited. Treatment includes pain relief with nonsteroidal anti-inflammatory agents and limiting activity. Pain relief coincides with degeneration of the infarcted, necrotic appendage, which typically occurs within

1 to 2 weeks.[69] Appendage torsion may recur, given appendage variability in both number and position.

FOURNIER'S GANGRENE

Fournier's gangrene should be considered in elderly, diabetic, or otherwise immune compromised males. Fournier's disease has also been reported in women and children.[70,71] Early surgical consultation and administration of broad-spectrum antibiotics is indicated in all suspected cases of Fournier's gangrene. Surgical debridement is imperative and remains the definitive treatment.[72,73] Computed tomography (CT) may be helpful in assessing the degree of extension.[74] However, delays in recognition and definitive surgical debridement can be life threatening, so imaging should not delay surgical consultation. Early intravenous broad-spectrum antibiotic therapy covering gram-positive, gram-negative, and anaerobic species is imperative. There is some literature to suggest a potent synergistic role of clindamycin along with β-lactam antimicrobials in combating necrotizing soft tissue infections, particularly when streptococcal species are involved.[75,76] Recommended empiric intravenous antimicrobials include ampicillin-sulbactam plus clindamycin plus ciprofloxacin, or clindamycin plus an aminoglycoside in individuals with known penicillin hypersensitivity.[77] The addition of vancomycin to either regimen for expanded gram-positive coverage is reasonable. The role of hyperbaric oxygen therapy has been suggested, although its utility remains the subject of much debate in the medical literature.[78,79]

INCARCERATED INGUINAL HERNIA

An inguinal hernia may occur when there is a defect in the anterior abdominal wall musculature. Alternatively, a persistent embryologic communication (patent processus vaginalis) between the peritoneal cavity and the tunica vaginalis may result in an indirect inguinal hernia. A reducible hernia occurs when abdominal contents can freely (or with simple manipulation) move between the abdomen and the hernia sac. An irreducible, or incarcerated, hernia cannot return to its normal site spontaneously or by simple manipulation. An irreducible hernia may become strangulated, where pressure on the hernial contents may compromise blood supply; this represents a surgical emergency. Both direct and indirect hernias may present when incarcerated or strangulated.

GENITOURINARY TRAUMA

Traumatic injury must be included in the differential of any GU complaint. Trauma to the GU system may be either blunt or penetrating (**Table 3**). The Société Internationale D'Urologie has published recommendations regarding the management of GU trauma.[80] Of importance, trauma-induced testicular torsion has been reported.[22] As such, consideration of testicular torsion in the differential diagnosis of blunt scrotal trauma is prudent.

Significant trauma to the scrotum and its associated structures occurs infrequently with minor blunt force mechanisms, owing to both testicular mobility and a protective cremasteric reflex.[80] In addition, each testicle is encapsulated by a fibrous tunica albuginea, which may protect the testicular parenchyma from injury. Blunt force injury may cause testicular contusion or, less frequently, rupture of the tunica albuginea. Traumatic dislocation of the testicle to an aberrant site outside of the scrotal compartment is possible with significant blunt-force trauma. All but the most superficial penetrating scrotal injuries will require specialty consultation for possible exploration.[81] Patients

Table 3
Scrotal trauma

Condition	Etiology, Presentation	Treatment
Testicular dislocation	Significant blunt-force mechanism (dislocation to the abdomen or to subcutaneous tissues surrounding the external inguinal ring)	Surgical intervention
Testicular rupture	Disruption of the tunica albuginea	Surgical intervention
Testicular contusion	Intratesticular hematoma; intact tunica albuginea	Typically conservative: ice, rest, elevation
Hematocele	Blood accumulation in the tunica vaginalis	Surgical drainage for large hematocele; conservative otherwise
Penetrating injury	Varies depending on cause	Typically surgical exploration/ intervention
Traumatic testicular torsion	Traumatically induced torsion has been reported	Surgical exploration/intervention

with either blunt or penetrating GU trauma may present with a hematocele, which is a painful, tender, ecchymotic scrotal mass resulting from the accumulation of blood within the tunica vaginalis. Ultrasonography is an invaluable tool in the evaluation of GU trauma.[82,83] In addition, CT imaging may be helpful in uncovering coexisting injuries.

SUMMARY

Male GU problems are frequently high-risk complaints from a medicolegal perspective.[84] Definitive diagnosis for the patient presenting with an acute scrotum is not always feasible in the ED setting. However, recognition of GU emergencies takes precedence. Identification of testicular torsion is critical given its implications for future fertility. Additional emergent conditions include Fournier's gangrene, incarcerated or strangulated inguinal hernia, and any form of GU trauma until proven otherwise. Other causes of the acute scrotum can typically be managed in the outpatient setting once these life threats or fertility threats have been reliably excluded.

There is no individual or combination of clinical features or diagnostic testing that can reliably rule out testicular torsion. The cremasteric reflex and testicular sonography are frequently used, yet imperfect, diagnostic tools. It is wise for the emergency practitioner to approach the acute scrotum with a "play not to lose" rather than a "play to win" mentality. It is prudent to maintain a high index of clinical suspicion and a low threshold for surgical consultation when evaluating for emergent conditions, particularly in the setting of ongoing pain. Armed with this knowledge, the acute scrotum can be skillfully and effectively managed in the ED setting.

ACKNOWLEDGMENTS

The authors wish to acknowledge Dr Robert Schneider, who is board certified in both emergency medicine and urology, for his contributions and mentorship.

REFERENCES

1. Lewis AG, Bukoswki TP, Jarvis PD, et al. Evaluation of the acute scrotum in the emergency department. J Pediatr Surg 1995;30(2):277–82.
2. Cavusoglu YH, Karaman A, Karaman I, et al. Acute scrotum—etiology and management. Indian J Pediatr 2005;72(3):201–3.
3. Primatesta P, Goldacre J. Inguinal hernia repair: incidence of elective and emergency surgery, readmission and mortality. Int J Epidemiol 1996;25(4): 835–9.
4. Ben-Chaim J, Leibovitch I, Ramon J, et al. Etiology of acute scrotum at surgical exploration in children, adolescents and adults. Eur Urol 1992;21(1):45–7.
5. Beni-Israel T, Goldman M, Bar Chaim S. Clinical predictors of testicular torsion as seen in the pediatric ED. Am J Emerg Med 2010;28:786–9.
6. Cummings JM, Boullier JA, Sekhon D, et al. Adult testicular torsion. J Urol 2002; 167(5):2109–10.
7. Mushtaq I, Fung M, Glasson MJ. Retrospective review of paediatric patients with acute scrotum. ANZ J Surg 2003;73(1–2):55–8.
8. Varga J, Zikovic D, Grebeldinger S, et al. Acute scrotal pain in children—ten years' experience. Urol Int 2007;78(1):73–7.
9. Sidler D, Brown RA, Millar AJ, et al. A 25-year review of the acute scrotum in children. S Afr Med J 1997;87(12):1696–8.
10. Kadish HA, Bolte RG. A retrospective review of pediatric patients with epididymitis, testicular torsion, and torsion of testicular appendages. Pediatrics 1998; 102(1):73–6.
11. McAndrew HF, Pemberton R, Kikiros CS, et al. The incidence and investigation of acute scrotal problems in children. Pediatr Surg Int 2002;18:435–7.
12. Corbett HJ, Simpson ET. Management of the acute scrotum in children. ANZ J Surg 2002;72(3):226–8.
13. Melekos MD, Asbach HW, Markou SA. Etiology of acute scrotum in 100 boys with regard to age distribution. J Urol 1988;139:1023–5.
14. Makela E, Lahdes-Vasama T, Rajakorpi H, et al. A 19-year review of paediatric patients with acute scrotum. Scand J Surg 2007;96(1):62–6.
15. Van Langen AM, Gal S, Hulsmann AR, et al. Acute idiopathic scrotal edema: four cases and a short review. Eur J Pediatr 2001;160(7):455–6.
16. Ciftci AO, Senocak ME, Tanyel FC, et al. Clinical predictors for differential diagnosis of acute scrotum. Eur J Pediatr Surg 2004;14(5):333–8.
17. Jefferson RH, Perez LM, Joseph DB. Critical analysis of the clinical presentation of acute scrotum: a 9-year experience at a single institution. J Urol 1997;158(3 Pt 2): 1198–200.
18. Likitnukul S, McCracken GH Jr, Nelson JD, et al. Epididymitis in children and adolescents. A 20-year retrospective study. Am J Dis Child 1987;141(1):41–4.
19. Knight PJ, Vassy LE. The diagnosis and treatment of the acute scrotum in children and adolescents. Ann Surg 1984;200:664–73.
20. Shun A, Puri P. Inguinal hernia in the newborn: a 15 year review. Pediatr Surg Int 1988;3:156–7.
21. Creagh TA, McDermott TE, McLean PA, et al. Intermittent torsion of the testis. BMJ 1988;297:525–6.
22. Seng YJ, Moissinac K. Trauma induced testicular torsion: a reminder for the unwary. J Accid Emerg Med 2000;17(5):381–2.
23. Vijayaraghavan SB. Sonographic differential diagnosis of acute scrotum: real-time whirlpool sign, a key sign of torsion. J Ultrasound Med 2006;25:563–74.

24. Kamaledeen S, Surana R. Intermittent testicular pain: fix the testes. BJU Int 2003; 91:406–8.
25. Caesar RE, Kaplan GW. The incidence of the cremasteric reflex in normal boys. J Urol 1994;152:779–80.
26. Rabinowitz R. The importance of the cremasteric reflex in acute scrotal swelling in children. J Urol 1984;132:89–90.
27. Caldamome AA, Valvo JR, Altebarmakian VK, et al. Acute scrotal swelling in children. J Pediatr Surg 1984;19:581–4.
28. Feldstein MS. Re: the importance of the cremasteric reflex in acute scrotal swelling in children. J Urol 1985;133:488.
29. Hughes ME, Currier SJ, Della-Giustina D. Normal cremasteric reflex in a case of testicular torsion. Am J Emerg Med 2001;19(3):241–2.
30. Nelson CP, Williams JF, Bloom DA. The cremasteric reflex: a useful but imperfect sign in testicular torsion. J Pediatr Surg 2003;38:1248–9.
31. Karmazyn B, Steinberg R, Kornreich L, et al. Clinical and sonographic criteria of acute scrotum in children: a retrospective study of 172 boys. Pediatr Radiol 2004; 35(3):302–10.
32. Van Glabeke E, Khairouni A, Larroquet M, et al. Acute scrotal pain in children: results of 543 surgical explorations. Pediatr Surg Int 1999;15(5–6):353–7.
33. Prehn CT. A new sign in the differential diagnosis between torsion of the spermatic cord and epididymitis. J Urol 1934;32:191–200.
34. Noske HD, Kraus SW, Altinkilic BM, et al. Historical milestones regarding torsion of the scrotal organs. J Urol 1998;159(1):13–6.
35. Dresner ML. Torsed appendage. Diagnosis and management: blue dot sign. Urology 1973;1(1):63–6.
36. Dunne PJ, O'Loughlin BS. Testicular torsion: time is the enemy. ANZ J Surg 2000; 70:441–2.
37. Centers for Disease Control and Prevention. Sexually transmitted disease treatment guidelines, 2010. MMWR Recomm Rep 2010;59(RR-12):67–9.
38. Visser AJ, Heyns CF. Testicular function after torsion of the spermatic cord. BJU Int 2003;92:200–3.
39. Sessions AE, Rabinowitz R, Hulbert WC, et al. Testicular torsion: direction, degree, duration, and disinformation. J Urol 2003;169(2):663–5.
40. Pepe P, Panella P, Pennisi M, et al. Does color Doppler sonography improve the clinical assessment of patients with acute scrotum? Eur J Radiol 2006;60(1): 120–4.
41. Expert Panel on Urologic Imaging. Acute onset of scrotal pain—without trauma, without antecedent mass. Available at: http://www.acr.org/SecondaryMainMenuCategories/quality_safety/app_criteria/pdf/ExpertPanelonUrologicImaging/AcuteOnsetofscrotalpainWithoutTraumaWithoutAntecedentMassDoc2.aspx. Reston (VA): American College of Radiology (ACR); 2005. Accessed February 20, 2008.
42. Kalfa N, Veyrac C, Lopez M, et al. Multicenter assessment of ultrasound of the spermatic cord in children with acute scrotum. J Urol 2007;177(1):297–301.
43. Arce JD, Cortes M, Vargas JC. Sonographic diagnosis of acute spermatic cord torsion. Rotation of the cord: a key to the diagnosis. Pediatr Radiol 2002;32: 485–91.
44. Kalfa N, Veyrac C, Baud C, et al. Ultrasonography of the spermatic cord in children with testicular torsion: impact on the surgical strategy. J Urol 2004;172: 1692–5.
45. Sidhu PS. Clinical and imaging features of testicular torsion: role of ultrasound. Clin Radiol 1999;54:343–52.

46. Haecker F-M, Hauri-Hohl A, von Schweinitz D. Acute epididymitis in children: a 4-year retrospective study. Eur J Pediatr Surg 2005;15:180–6.
47. Sakellaris GS, Charissis GC. Acute epididymitis in Greek children: a 3-year retrospective study. Eur J Pediatr 2008;167(7):765–9.
48. Yang DM, Lim JW, Kim JE, et al. Torsed appendix testis. Gray scale and color Doppler sonographic findings compared with a normal appendix testis. J Ultrasound Med 2005;24:87–91.
49. Blaivas M, Sierzenski P, Lambert M. Emergency evaluation of patients presenting with acute scrotum using bedside ultrasonography. Acad Emerg Med 2001;8(1): 90–3.
50. Burks DD, Markey BJ, Burkhard TK, et al. Suspected testicular torsion and ischemia: evaluation with color Doppler sonography. Radiology 1990;175: 815–21.
51. Ingram S, Hollman AS, Azmy A. Testicular torsion: missed diagnosis on color Doppler sonography. Pediatr Radiol 1993;23:483.
52. Steinhardt GF, Boyarsky S, Mackey R. Testicular torsion: pitfalls of color Doppler sonography. J Urol 1993;150:461–2.
53. Yazbeck S, Patriquin HB. Accuracy of Doppler sonography in the evaluation of acute conditions of the scrotum in children. J Pediatr Surg 1994;29(9):1270–2.
54. Allen TD, Elder J. Shortcomings of color Doppler sonography in diagnosis of testicular torsion. J Urol 1995;154(4):1508–10.
55. Stehr M, Boehm R. Critical validation of color Doppler ultrasound in diagnostics of acute scrotum in children. Eur J Pediatr Surg 2003;13:386–92.
56. Frauscher F, Klauser A, Radmayr C. Ultrasonographic assessment of the scrotum. Lancet 2001;357:721–2.
57. Baud C, Veyrac C, Couture A, et al. Spiral twist of the spermatic cord: a reliable sign of testicular torsion. Pediatr Radiol 1998;28:950–4.
58. Frush DP, Babcock DS, Lewis AG, et al. Comparison of color Doppler sonography and radionuclide imaging in different degrees of torsion in rabbit testes. Acad Radiol 1995;2:945–51.
59. Nussbaum AR, Bulas D, Shalaby-Rana E, et al. Color Doppler sonography and scintigraphy of the testis: a prospective, comparative analysis in children with acute scrotal pain. Pediatr Emerg Care 2002;18(2):67–71.
60. Terai A, Yoshimura K, Ichioka K, et al. Dynamic contrast-enhanced subtraction magnetic resonance imaging in the diagnostics of testicular torsion. Urology 2006;67:1278–82.
61. Wanatabe Y, Dohke M, Ohkubo K, et al. Scrotal disorders: evaluation of testicular enhancement patterns at dynamic contrast enhanced subtraction MRI imaging. Radiology 2000;217(1):219–27.
62. Lam WW, Yap T, Jacobsen AS, et al. Colour Doppler ultrasonography replacing surgical exploration for acute scrotum: myth or reality? Pediatr Radiol 2005; 35(6):597–600.
63. Garel L, Dubois J, Azzie G, et al. Preoperative manual detorsion of the spermatic cord with Doppler ultrasound monitoring in patients with intravaginal testicular torsion. Pediatr Radiol 2000;30:41–4.
64. Centers for Disease Control and Prevention (CDC). Update to CDC's sexually transmitted diseases treatment guidelines, 2006: fluoroquinolones no longer recommended for treatment of gonococcal infections. MMWR Morb Mortal Wkly Rep 2007;56(14):332–6.
65. Klin B, Zlotkevich L, Horne T, et al. Epididymitis in childhood: a clinical retrospective study over 5 years. Isr Med Assoc J 2001;3:833–5.

66. Lau P, Anderson PA, Giacomantonio JM, et al. Acute epididymitis in boys: are antibiotics indicated? Br J Urol 1997;79:797–800.
67. Somekh E, Gorenstein A, Serour F. Acute epididymitis in boys: evidence of a post-infectious etiology. J Urol 2004;171(1):391–4.
68. Gatti JM, Murphy JP. Current management of the acute scrotum. Semin Pediatr Surg 2007;16(1):58–63.
69. Skoglund RW, McRoberts JW, Ragde H. Torsion of testicular appendages: presentation of 43 new cases and a collective review. J Urol 1970;104(4): 598–600.
70. Adams JR, Mata JA, Venable DD, et al. Fournier's disease in children. Urology 1990;35(5):439–41.
71. Eke N. Fournier's gangrene: a review of 1726 cases. Br J Surg 2000;87(6): 718–28.
72. Corman JM, Moody JA, Aronson WJ. Fournier's gangrene in a modern surgical setting: improved survival with aggressive management. BJU Int 1999;84:85–8.
73. Basoglu M, Ozbey I, Selcuk Atamanalp S, et al. Management of Fournier's gangrene: review of 45 cases. Surg Today 2007;37:558–63.
74. Rajan DK, Scharer KA. Radiology of Fournier's gangrene. AJR Am J Roentgenol 1998;170(1):163–8.
75. Sriskandan S, McKee A, Hall L, et al. Comparative effects of clindamycin and ampicillin on superantigenic activity of *Streptococcus pyogenes*. J Antimicrob Chemother 1997;40:275–7.
76. Zimbelman J, Palmer A, Todd J. Improved outcome of clindamycin compared with beta-lactam antibiotic treatment for invasive Streptococcus pyogenes infection. Pediatr Infect Dis J 1999;18(12):1096–100.
77. Stevens DL, Bisno AL, Chambers HF, et al. Practice guidelines for the diagnosis and management of skin and soft-tissue infections. Clin Infect Dis 2005;41(10): 1373–406.
78. Mindrup SR, Kealey GP, Fallon B. Hyperbaric oxygen for the treatment of Fournier's gangrene. J Urol 2005;173(6):1975–7.
79. Jallali N, Withey S, Butler PE. Hyperbaric oxygen as adjuvant therapy in the management of necrotizing fasciitis. Am J Surg 2005;189:462–6.
80. Morey AF, Metro MJ, Carney KJ, et al. Consensus on genitourinary trauma: external genitalia. BJU Int 2004;94:507–15.
81. Van Der Horst C, Martinez Portillo FJ, Seif C, et al. Male genital injury: diagnostics and treatment. BJU Int 2004;93:927–30.
82. Lee SH, Bak CW, Choi MH, et al. Trauma to male genital organs: a 10-year review of 156 patients, including 118 treated by surgery. BJU Int 2008;101(2):211–5.
83. Buckley JC, McAninch JW. Use of ultrasonography for the diagnosis of testicular injuries in blunt scrotal trauma. J Urol 2006;175:175–8.
84. Matteson JR, Stock JA, Hanna MK, et al. Medicolegal aspects of testicular torsion. Urology 2001;57(4):783–7.

Penile Emergencies

Jeffrey Dubin, MD, MBA*, Jonathan E. Davis, MD

KEYWORDS

• Penis • Priapism • Paraphimosis • Fracture • Entrapment
• Pain • Emergency

The penis is a very sensitive organ and even minor injury or discomfort may cause a patient to seek emergency evaluation. Emergency practitioners must be most concerned with the entities that, if left untreated, can result in ischemia and necrosis of the penis: ischemic priapism, paraphimosis, and entrapment injury. Any penile trauma should be considered an emergency until proven otherwise. This article discusses emergent penile complaints in adults, with emphasis on the most serious and common conditions.

ANATOMY

The penis consists of the paired corpora cavernosa, or erectile bodies, that lie dorsal to the corpus spongiosum (**Fig. 1**). The corpus spongiosum surrounds the penile urethra. The corpora cavernosa and corpus spongiosum are wrapped in a thin connective tissue layer, the tunica albuginea. The glans is the distal head of the penis. The distal foreskin, or prepuce, in uncircumcised men lies over the glans and can be retracted proximally to expose the glans. The coronal sulcus distinguishes the glans penis from the penile shaft.

EMERGENT CONDITIONS

Priapism

Priapism is defined as prolonged erection of the penis, generally lasting more than 4 hours, in the absence of sexual desire or stimulation. This medical condition was named after Priapus, an ancient Greek god of fertility and horticulture who was endowed with oversized genitalia.[1] Ironically, one cause of priapism is prolonged effects of erectile dysfunction medications, making a pleasurable emulation of Priapus a painful one. More than one-third of patients with severe priapism may experience permanent erectile dysfunction despite treatment, resulting in obvious infertility or other emotional or functional sequelae.[2]

The authors have nothing to disclose.

Department of Emergency Medicine, Washington Hospital Center, Georgetown University School of Medicine, 110 Irving Street, NW, Washington, DC 20010, USA
* Corresponding author.
E-mail address: Jeffrey.s.dubin@medstar.net

Emerg Med Clin N Am 29 (2011) 485–499
doi:10.1016/j.emc.2011.04.006 emed.theclinics.com
0733-8627/11/$ – see front matter

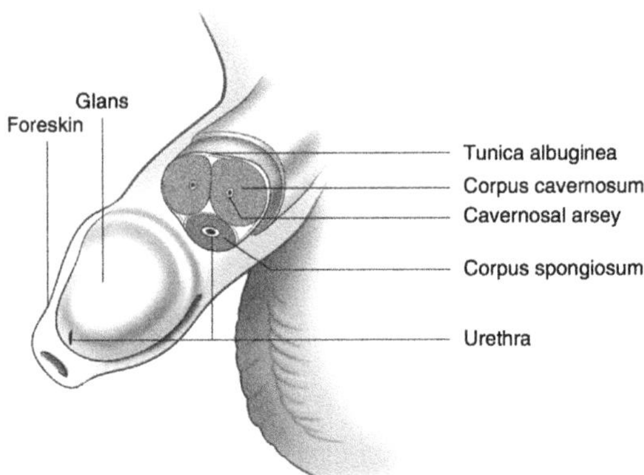

Fig. 1. Anatomy of the penis. (*From* Davis JE. Penile complaints. In: Amieva-Wang NE, editor. A practical guide to pediatric emergency medicine: caring for children in the emergency department. Cambridge (United Kingdom): Cambridge University Press; 2011. p. 700; with permission.)

Priapism can be divided into two main categories. Ischemic priapism, also known as low-flow priapism, is the most commonly seen variant and is caused by painful venous engorgement of the corpora cavernosa and requires emergency treatment. Nonischemic (high-flow) priapism is rare and is often painless. It is caused by increased arterial inflow to the penis from traumatic arterial-cavernosal fistulae and does not require urgent treatment.

Ischemic priapism can be considered a compartment syndrome of the penis.[3] The corpora cavernosa become engorged with stagnant, oxygen-depleted venous blood from either an intraluminal obstruction of venous blood flow or an inability of the penile muscle tissue to adequately contract and augment venous outflow.[2] The causes of ischemic priapism are multiple and varied (**Table 1**).

The corporal smooth muscle dysfunction resulting in ischemia is most frequently caused by vasoactive medications or nerve dysfunction. Erectile dysfunction treatments inhibit the contraction of the smooth muscles of the corpora cavernosa.[3] Injectable drugs, such as papaverine, and oral medications, such as sildenafil citrate or similar, can potentially be "too much of a good thing" and may cause permanent erectile dysfunction. α-Adrenergic blocking agents such as tamsulosin can also affect the smooth muscles of the cavernosa, resulting in complete or even partial priapism. Segmental thrombosis of single corpus cavernosa causing focal and unilateral priapism has been reported as a result of tamsulosin use.[4]

Other antihypertensive drugs, such as prazosin and labetolol, have been associated with priapism through similar mechanisms.[5] Antidepressant and antipsychotic medications, both older and newer, may cause ischemic priapism. Atypical antipsychotic drugs, such as ziprasidone, have been shown to cause ischemic priapism, presumably through the same α-receptor mechanism.[6] Other drugs that have also been associated with priapism include anticoagulants, testosterone, immunosuppressants (eg, tacrolimus), recreational drugs (eg, cocaine, marijuana), and alcohol.[3]

Neurologic causes of ischemic priapism are believed to include the inhibition or dysfunction of the autonomic smooth muscles of the corpora cavernosa. Spinal cord injuries, stroke, cauda equine syndrome, spinal disc disease, epidural anesthesia, and neurosyphilis have been known to cause priapism.[3] Ischemic priapism has even been reported after hip arthroplasty, presumably caused by intraoperative nerve injury.[7]

Table 1
Selected etiologies of ischemic (low-flow) priapism

Category	Examples
Medications	
Impotence agents	Intracavernosal therapies (prostaglandin E1, papaverine, phentolamine) Oral agents (ie, sildenafil)
Antihypertensives	Hydralazine, prazosin, doxazosin
Antidepressants	Trazadone, fluoxetine, sertraline, citalopram
Antipsychotics	Phenothiazines, atypical antipsychotics
Illicit substances	Cocaine, marijuana
General anesthetics	
Miscellaneous	Hydroxyzine, metoclopramide, omeprazole, total parenteral nutrition
Hematologic disorders	
Sickle cell disease	
Leukemia	
Myeloma	
Central nervous system	
Brain	Cerebrovascular accident
Spinal cord	Spinal stenosis, spinal cord injury, lumbar disc herniation
Others	
Infections	Malaria, rabies
Toxins	Black widow, scorpion
Carbon monoxide	
Hypertriglyceridemia	
Idiopathic	

From Davis JE. Male genitourinary emergencies. In: Adams JG, Barton ED, Collings JL, et al, editors. Emergency medicine. New York: Elsevier; 2008. p. 1210; with permission.

Intraluminal obstruction is the cause most often seen in patients with sickle cell disease. Clumping of sickle cells causes venous outflow obstruction, leading to a painful, engorged penis. Over one-third of men with sickle cell anemia may develop ischemic priapism at least once during their lifetime.[8] Additional conditions that cause ischemic priapism in a similar manner of hyperviscosity or red cell or platelet aggregation include other hemoglobinopathies and blood dyscrasias, parental nutrition, and heparin-induced thrombocytopenia.[3] Obstruction of the venous outflow to the corpora cavernosa can also occur from local invasion of, or metastasis from, genitourinary and rectal cancers.[9,10]

A subtype of ischemic priapism is known as *stuttering priapism*. This entity is typically observed in patients with sickle cell disease. Patients experience recurrent episodes of priapism that often last less than 3 hours and often do not require emergency treatment unless symptoms become markedly prolonged.[11]

Whether from intraluminal vaso-occlusion or penile vascular bed smooth muscle dysfunction, the resulting ischemic priapism can quickly cause permanent damage to the penis if left untreated. However, even with effective treatment, future erectile dysfunction is still a possibility. After 4 hours of persistent priapism, a heightened release of inflammatory cytokines occurs in the acidotic and hypoxic corpora cavernosa. Inflammation may include smooth muscle changes, including cell death and fibrosis, which may cause permanent erectile dysfunction.[12]

Evaluation of the patient with priapism may involve several steps before a final cause can be identified. Patient history can help differentiate between ischemic and nonischemic priapism. Ischemic priapism is painful, nontraumatic, and may be associated with a history of priapism, hemoglobinopathy, or vasoactive drug use, whereas nonischemic priapism is typically painless and caused by traumatic injury. Patients with ischemic priapism often present shortly after onset of symptoms because of pain, whereas patients with nonischemic priapism may present after several hours or days of symptoms. On physical examination, ischemic priapism will present with a rigid penile shaft but soft glans. Patients with nonischemic priapism will often have a partial erection, but the entire penis, including the glans, will be firm. The presence of the "peisis sign," which is partial or complete resolution of the erection during compression of the perineum, may also help support the diagnosis of nonischemic priapism.[13] Any patient presenting with the first episode of priapism and who is not known to have sickle cell disease should have a sickle cell preparation and a complete blood cell count, regardless of ethnicity.

Aspiration of the corpora cavernosa is helpful in distinguishing ischemic from nonischemic priapism. The blood gas of ischemic priapism will be grossly dark in color and have a pH less than 7.25, a Pao_2 less than 30 mm Hg, and a Pco_2 greater than 60 mm Hg. In contrast, corporal blood gas from nonischemic priapism will appear much closer to normal arterial blood gas, typically with a pH greater than 7.30, Pao_2 greater than 50, and Pco_2 less than 40. Finally, color duplex ultrasound of the penis and perineum may be useful in assessing for the presence or absence of blood flow through the cavernosal arteries. Absent blood flow will confirm the diagnosis of ischemic priapism. Normal or increased blood flow will support the diagnosis of nonischemic priapism. Arteriography may be indicated for nonischemic priapism, but it is often performed when embolization treatment is planned rather than as an initial diagnostic modality.[2,3]

A urologic surgeon typically manages treatment of acute priapism. However, treatment for ischemic priapism will frequently need to be initiated in the emergency setting while awaiting specialty consultation. The classic teaching is that the initial treatment—oral (or subcutaneous) terbutaline—is the same regardless of inciting cause, although its efficacy is debated.[14–16] Terbutaline, a β_2-adrenergic agonist, is thought to increase venous outflow from the engorged corpora through relaxation of venous sinusoidal smooth muscle. Terbutaline has an unproven benefit; however, given its limited propensity for adverse effects, a trial is reasonable in select circumstances while awaiting specialty consultation.[17]

If terbutaline fails to work rapidly, the next step in the treatment of priapism is corporal blood aspiration, saline irrigation, and injection of an α-adrenergic receptor agonist such as dilute phenylephrine. Phenylephrine should be diluted in normal saline to a concentration of 0.1 to 0.5 mg/mL, and 1-mL injections made every 3 to 5 minutes for 1 hour. Lower concentrations in smaller volumes should be used in children and patients with severe cardiovascular disease.[16] Use of a preprocedure penile block is essential.

In addition to the treatment directed at acutely relieving the tumescence, other underlying causes, if they exist, should be treated. For example, patients with sickle cell disease may benefit from intravenous fluids and supplemental inhaled oxygen. However, recent literature debunks prior recommendations regarding blood transfusion for patients with priapism caused by sickle cell anemia, and thus routine transfusion is no longer recommended.[18] Certainly any potentially offending medications should be discontinued, if possible, and in rare cases of priapism caused by malignancy, further treatment such as local radiation should be considered.[10]

Treatment of stuttering priapism includes preventative daily antiandrogen therapy, such as cyproterone acetate, or gonadotropin-releasing hormone drugs, such as leuprolide, which paradoxically reduce the frequency of priapism but do not inhibit sexual activity. A promising new treatment is daily treatment with low-dose inhibitors of the enzyme phosphodiesterase type 5. These agents may reduce cellular nitric oxide action and decrease vasodilation, thus reducing erection duration. However, even patients with stuttering priapism may require emergency treatment for typical ischemic priapism in the setting of particularly severe symptoms or a markedly prolonged erection.[11]

Regardless of the precipitating cause of ischemic priapism, surgical shunt procedures are used as a last resort in patients with low-flow priapism unresponsive to the aforementioned treatments.[2,3]

Treatment of nonischemic priapism requires less urgency. No risk of long-term damage is associated with the absence of immediate treatment and, although the condition is distressing, pain is not a prominent feature. Conservative therapies, such as rest, ice packs, and observation for several days, will help resolve the inciting arteriovenous fistulae in more than 60% of cases; however, of those who improve (detumescence), nearly one-third may still experience erectile dysfunction.[19] If conservative management fails or is otherwise nonfeasible, embolization is the next step. Embolization has a greater than 90% success rate in treating priapism, but still nearly 10% of patients may have erectile dysfunction after this procedure.[20] Surgical ligation of the cavernosal artery or ligation of the fistula may be required if embolism fails.[21] However, after ligation, close to half of patients experience erectile dysfunction.[19] Alternative methods to treat nonischemic priapism include injection of thrombin or methylene blue into the corpora cavernosa in an effort to occlude the arteriovenous fistula, but these should be considered less favored alternatives to embolization.[3]

Paraphimosis

Paraphimosis is the inability to completely reduce the penile foreskin distally back to its natural position overlying the glans penis. This condition occurs in uncircumcised men. The entrapped distal foreskin forms a constricting band on the penile shaft. Compression inhibits venous drainage of the glans and results in a vicious circle of progressive glans edema that further prevents reduction foreskin distally. Glans edema may become so severe that arterial inflow is compromised and may result in necrosis and gangrene of the glans, which rarely may even be complicated by the development of necrotizing fasciitis.[22] Patients will present with a red, painful, and swollen glans penis associated with an edematous, proximally retracted foreskin that forms a circumferential constricting band. The penile shaft proximal to the constricting band is typically soft.

Paraphimosis often occurs in the extremes of life. It may commonly occur in elderly patients after urinary catheterization or medical examination if the foreskin is not returned to its natural location over the glans, termed *iatrogenic paraphimosis*. Poor hygiene and balanoposthitis (see later sections on Balanitis and Posthitis) at any age are also associated with development of paraphimosis. Inflammation can result in contracture of the distal foreskin. Later when the foreskin is retracted proximally over the compressible glans, the contracted foreskin forms a constrictive band and gets "stuck" in the retracted position. One theory regarding the predisposition of elderly men to paraphimosis is decreased frequency of erections from dysfunction, reduced libido, or other factors causes natural dilation of the preputial orifice to occur less frequently, elevating the entrapment risk.[23]

Paraphimosis may also occur after intercourse or other sexual activity.[24] Paraphimosis has even been observed after prolonged erections experienced during cultural celebrations involving many hours of erotic dancing.[25] Uncircumcised men must be vigilant about foreskin replacement after sexual activity, and should be instructed to seek care immediately if a paraphimosis develops.[26] Trauma and purposeful and accidental tourniquets may cause paraphimosis (see later section on Penile Trauma, Entrapment, and Foreign Body). Some uncommon causes of paraphimosis include genital piercings,[27] plasmodium falciparum,[28] chancroid,[29] lichen sclerosis, and contact dermatitis.[24] Special consideration should be given to the care and evaluation of developmentally disabled men who require assistance with genital hygiene. Patients and their caregivers may be unaware of the potential for or the development of paraphimosis and the need to treat it emergently.[30]

Paraphimosis is a urologic emergency that must be treated promptly to prevent glans necrosis. Paraphimosis can frequently be managed in the emergency department without the need for emergent specialty consultation. Many methods for successful paraphimosis reduction have been reported; however, the most commonly used initial maneuver involves manual compression of the distal glans penis to decrease edema, followed by reduction of the glans penis back through the proximal constricting band of foreskin.[31]

Glans edema must be reduced so that the edematous foreskin can be moved distally, back to its natural position. Typically this is performed with manual pressure on the glans to decrease the edema; the foreskin may then be pulled distally into the normal position (**Fig. 2**). This technique can be difficult and painful, and therefore many adjunctive methods have been reported to first help reduce glans swelling. Routinely used maneuvers include the application of ice packs (filling the tip of an examining glove with ice is often recommended) or wrapping the glans in compressive bandages. Alternatively, techniques focusing on reducing foreskin edema have been advocated. The Dundee technique involves making multiple micropunctures of the edematous foreskin and then squeezing out the edema fluid.[32]

Hyaluronidase has been reported to result in rapid reduction of prepuce edema, which facilitates manual reduction of the foreskin. This enzyme, when injected into

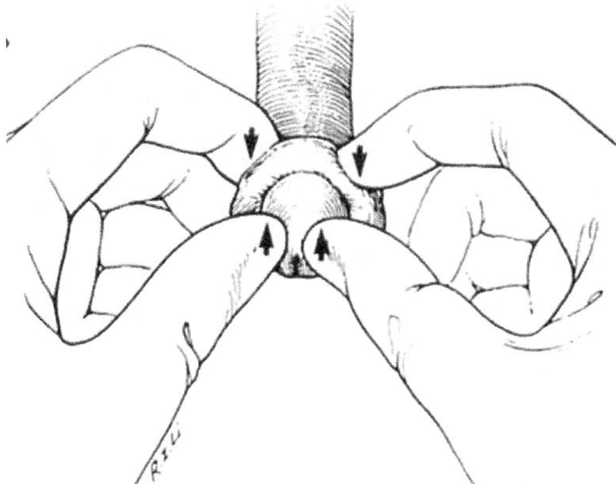

Fig. 2. Paraphimosis reduction. (*From* Barone JG, Fleisher MH. Treatment of paraphimosis using the "puncture" technique. Ped Emerg Care 1993;9(5):299; with permission.)

the swollen retracted foreskin, causes hydrolysis of hyaluronic acid that in turn increases tissue permeability so that the edema in the foreskin is diffused out into the surrounding tissue of the penis.[33] There have even been advocates of a completely noninvasive way to reduce the foreskin edema through applying granulated sugar to the penis. This sugar forms an osmotic gradient that draws out the fluid to reduce the edema, but this may take several hours.[34] Publications on these procedures are generally observational in design and involve small numbers of patients, such as case reports. No large studies of comparative effectiveness have been conducted, and therefore recommending any one method over another is difficult.[35]

Despite these various minimally or noninvasive methods to treat paraphimosis, sometimes a dorsal slit procedure or even formal circumcision is required emergently for resistant cases.[31] Referral to a urologic surgeon for routine follow-up is prudent after successful paraphimosis reduction, because patients may benefit from elective circumcision to prevent recurrence. A condition of chronic paraphimosis was recently described, in which patients present 1 week or more after the onset of paraphimosis.[36] A mildly constricting yet irreducible fibrous band of foreskin is present, but glans edema or necrosis is absent. Pain only develops with erections, and therefore treatment is frequently delayed. Patients diagnosed with chronic paraphimosis require modified or formal circumcision for treatment.[36]

Penile Trauma, Entrapment, and Foreign Body

Penile trauma, entrapment, and foreign bodies are frequently painful and distressing conditions for patients. Genitourinary injury or trauma should be considered an emergency requiring urologic surgical consultation until proven otherwise. Significant trauma, such as penile amputation, deep laceration, or urethral injury, frequently requires emergent surgical evaluation and management. However, most minor injuries can be safely managed in the emergency setting without the need for subspecialty consultation.

Burns to the penis require referral to a dedicated burn unit with experience in treating these injuries.[37] With appropriate care, even deep partial-thickness penile burn injuries can have favorable functional outcomes without deep scaring and contractures. Skin matrix substitutes placed after burn debridement function as scaffolding for new dermis growth before skin grafting and may serve as an effective barrier to infection.[38]

Zipper injuries are more common in children than adults. Often the patient is uncircumcised and the foreskin gets caught and crushed when the zipper is closed. Lubricants such as mineral oil can be used to free the skin from the zipper, but this does not always work. Cutting the median bar of the zipper will separate the zipper, allowing the two sides of the zipper to fall apart. The median bar is the small piece of metal that connects the anterior and posterior plates of the zipper. A bone or wire cutter is needed to divide the median bar (**Fig. 3**).[39] If these tools are unavailable, another method is to grasp opposite sides of the zipper, one inferior and one superior to the site of zipper entrapment, and slowly separate the teeth by pulling in opposite directions. Local anesthesia is recommended before using this method.[40] If these methods fail to release the entrapped foreskin, emergent partial or complete circumcision to separate the prepuce from the zipper may be necessary.

Glans edema mimicking paraphimosis can occur in circumcised or uncircumcised men in penile entrapment injuries. In these instances, external objects may constrict the mid to distal shaft, leading to the same pathophysiologic derangements seen

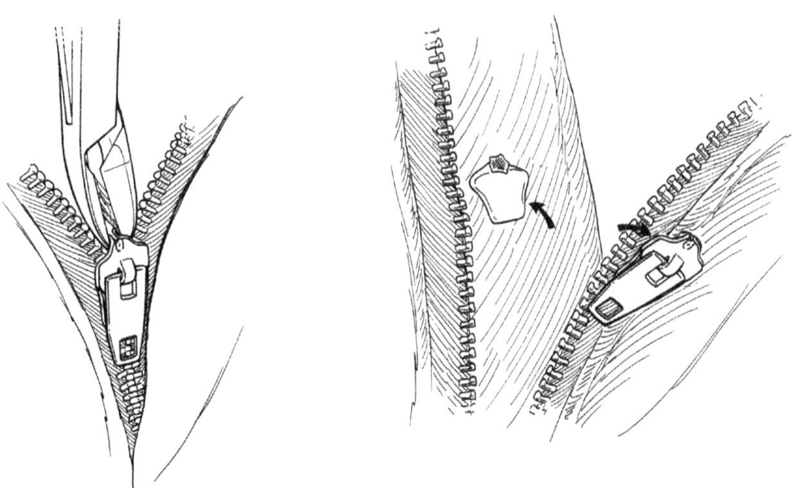

Fig. 3. Zipper removal. (*From* Vilke GM. Zipper removal. In: Rosen P, Chan TC, Vilke GM, et al, editors. Atlas of emergency procedures. St Louis (MO): Mosby; 2001. p. 137; with permission.)

with paraphimosis. Objects may either be placed intentionally for sexual stimulation or may occur sporadically, as in the case of a hair tourniquet in male infants. Hair tourniquets may be particularly difficult to diagnose, because the offending hair may be nearly invisible within an engorged and edematous coronal sulcus. An occult hair tourniquet should be considered, along with testicular torsion, in male infants who are crying inconsolably.

In adolescent or adult men, rings or other constricting bands may be used for self-stimulation or to maintain an erection.[41] Depending on the object and degree of entrapment and distal edema, release may be challenging. Occasionally, constricting objects may be removed without the need for cutting or sawing. One method is the string method.[42] Similar to that used to remove a ring from a finger, a flat string is passed under the ring so that it protrudes proximally. Then the distal end of the string is wound around the penis and when the proximal end of the string is pulled up and distally, with luck the ring will move distally, little by little, until it is removed. Glass saws may be helpful for removing glass bottles, but plastic bottles are not easily cut by a glass saw or scalpel. Rather, an oscillating cast saw is recommended for an entrapped plastic bottle. Using a splint device, such as a wooden tongue depressor blade, between the bottle and the skin of the penis is recommended.[43]

Metal devices may be removed with ring cutters, but may require heavy equipment such as pneumatic saws used by fire department personnel to extricate victims from crushed automobiles. One challenge in using these machines is that the skin entrapped under the device must be protected from the blade. In some cases, aspiration of blood from the entrapped corpora cavernosa may relieve enough edema so that a protective device can be placed before engaging the saw.[44] Because a great deal of heat is often generated from these saws, continuous irrigation of the area with cold water or saline is also necessary to protect the penis from thermal injury.[45] Time is critical when removing entrapped objects. With prolonged duration of entrapment, ischemia or gangrene of the distal penis may occur, in the most severe cases placing the penis at risk for possible amputation.[46]

In addition to foreign bodies placed around the penis shaft, foreign bodies are sometimes placed in the urethra or directly into the penis or scrotum. These objects are not always placed for sexual gratification. In one reported case, an elderly man was seen after complications occurred from placing a bean in his urethra as a plug to treat incontinence.[47] When faced with a urethral foreign body, the object may be grasped with a needle holder or clamp and removed with gentle traction. However, the goal is to remove the object without causing further damage and propelling the object further proximally. If the object cannot be readily removed, then specialty consultation will be necessary. A retrograde urethrogram is often unnecessary if the object is smooth and can be readily visualized at the meatus.[48] Foreign bodies identified in the penile shaft or scrotum should not be assumed to be the only embedded objects, because patients who place items in their genitalia may have multiple foreign bodies from prior insertions.[49] Patients with foreign bodies in their penis may present early because of pain and bleeding or late as a result of infection. Men may inject items such as petroleum jelly, oil, silicon, or paraffin directly into the penile shaft in an attempt to enlarge the penis or enhance sexual stimulation. Unfortunately, these patients may seek emergency care for pain or infection. Injections may result in chronic abscesses and fistulas, pain with erection, swelling, or phimosis. A granulomatous reaction to the foreign material can occur, often necessitating surgery to remove the injected substances.[50] This surgical cure is invasive and skin grafting is frequently necessary to close the wounds.[51]

OTHER CONDITIONS

Phimosis

Phimosis is a condition in which the prepuce cannot be retracted proximally over the glans. Similar to paraphimosis, phimosis occurs in uncircumcised men. However, unlike paraphimosis, it seldom requires emergency treatment. Phimosis is typically a chronic condition that may present acutely when a patient is unable to void spontaneously as a result of distal urethral obstruction. Phimosis occurs naturally in newborns and is caused by physiologic adherence between the epithelial lining of the glans and distal foreskin, leading to a nonretractile foreskin. By 3 years of age, fewer than 10% of foreskins remain nonretractile, with nearly all becoming retractile by late adolescence.[52]

Pathologic phimosis exists when the failure to retract results from distal scarring of the prepuce. A white fibrous band may even be visible around the distal preputial orifice.[53] Severe balanitis and posthitis may result in pathologic phimosis. Complications of phimosis include preputial stone formation or urine obstruction, which may require emergency treatment with a dorsal slit procedure to allow for free urine flow.[54]

Balanitis and Posthitis

Balanitis is inflammation of the glans penis, and posthitis is inflammation of the penile foreskin. Often both the glans and foreskin are inflamed, termed *balanoposthitis*. Glans or prepuce inflammation is often caused by infection. Uncircumcised men are at risk for developing infection because the tight foreskin, together with poor hygiene and smegma buildup, creates an environment conducive to the development of inflammation. Patients with this condition typically complain of a red, edematous glans or foreskin, often with discharge. Determining the causal agent may be challenging. *Candida albicans* is the causal agent in nearly one-third of balanitis cases.[55] The typical findings of candidiasis are erythema and papules with "satellite" lesions. Burning and pruritis may also be present. Candida can be contracted from sexual activity with an infected partner. Diabetics or other immunosuppressed patients are at risk for candidal balanitis or posthitis. Treatment with topical azole antifungal agents and effective hygiene typically is sufficient, but in severe cases a single oral dose of 150 mg of fluconazole may be necessary.[55] Other common infectious causes include streptococcal and staphylococcal species, which typically require oral antimicrobial treatment. Sexually transmitted diseases, including chlamydia and syphilis, may also cause balanitis and posthitis. Therefore, cultures or other diagnostic testing for suspected causal agents may be necessary to help guide treatment.[56] Balanoposthitis may be complicated by phimosis, cellulitis of the penile shaft, or abscess formation.[57]

Noninfectious causes of balanoposthitis occur less frequently overall, yet remain important considerations.[58] Contact dermatitis may occur from condoms, spermicidals, or lubricating gels associated with condom use.[59] Lichen planus is an inflammatory dermatosis that affects only the glans (balanitis), causing itchy red and whitish plaques. It is treated with high-potency topical steroids.[60] Balanitis xerotica obliterans is a rare condition of unknown origin that causes chronic inflammation of the glans, dry skin, and pruritis, and may be associated with endarteritis.[61]

Sexually Transmitted Disease

Several sexually transmitted diseases are associated with penile findings or discomfort. Urethritis may result in symptoms of dysuria, penile discharge, and urethral pruritis. Confirmatory testing is helpful in targeting treatment. Alternatively, empiric treatment for both gonorrhea and chlamydia is an accepted common practice. Current Centers for Disease Control and Prevention treatment recommendations are for 250 mg of ceftriaxone intramuscularly for gonorrhea treatment, plus 1 g of azithromycin orally or 100 mg of doxycycline orally twice daily for 7 days for chlamydia treatment. Patients should be encouraged to notify all sexually partners, because contacts also require evaluation and treatment.[62]

Chancroid is caused by infection with *Haemophilus ducreyi* and results in a painful, friable, nonindurated, necrotic ulcer that may form anywhere on the penis. Chancroid ulceration on the prepuce may result in balanoposthitis or phimosis. Treatment involves 1 g of azithromycin orally or 250 mg of ceftriaxone intramuscularly. Although primary syphilis can cause a genital ulcer (chancre), it is often a painless lesion in contrast to chancroid.[63]

Herpes simplex virus (HSV) types 1 and 2 cause lifelong recurrent infections. HSV-2 is the causal agent in nearly all outbreaks of genital herpes. Crops of papules or vesicles, progressing to pustules or ulcers, characterize this painful condition. A burning sensation or pruritis with genital herpes may be present, and patients with initial infection may develop urinary retention. Empiric treatment should not be delayed while awaiting results of confirmatory diagnostic studies. Treatment for the first outbreak of genital herpes is 400 mg of acyclovir orally 3 times daily for 7 to 10 days. For recurrent herpes, the treatment is shortened to five days.[42,64]

Penis Fracture

Fracture of the penis is a rare urologic emergency. Injury to the corpus cavernosum typically occurs during vigorous sexual intercourse when the penis may slip out and be pushed against the partner's perineum, during masturbation, or rarely from rolling over in bed with an erect penis.[65] Penis fracture during masturbation may occur if an erect penis is forcefully bent in attempt to quickly reduce the erection.[66] Classic historical features of penile fracture include a cracking sound followed by pain, rapid detumescence, swelling, and ecchymosis. The penis will often be deformed and bent in the direction of the uninjured corpora cavernosum.[67] The injury is caused by an acute tear of the tunica albuginea, which becomes very thin during erection and is easily torn with sudden bending.[68] Usually one corpora cavernosa is torn, but bilateral cavernosal injuries may occur simultaneously. Potential coexisting injuries include those to the penile urethra, corpus spongiosum, or dorsal vein of the penis.[69] The dorsal vein of the penis becomes stretched during erection and may tear in a similar manner to the tunica albuginea. In isolated dorsal vein injury, pain and ecchymosis will be present, but the classic cracking sound and sudden detumescence will be absent.[70] Patients with urethral injuries are at risk for developing urethral strictures.

Emergency surgical exploration and repair are recommended to treat penile fractures. However, the option of delaying surgical repair for 7 to 12 days has been suggested, particularly in patients presenting more than 24 hours after fracture and without coexisting urethral injury.[71,72] If blood is present at the urethral meatus, a preoperative urethrogram should be performed. Alternatively, the urethra can be explored during surgery.[69] Some authors recommend MRI before surgery to delineate the extent of injury and help direct where the incision should be made.[66] In some cases, MRI may prevent unnecessary surgery if imaging shows only a hematoma rather than a tear of the tunica albuginea.[66] Most patients recover well after surgical repair, but roughly 10% will have permanent curvature of the penis and some will experience pain during intercourse.[69] Erectile dysfunction after repair is rare. One long-term follow-up study showed that fewer than 2% of patients become impotent.[73]

Peyronie's Disease

Peyronie's disease was first reported in 1743. It is a connective tissue disorder in which plaques or scars form in the tunica albuginea, resulting in penile pain, induration, palpable plaques on the shaft that cause abnormal curvature of the erect penis, and ultimately erectile dysfunction. The characteristic scar formation can occur after major trauma and minor "microtrauma" during intercourse. In many cases, patients will not recall any distinct precipitating traumatic event. Patients with Peyronie's disease are thought to have a genetic predisposition for abnormal scar formation. Patients should be referred for nonurgent urologic surgery follow-up. Typical therapies range from tocopherol (vitamin E) pills to plaque injections with interferon α.[74]

Penile Calciphylaxis

Penile calciphylaxis is a rare disorder. Patients may present with severe penile pain from ischemia caused by calcification and fibrosis of the penile arteries. In its most extreme form, it may progress to gangrene, requiring penectomy. The underlying cause is often secondary hyperparathyroidism associated with end stage renal disease. Affected patients may also have concurrent calciphylaxis of the limbs. Emergency urologic surgical consultation is needed for infection or necrosis requiring debridement.[75]

SUMMARY

Of the various penile conditions discussed, emergency practitioners must be most concerned with the entities that, if left untreated, can result in ischemia and necrosis of the penis, namely ischemic priapism, paraphimosis, and entrapment injuries. In addition, any penile trauma should be considered an emergency until proven otherwise. Emergency clinicians must be able to recognize these emergent conditions, begin treatment, and obtain timely urology consultation if necessary. Many other penile conditions can be safely and effectively managed without the need for emergent specialty consultation, and thus can be referred for urgent outpatient follow-up.

REFERENCES

1. Papadopoulos I, Kelami A. Priapus and priapism from mythology to medicine. Urology 1988;32(4):385–6.
2. Burnett B, Bivalacqua T. Priapism: current principles and practice. Urol Clin North Am 2007;34:631–42.
3. Huang YC, Harraz A, Shindel A, et al. Evaluation and management of priapism: 2009 update. Nat Rev Urol 2009;6:262–71.
4. Kilinc M, Piskin S, Guven R, et al. Partial priapism secondary to tamsulosin: a case report and review of the literature. Andrologia 2009;21:199–201.
5. Cherian J, Rao A, Thwaini A, et al. Medical and surgical management of priapism. Postgrad Med J 2006;82:89–94.
6. Sood S, James W, Bailon M. Priapism associated with atypical antipsychotic medications: a review. Int Clin Psychopharmacol 2008;23:9–17.
7. Hishmeh S, DiMaio F. Priapism as a complication after total hip arthroplasty. Orthopedics 2008;31(4):397.
8. Edmond A, Holman R, Hayes R, et al. Priapism and impotence in homozygous sickle cell disease. Arch Intern Med 1980;140(11):1434–7.
9. Cherrie R, Brosman S. Case profile: priapism secondary to metastatic adenocarcinoma of the rectum. Urology 1985;25(6):655.
10. Chan P, Begin L, Arnold M, et al. Priapism secondary to penile metastasis: a report of two cases and a review of the literature. J Surg Oncol 1998;68:51–9.
11. Muneer A, Minhas S, Arya M, et al. Stuttering priapism—a review of the therapeutic options. Int J Clin Pract 2008;62(8):1265–70.
12. Bivalacqua T, Burnett A. Priapism: new concepts in the pathophysiology and new treatment strategies. Curr Urol Rep 2006;7:497–502.
13. Caumartin Y, Lacoursiere L, Naud A. High-flow priapism: an overview of diagnostic and therapeutic concepts. Can J Urol 2006;13(5):3238–90.
14. Lowe JC, Jarow JP. Placebo-controlled study of oral terbutaline and pseudoephedrine in management of prostaglandin E_1-induced prolonged erections. Urology 1993;42:51–4.
15. Govier FE, Jonsson E, Kramer-Levin D. Oral terbutaline for the treatment of priapism. J Urol 1994;151:878–9.
16. The management of priapism. U.S. Department of Health & Human Services: Agency for Healthcare Research and Quality Web site. Available at:http://guidelines.gov/content.aspx?id=3741. Accessed January 5, 2011.
17. Priyadarshi S. Oral terbutaline in the management of pharmacologically induced prolonged erection. Int J Impot Res 2004;16:424–6.
18. Merritt A, Haiman C, Henderson S. Myth. Blood transfusion is effective for sickle cell anemia-associated priapism. CJEM 2006;8(2):119–22.
19. Montague D, Boderick G, Dmochowski R, et al. American urological association guideline on the management of priapism. J Urol 2003;170:1318–24.
20. Kojima H, Tanigawa N, Kariya S, et al. High-flow priapism undergoing arterial embolization: review of literature following the American urological association guideline on the management of priapism. Minim Invasive Ther Allied Technol 2009;18:1–5.
21. Shapiro R, Berger R. Post-traumatic priapism treated with selective cavernosal artery ligation. Urology 1997;49:638–43.

22. Ahmed J, Mallick I. Paraphimosis leading to Fournier's gangrene. J Coll Physicians Surg Pak 2009;19(3):203–4.
23. Williams J, Morris P, Richardson J. Paraphimosis in elderly men. Am J Emerg Med 1995;13(3):351–4.
24. Berk D, Lee R. Paraphimosis in a middle-aged adult after intercourse. Am Fam Physician 2004;69(4):807–8.
25. Ramdass M, Naraynsingh V, Kuruvilla T, et al. Case report: paraphimosis due to erotic dancing. Trop Med Int Health 2000;5(12):906–7.
26. Raman S, Kate V, Ananthakrishnan N. Coital paraphimosis causing penile necrosis. Emerg Med J 2008;25(7):454.
27. Jones S, Flynn R. An unusual (and somewhat piercing) cause of paraphimosis. Br J Urol 1996;78:803–4.
28. Gozal D. Paraphimosis apparently associated with plasmodium falciparum infection. Trans R Soc Trop Med Hyg 1991;85:443.
29. Harvey K, Biship L, Silver D, et al. A case of chancroid. Med J Aust 1977;1:956–7.
30. Wilson N, Cumella S, Parmenter T, et al. Penile hygiene: puberty, paraphimosis and personal care for men and boys with an intellectual disability. J Intellect Disabil Res 2009;53(2):106–14.
31. Choe JM. Paraphimosis: current treatment options. Am Fam Physician 2000;62: 2623–6.
32. Reynard J, Barua J. Reduction of paraphimosis the simple way - the Dundee technique. BJU Int 1999;83(7):859–60.
33. DeVries C, Miller A. Reduction of paraphimosis with hyaluronidase. Urology 1996; 48(3):464–5.
34. Kerwat R, Shandall A, Stephenson B. Reduction of paraphimosis with granulated sugar. Br J Urol 1998;82(5):755.
35. Mackway-Jones K. Ice, pins, or sugar to reduce paraphimosis. Emerg Med J 2004;21:77–8.
36. Rangarajan M, Jayakar S. Paraphimosis revisited: is chronic paraphimosis a predominantly third world condition? Trop Doct 2008;38:40–2.
37. American College of Surgeons, Committee on Trauma. Resources for the optimal care of the injured patient. Chicago: American College of Surgeons; 2006.
38. Jaskille A, Shupp J, Jeng J, et al. Use of Integra in the treatment of third degree burns to the penile shaft: a case series with 6-month follow-up. J Burn Care Res 2009;30:524–8.
39. Nakagawa T, Toguri A. Penile zipper injury. Med Princ Pract 2006;15:3003–304.
40. McCann P. Case report: a novel solution to penile zipper injury—the needle holder. ScientificWorldJournal 2005;5:298–9.
41. Massoud W, Pascal H, Awad A, et al. External genitalia entrapment a case report. Urol J 2010;7:136–7.
42. Noh J, Kang TW, Heo T, et al. Penile strangulation treated with the modified string method. Urology 2004;644:591.
43. May M, Gunia S, Helke C, et al. Penile entrapment in a plastic bottle—a case for using an oscillating splint saw. Int Urol Nephrol 2006;38:93–5.
44. Kimber RM, Mellon J. The role of special cutting equipment and corporeal aspiration in the treatment of penile incarceration with a barbell retaining collar. J Urol 2004;172:975.
45. Xu T, Gu M, Wang H. Emergency management of penile strangulation: a case report and review of the Chinese literature. Emerg Med J 2009;26(1):73–4.
46. Nuhu A, Edino S, Agbese G, et al. Penile gangrene due to strangulation by a metallic nut: a case report and review of the literature. Internet J Surg 2009;21(2):1–9.

47. Patel A. Dry haricot bean: a new continence aid for elderly men? BMJ 1990;301: 1432–3.
48. Thomas S, White B. Foreign bodies. In: Marx J, Hockberger R, Walls R, et al, editors. Rosen's emergency medicine concepts and clinical practice. 7th edition. Philadelphia: Mosby; 2009. p. 731.
49. Blake-James B, Hussain M, Peters L. Genital foreign bodies: more than the eye can see. Eur J Emerg Med 2007;12:53–5.
50. Wiwanitkit V. Penile injection of foreign bodies in eight Thai patients. Sex Transm Infect 2004;80:546.
51. Nylrady P, Kelemen Z, Kiss A, et al. Treatment and outcome of Vaseline-induced sclerosing lipogranuloma of the penis. Urology 2008;71:1132–7.
52. McGregor TB, Pike JG, Leonard MP. Pathologic and physiologic phimosis: approach to the phimotic foreskin. Can Fam Physician 2007;53:445–8.
53. McGregor T, Pike J, Leonard M. Phimosis—a diagnostic dilemma? Can J Urol 2005;12(2):2598–602.
54. Ho K, Segura J. Lower urinary tract calculi. In: Wein AJ, editor. Campbell-Walsh urology. 9th edition. Philadelphia: Saunders; 2007. p. 2672–3.
55. Janik M, Heffernan M. Yeast infections: candidiasis and tinea (pityriasis) versicolor. In: Wolff K, Goldsmith LA, Katz SI, et al, editors. Fitzpatrick's dermatology in general medicine. 7th edition. New York: McGraw Hill; 2008. p. 1824–8.
56. Lisboa C, Ferreira A, Resende C, et al. Infectious balanoposthitis: management, clinical and laboratory features. Int J Dermatol 2009;48:121–4.
57. Mahler S, Manthey D. Diagnosis of a preputial cavity abscess with bedside ultrasound in the Emergency Department. J Emerg Med 2008;35(3):273–6.
58. Lisboa C, Ferreira A, Resende C, et al. Noninfectious balanitis in patients attending a sexually transmitted diseases clinic. Int J Dermatol 2009;48:445–6.
59. Muratore L, Calogiuri G, Foti C, et al. Contact allergy to benzocaine in a condom. Contact Derm 2008;59:173–4.
60. Lehman J, Tollefson M, Gibson L. Lichen planus. Int J Dermatol 2009;48:682–94.
61. Sakti D, Gurunadha HS, Tunuguntla R. Balanitis xerotica obliterans—a review. World J Urol 2000;18:382–7.
62. Centers for Disease Control and Prevention. Sexually transmitted diseases treatment guidelines. MMWR Morb Mortal Wkly Rep 2010;59(RR-12):40–51.
63. Sehgal V, Srivastava G. Chancroid: contemporary appraisal. Int J Dermatol 2003; 42:182–90.
64. Gupta R, Warren T, Wald A. Genital herpes. Lancet 2007;370:2127–37.
65. Ghilan A, Al-Asbahi W, Ghafour M, et al. Management of penile fractures. Saudi Med J 2008;29(10):1443–7.
66. Abolysor A, Moneim A, Abdelatif A, et al. The management of penile fracture based on clinical and magnetic resonance imaging findings. BJU Int 2005;96: 373–7.
67. Khan R, Malik M, Jamil M, et al. Penile fracture: experience at Ayub teaching hospital. J Ayub Med Coll Abbottabad 2008;20(4):49–50.
68. Pandyan G, Zaharani A, Al Rashid M. Fracture penis: an analysis of 26 cases. ScientificWorldJournal 2006;6:2327–33.
69. Atat R, Sfaxi M, Benslama M, et al. Fracture of the penis: management and long term results of surgical treatment. Experience in 300 cases. J Trauma 2008;64: 121–5.
70. Perlmutter A, Roberts L, Farivar-Mohseni H, et al. Ruptured superficial dorsal vein of the penis masquerading as a penile fracture: case report. Can J Urol 2007; 14(4):3651–2.

71. Naraynsingh V, Ramdass MJ, Thomas D, et al. Delayed repair of a fractured penis: a new technique. Int J Clin Pract 2003;57(5):428–9.
72. Nasser TA, Mostafa T. Delayed surgical repair of penile fracture under local anesthesia. J Sex Med 2008;5(10):2464–9.
73. Zargooshi J. Sexual function and tunica albuginea wound healing following penile fracture: an 18-year follow-up study of 352 patients from Kermanshah, Iran. J Sex Med 2009;6(4):1141–50.
74. Hellstrom W. Medical management of Peyronie's disease. J Androl 2009;30(4):397–405.
75. Karpman E, Das S, Kurzrock E. Penile calciphylaxis: analysis of risk factors and mortality. J Urol 2003;169(6):2206–9.

Genitourinary Trauma

Sanjay Shewakramani, MD*, Kevin C. Reed, MD

KEYWORDS

• Genitourinary • Urologic • Trauma • Emergency • Renal

Injury to the genitourinary (GU) tract occurs in up to 10% of patients presenting with abdominal trauma.[1] GU injuries often occur in the setting of polytrauma and may be overlooked.[2] Although GU trauma does not often cause significant shock alone, it can lead to significant morbidity and mortality if not recognized early.[3,4] Blunt trauma accounts for around 90% of injuries.[5] However, penetrating trauma seems to be increasing in frequency and is the cause of up to 20% of GU trauma in urban settings.[6] The kidney is the most frequently injured organ, with injuries occurring in 1% to 5% of all trauma cases,[7] followed by the urethra and bladder.[8] Anatomic differences between external genitalia as well as the higher incidence of violence amongst men account for the male predominance of urologic trauma.[9]

Plain radiography, ultrasonography, computed tomography (CT), and magnetic resonance imaging (MRI) have all been used effectively to diagnose urologic trauma.[10] The treatment of GU trauma is often conservative, but it is important to be aware of situations in which emergent therapy is indicated.[11] Because the pathophysiology, diagnostic approach, and management of GU trauma vary greatly depending on the involved organ, each entity should be considered individually when discussing urologic trauma.

ANATOMY

The upper segment of the GU system includes the kidneys, ureters, and renal pedicle (composed of the renal artery and vein). The kidney is a retroperitoneal structure and lies within the paravertebral gutter, extending from the 12th rib to the 3rd lumbar vertebra. Because of the large size of the liver, the right kidney lies slightly inferior to the left kidney. The ureters measure 25 to 30 cm in length and travel along the anterior aspect of the psoas muscle, connecting the renal pelvis to the bladder.

The bladder and urethra are located in the pelvis and form the lower GU tract. The male and female urethrae differ significantly in length (20 and 4 cm, respectively),

The authors have nothing to disclose.
Department of Emergency Medicine, Georgetown University Hospital, 3800 Reservoir Road, Washington, DC 20007, USA
* Corresponding author.
E-mail address: sanjay.shewakramani@medstar.net

Emerg Med Clin N Am 29 (2011) 501–518
doi:10.1016/j.emc.2011.04.009 emed.theclinics.com

which partially accounts for the increased incidence of urethral trauma in men. The external portion of the GU system includes the anterior urethra, penis, scrotum, and testicles in men and the labia, clitoris, and hymen in women.[12]

BLADDER

Bladder injures caused by blunt or penetrating trauma are rarely isolated injuries. About 80% to 94% of patients have significant associated nonurologic injuries, with mortality rates of 8% to 44%.[13–20] Pelvic fractures are the most common associated injury; however, bladder injury occurs in only 5% to 10% of patients with pelvic fractures.[16,19,21–24]

The bladder is located deep in the bony pelvis, affording some protection from external trauma. Most blunt bladder injuries are caused by rapid deceleration during motor vehicle accidents. Injury may also occur secondary to falls, crush injuries, assault, and blows to the lower abdomen. Disruption of the bony pelvis tends to tear the bladder at its fascial attachments, whereas bone fragments may lacerate the organ directly. Bladder laceration may also arise from penetrating trauma.[25]

Bladder contusions are defined as mucosal or muscularis injury when there is no loss of wall continuity. Full-bladder rupture may be either extraperitoneal or intraperitoneal. Extraperitoneal injury is usually associated with pelvic fracture. Although intraperitoneal injury may also occur because of pelvic fracture, it occurs more commonly from penetrating or burst injury at the dome because of sudden elevated pressures in a full bladder resulting from a direct blow.[25]

Appropriate diagnosis and grading are important for ultimate management. Associated abdominal and pelvic injuries may mask or confuse bladder symptoms, such as suprapubic or nonspecific abdominal pain or the inability to void. Physical examination findings suggesting possible bladder injury include suprapubic tenderness, lower abdominal bruising, muscle guarding or rigidity, and diminished bowel sounds.[25] If bladder injury is suspected, a spontaneously voided or urinary catheter specimen is essential. The most reliable sign of bladder injury is gross hematuria, present in 93% to 100% of cases.[15,16,26,27] However, if blood is noted at the meatus or if the urinary catheter does not pass easily, urgent assessment of urethral integrity with retrograde urethrography (RUG) should be performed because concomitant bladder and urethral injuries occur in 10% to 29% of patients.[21,28]

Imaging of the bladder should be performed on the basis of clinical suspicion, physical examination findings, and presence of hematuria or pelvic fracture. An absolute indication for immediate cystography after blunt trauma is gross hematuria associated with a pelvic fracture because bladder rupture is present in up to 29% of patients with this combination of findings. Relative indications for cystography after blunt trauma include gross hematuria without a pelvic fracture, microhematuria with pelvic fracture, and isolated microscopic hematuria.[22] Although the diagnosis of bladder rupture is extremely low in these groups (eg, 0.6% in patients with pelvic fracture and microhematuria),[25] it is prudent to maintain a high index of suspicion if associated clinical indicators of potential bladder injury are present (**Box 1**). In addition, penetrating injuries of the buttock, pelvis, or lower abdomen with any degree of hematuria warrant urgent cystography.

Retrograde cystography is nearly 100% accurate for bladder injury if it is performed correctly.[25] The bladder should be filled with a water-soluble contrast in cooperative patients till either a sense of discomfort or to a maximum of 350 mL. Bladder distention is needed to visualize small tears because false-negative results have been reported with retrograde instillation of 250 mL. A 3-film technique is recommended, including

Box 1
Clinical indicators of potential bladder injury

- Suprapubic pain or tenderness
- Free intraperitoneal fluid on CT or ultrasonographic examination
- Inability to void or low urine output
- Clots in urine
- Signs of perineal or genital trauma
- Unresponsive, intoxicated, or altered sensorium
- Preexisting bladder disease or urologic surgery
- Abdominal distention or ileus

Data from Morey F, Rozanski TS. Genital and lower urinary tract trauma. In: Wein AJ, editor. Campbell-Walsh Urology. 9th edition. Philadelphia: WB Saunders; 2007.

a film before administration of the contrast agent, an anteroposterior full bladder film, and a drainage film.[23,29] Although upper and lower urinary tract injuries rarely coincide (0.4%), hematuria and mechanism of injury mandate consideration of upper tract imaging studies as well.[25] Dense flame-shaped collections of contrast material in the pelvis is classic for extraperitoneal extravasation, which may extend to the retroperitoneum, scrotum, phallus, thigh, or anterior abdominal wall. Intraperitoneal extravasation is identified when contrast material outlines the loops of the bowel.[25]

CT cystography is often preferred over plain film cystography to assess bladder integrity. CT cystography is considered as accurate as plain film cystography as long as the bladder is filled in retrograde fashion with diluted contrast material to a volume of 350 to 400 mL.[15,25,30] Drainage films are not required because the retrovesical space can be well visualized on routine CT imaging.[29] Simply clamping the urethral catheter to allow anterograde filling and distention of the bladder from intravenous contrast is inadequate for diagnosis of bladder rupture. Conventional abdominal CT imaging of the trauma patient (without cystography) may show findings suggestive of bladder injury but cannot rule out the diagnosis.[15,31,32]

Uncomplicated extraperitoneal bladder rupture is typically managed conservatively with large-bore (eg, 22F) urethral catheter drainage alone. However, several investigators have reported fewer complications, such as fistula, failure to heal, clot retention, or sepsis, with open repair (5% overall) versus conservative management (12% overall).[21,33]

Blunt extraperitoneal injuries with any complicating features warrant immediate open repair to prevent complications such as fistula, abscess, or prolonged leak. Complicating features include concomitant vaginal or rectal injury, failure of the urethral catheter to provide adequate drainage, bladder neck injuries, and need for internal fixation of pelvic fractures.[34] For this reason, if a stable patient is undergoing exploratory laparotomy for other associated injuries, repair of the extraperitoneal rupture is recommended during the initial surgery. In addition, immediate repair is indicated when internal fixation of pelvic fractures is performed, which may prevent urine leakage onto the orthopedic fixative hardware and subsequent infection.[25] Indications for immediate repair of bladder injury are listed in **Box 2**.

All penetrating or intraperitoneal injuries resulting from external trauma should also be managed by immediate operative repair because these injuries are often larger than suggested on cystography and are unlikely to heal spontaneously.[25] In patients

Box 2
Indications for immediate repair of bladder injury

- Extraperitoneal bladder injury with complicating features
- Extraperitoneal bladder injury in a stable patient undergoing exploratory laparotomy for other associated injuries
- Intraperitoneal bladder injury from external trauma
- Penetrating bladder injury from external trauma
- Inadequate bladder drainage or clots in urine
- Bladder neck injury
- Rectal or vaginal injury
- Open pelvic fracture
- Pelvic fracture requiring open reduction and internal fixation
- Selected stable patients undergoing laparotomy for other reasons
- Bone fragments projecting into the bladder

From Morey F, Rozanski TS. Genital and lower urinary tract trauma. In: Wein AJ, editor. Campbell-Walsh Urology. 9th edition. Philadelphia: WB Saunders; 2007; with permission.

with intraperitoneal rupture, antimicrobials should be administered for at least 3 days, and a cystogram should be obtained 7 to 10 days after surgery.[19] In cases of isolated bladder injury, suprapubic tube drainage provides no benefit over urethral catheter drainage alone.[14,16,20]

Prompt diagnosis and appropriate management of bladder injuries typically lead to excellent results and minimal morbidity; thus, early identification of these injuries is key. Unrecognized bladder injuries can manifest clinically in many ways, including acidosis, azotemia, fever and sepsis, low urine output, peritonitis, ileus, urinary ascites, or respiratory difficulties. Unrecognized bladder neck, vaginal injury, or rectal injury associated with bladder rupture can result in incontinence, fistula, stricture, and compromise outcomes for delayed major reconstruction. Despite timely and appropriate bladder repair, neurologic injury caused by severe pelvic fractures may result in voiding difficulties.[25]

URETER

Ureteral injuries (**Table 1**) after trauma are rare, occurring in less than 4% of penetrating trauma and less than 1% of blunt trauma cases. A significant percentage (10%–28%) of patients with ureteral injuries have associated renal injuries, whereas a much smaller percentage (5%) have associated bladder injuries.[35–37]

Penetrating trauma may transect the ureter, causing disruption of the delicate intramural blood supply and subsequent necrosis.[38] Patients with blunt trauma presenting with ureteral injury typically have been subject to extreme forces applied over a larger region of the body. Although a relatively uncommon injury, a fractured lumbar lateral vertebral process or thoracolumbar spinal dislocation should always increase the level of suspicion for ureteral injury.[35]

Individuals with penetrating trauma with any degree of hematuria or a wound pattern that suggests the possibility of GU injury should undergo imaging.[35] Because many (25%–45%) cases of ureteral injury do not show microscopic hematuria,[36,39–41] a high

Table 1
The American Association for the Surgery of Trauma Organ Injury Severity Scale for the ureter

Grade[a]	Type	Description
I	Hematoma	Contusion or hematoma without devascularization
II	Laceration	<50% transection
III	Laceration	≥50% transection
IV	Laceration	Complete transection with <2 cm devascularization
V	Laceration	Avulsion with >2 cm devascularization

[a] Advance one grade for bilateral up to grade III.

Data from Moore EE, Cogbill TH, Jurkovich GJ, et al. Organ injury scaling. III: chest wall, abdominal vascular, ureter, bladder, and urethra. J Trauma 1992;33:338; and *Reproduced from* McAninch JW, Santucci RA. Renal and ureteral trauma. In: Wein AJ, editor. Campbell-Walsh Urology. Philadelphia: WB Saunders; 2007; with permission.

index of suspicion is required in cases of potential ureteral injury after penetrating trauma. Attention to the course of the bullet, knife, or other penetrating object, combined with judicious use of imaging, may decrease the rate of delayed diagnosis. Patients with blunt trauma with gross or microscopic hematuria, hypotension, a history of significant deceleration mechanism, or significant associated injuries should undergo imaging as well.[42]

Although rare, ureteropelvic junction (UPJ) disruption secondary to blunt trauma is often missed because hematuria may be absent. Therefore, a high index of suspicion for this injury should be maintained when there is a history of a rapid deceleration mechanism. Delayed presentation of ureteral injuries is most commonly associated with fever, leukocytosis, and local peritoneal irritation. Such findings should always prompt radiographic imaging.[35]

Preoperative intravenous pyelography (IVP) may be nondiagnostic in 33% to 100% of cases.[36,40,41] As such, IVP is considered a second-line diagnostic choice. Despite its limitations, a single intraoperative IVP is generally recommended for patients requiring emergency surgery for other injuries before alternative urinary system imaging.[35] CT seems promising in detecting ureteral injuries because it allows visualization of the entire course of the ureters, but research assessing its accuracy is limited.[43] The absence of contrast in the ureter on delayed images suggests ureteral injury.[35] Urinary extravasation from ureteral injury is helpful if visualized, although it may be at least partially contained by surrounding fascia, potentially obscuring an injury. UPJ disruption is typically associated with an unusual pattern of either medial or circumrenal contrast extravasation.[44]

Because modern helical CT scanners often obtain images before intravenous contrast dye is excreted in the urine, delayed images should be obtained (5–20 minutes after contrast injection) to allow contrast material to extravasate from the injured collecting system, renal pelvis, or ureter.[45,46] In one study, all patients with significant ureteropelvic lacerations had either medial extravasation of contrast material or nonopacification of the ipsilateral ureter on delayed CT.[43] Such findings should always raise suspicion for ureteral injury. Periureteral urinoma seen on delayed CT imaging can be diagnostic.[47] Retrograde ureterograms are used in some centers as a primary diagnostic technique to detect acute ureteral injuries, but less-invasive methods, such as delayed CT imaging, may be preferred. Delayed diagnosis of ureteral injury (more than 48 hours after initial trauma) is best accomplished with retrograde ureterography rather than CT imaging.[35]

Ureteral contusions, although considered minor ureteral injuries, often heal with stricture or breakdown if microvascular injury results in ureteral necrosis. Therefore, severe or large areas of contusion require surgical intervention. Minor ureteral contusions can be treated with stent placement.[35]

Ureteral avulsion from the renal pelvis or a proximal ureteral injury can be managed by reimplantation of the ureter directly into the renal pelvis. Typically, these injuries are treated by open surgery (especially when not discovered immediately) or laparoscopically.[48] Ureteroureterostomy, or end-to-end repair, is used in injuries to the upper two-thirds of the ureter. This technique is commonly performed and has reported success rates as high as 90%.[35] However, complications, including urine leakage, abscess, and fistula, occur in up to 24% of patients.[36,37,49,50] Delayed ureteral repairs, especially when a very long segment of ureter is damaged, can also be performed by the creation of a ureteral conduit out of the ileum with success rates ranging from 81% to 100% reported in the literature.[51–53]

Multiple surgical techniques are described in the urology literature for the repair of middle and lower ureteral injuries. Urology surgery consultation is required to plan further care, management, and ultimate disposition in these cases. In cases of severe multisystem trauma, it is sometimes necessary to defer definitive treatment of ureteral injuries. In cases of severe hemorrhagic shock, uncontrollable intraoperative bleeding, significant colon injury (especially those requiring colectomy), or severe associated injury to the ipsilateral kidney, ureteral repair should be avoided in favor of nephrectomy or staged repair.[50,54] An algorithm for the management of suspected ureteral injuries can be found in **Fig. 1**.

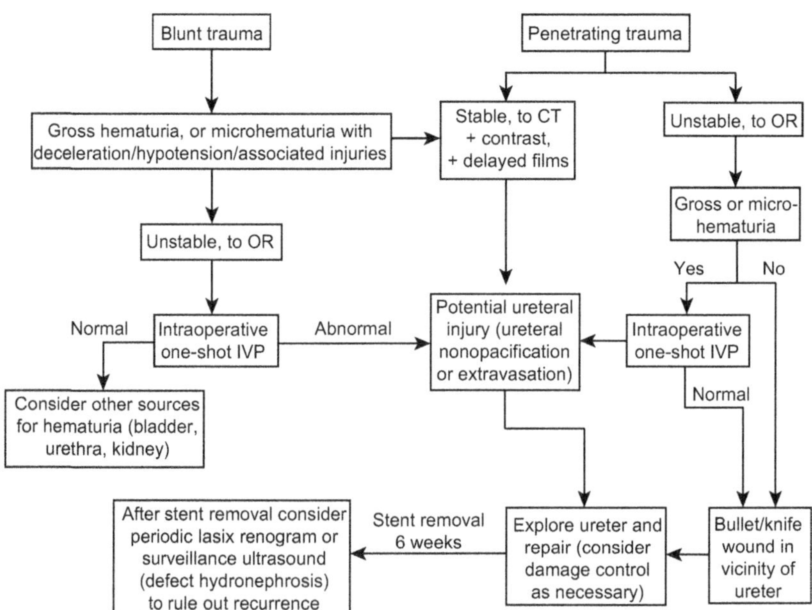

Fig. 1. Algorithm for the diagnosis and treatment of ureteral injuries from external violence. (*From* McAninch JW, Santucci RA. Renal and ureteral trauma. In: Wein AJ, editor. Campbell-Walsh Urology. Philadelphia: WB Saunders; 2007. p. 1290; with permission.)

KIDNEY

The kidney is the most commonly injured portion of the GU system. Blunt renal injury most commonly results from motor vehicle collision, fall from a height, or assault. Penetrating renal injury typically occurs secondary to gunshot or stab wounds. In a large reported series, the incidence of renal injuries inflicted by gunshot wounds was 4%.[55]

In blunt trauma, it is crucial to determine the degree of deceleration involved. Rapid deceleration can cause vascular damage to the renal vessels, including renal pedicle avulsion, renal artery thrombosis, or renal vein disruption. The mobility of the kidney results in a stretch on the renal artery, which in turn may cause disruption of the relatively inelastic arterial intima. Subsequent thrombus may occlude the vessel, leading to renal ischemia.[35]

Gunshot or stab wounds to the upper abdomen or lower chest should alert the physician to possible renal injury. Bullet velocity has the greatest effect on soft tissue damage. High-velocity weapons create large temporary cavities causing extensive destruction.[56] Handguns generally are considered low-velocity weapons (<2000 ft/s).[35] Stab wounds to the upper abdomen, flank, and lower chest commonly result in renal injury. A weapon's dimensions are important because the length and width give valuable information on its penetrating and destructive characteristics.[35]

A thorough physical examination of the abdomen, chest, and back must be performed in both blunt and penetrating traumas. Any suspected fractures of the lower ribs and lower thoracic and upper lumbar vertebrae raise the risk of associated renal injuries. Gunshot wounds can be misleading because small-entrance wounds may not reveal the extent of tissue damage. When radiographs are taken of the chest and abdomen, the placement of a small metallic object (eg, a paper clip) at the entrance and exit sites helps to define the locations of these wounds.[35]

The presence of either microscopic or gross hematuria raises the concern for renal injury.[35] However, this condition is not seen in all cases because hematuria can be absent in up to 36% of renal vascular injuries from blunt trauma.[57] Microscopic hematuria may be present in a wide range of renal injuries. In patients with blunt trauma and microscopic hematuria who are in shock, there is a higher incidence of significant renal injuries.[58] The first urine specimen obtained either by catheterization or by spontaneous voiding should be used to determine the presence of hematuria because later urine samples are often diluted by diuresis, causing an underestimation or absence of hematuria.[35]

Many clinicians accept that more than 5 red blood cells per high-power field indicate the need for renal imaging in blunt trauma. However, the use of this threshold for imaging has been associated with a low incidence of renal abnormalities.[35] A multiyear study based at the San Francisco General Hospital sought to define better criteria for renal imaging after blunt trauma.[58] The results suggest that all patients with blunt trauma with gross hematuria or patients with microscopic hematuria and shock should undergo renal imaging. Patients with microscopic hematuria without shock have been shown to rarely have a significant injury.[58] However, in cases in which a high suspicion for renal injury exists based on history taking and examination, imaging should be performed regardless of urine examination. For example, patients sustaining blunt trauma from rapid deceleration (eg, head-on or high-speed motor vehicle collisions or falls from great heights) are at risk for vascular injury, which can occur in the absence of microscopic hematuria. Penetrating injuries with any degree of hematuria should be imaged because the presence of shock, degree of hematuria, location of the entry wound, and type of injury are unreliable predictors of significant injury.[35]

Although ultrasonography is being used with a greater frequency to confirm the presence of retroperitoneal hematoma, sonograms cannot clearly delineate parenchymal lacerations, vascular injuries, or collecting system injuries and cannot accurately detect urinary extravasation.[35] The preferred imaging study for renal trauma is contrast-enhanced CT because its high sensitivity and specificity provides the most definitive grading information. The major disadvantage of modern spiral CT imaging is in the diagnosis of renal parenchymal injury. Contrast material has often not had sufficient time to be excreted into the parenchyma and collecting system to adequately detect parenchymal lacerations and urinary extravasation.[45] Repeat imaging 10 minutes after injection of contrast material demonstrates both parenchymal and collecting system injuries with greater accuracy. Findings on CT that suggest major injury include medial hematoma (vascular injury), medial urinary extravasation (renal pelvis or UPJ avulsion injury), and lack of contrast enhancement of the parenchyma (arterial injury).[35]

The exception for using IVP over CT is the single-shot intraoperative IVP when clinical circumstances mandate immediate operative intervention for other injuries, precluding CT imaging. Similarly, the use of arteriography (based on institutional preference and availability) is limited to localized arterial injuries suspected on CT imaging that may be amenable to selective embolization.[35]

Numerous classifications schemas for renal injuries exist, but the most widely accepted and utilized classification is shown in **Table 2**.

Patients with gross hematuria who have well-defined injuries with appropriate imaging should be admitted for bed rest.[35] More concerning injuries that may require intervention are found in only 5.4% of renal trauma cases.[59] A hemodynamically stable patient with blunt trauma can usually be managed without renal exploration; overall, 95% of blunt renal injuries can be managed nonoperatively.[60] Grade IV and V injuries more often require surgical exploration, but selected cases can be managed nonoperatively (**Fig. 2**).[61,62] Penetrating trauma to the kidney may also be managed nonoperatively, although this trauma occurs less commonly than blunt trauma.

Trauma patients with higher-grade injuries selected for nonoperative management should be closely monitored for bleeding, with frequent monitoring of vital signs, serial hemoglobin/hematocrit readings, and possibly repeat abdominal CT imaging.[35,63]

Table 2
The American Association for Surgery of Trauma Organ Injury Severity Scale for kidney

Grade[a]	Type	Description
I	Contusion	Microscopic or gross hematuria, urologic study results normal
	Hematoma	Subcapsular, nonexpanding hematoma without parenchymal laceration
II	Hematoma	Nonexpanding perirenal hematoma confined to renal retroperitoneum
	Laceration	<1 cm parenchymal depth of renal cortex without urinary extravasation
III	Laceration	>1 cm parenchymal depth of renal cortex without collecting system rupture or urinary extravasation
IV	Laceration	Parenchymal laceration extending through renal cortex, medulla, and collecting system
	Vascular	Main renal artery or vein injury with contained hemorrhage
V	Laceration	Completely shattered kidney
	Vascular	Avulsion of renal hilum, devascularizing the kidney

[a] Advance one grade for bilateral injuries up to grade III.

Data from Moore EE, Shackford SR, Pachter HL, et al: Organ injury scaling: spleen, liver, and kidney. J *Trauma* 1989;29:1665–6; and *Reproduced from* McAninch JW, Santucci RA. Renal and ureteral trauma. In: Wein AJ, editor. Campbell-Walsh Urology. Philadelphia: WB Saunders; 2007; with permission.

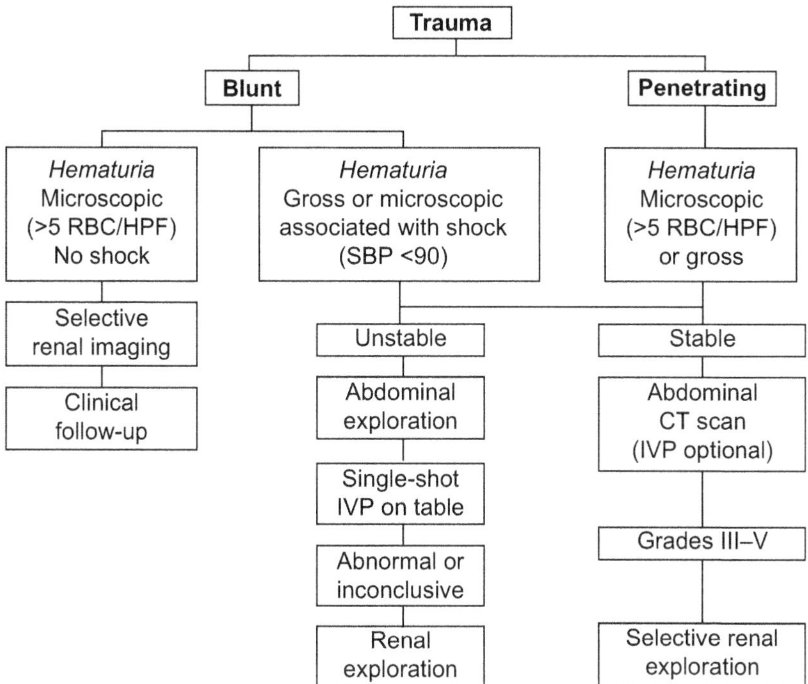

Fig. 2. Flow chart for adult renal injuries to serve as a guide for decision making. RBC/HPF, red blood cells per high-power field; SBP, systolic blood pressure. (*From* McAninch JW, Santucci RA. Renal and ureteral trauma. In: Wein AJ, editor. Campbell-Walsh Urology. Philadelphia: WB Saunders; 2007. p. 1278; with permission.)

However, no clear consensus exists on the routine role and timing of reimaging patients with renal injuries. If bleeding persists or delayed bleeding occurs, angiography with embolization may reduce or prevent the need for surgical intervention. If urinary extravasation is present, serial renal CT imaging should be instituted and internal ureteral stent drainage may be required.[35]

Absolute and relative indications for renal exploration have been delineated to aid in management. Absolute indications include evidence of persistent renal bleeding, expanding perirenal hematoma, and pulsatile perirenal hematoma. Relative indications include nonviable tissue, urinary extravasation, delayed diagnosis of arterial injury, segmental arterial injury, and incomplete staging. If a patient's critical condition necessitates surgical intervention before appropriate imaging studies (incomplete staging) and if renal injury on exploration is obvious (perirenal hematoma or gross hematuria), single-shot intraoperative IVP should be performed to assess for other injuries.[35]

Immediate renal exploration is recommended in cases of main renal artery thrombosis in an attempt to salvage the kidney. With delayed diagnosis (>8 hours), the kidney typically cannot be salvaged.[57] However, case reports of successful renal revascularization via endovascular stents offer a more recent and promising approach to renal artery thrombosis due to an intimal flap dissection (tear).[64]

Many patients with renal vascular injury are critically injured, with numerous associated organ injuries. Time constraints may limit attempts at vascular repair; therefore, a nephrectomy is typically performed.[35] More recently, the benefit of damage control to improve renal salvage has been documented.[65] The wound and area around the injured kidney are packed with laparotomy pads to control bleeding, with a planned return to the operating room in 24 hours to explore and evaluate the extent of injury.

URETHRA

Male and female urethrae differ significantly from an anatomic perspective. The female urethra, which is approximately 4 cm in length, lies posterior to the symphysis pubis and travels within the anterior wall of the vagina. Given its short length, injury to the female urethra is rare, but injury can occur as a result of pelvic fracture.[66] The male urethra, measuring approximately 20 cm in length, is divided into posterior (prostatic and membranous) and anterior (bulbar and pendulous) segments (**Fig. 3**). The pendulous urethra, also known as the penile urethra, travels within the corpus spongiosum. The anterior and posterior segments are separated by the urogenital diaphragm.[12] Because of its relative predominance in injury, this discussion focuses primarily on the male urethra.

Distinguishing between the anterior and posterior segments is important because the etiology, diagnosis, and management of injury differ significantly. Most anterior urethral injuries arise from direct trauma, either blunt or penetrating, to the perineum. These injuries are often not detected initially and present years later when complicated

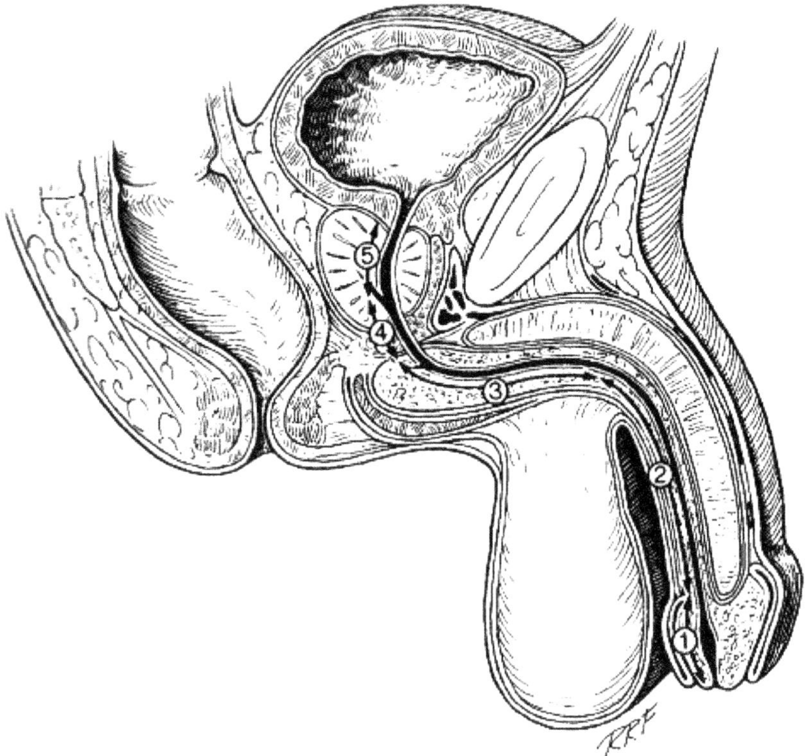

Fig. 3. Anatomy of the male urethra. (1) Fossa navicularis, (2) pendulous urethra, (3) bulbous urethra, (4) membranous urethra, and (5) prostatic urethra. (*From* Jordan GH, Schellhammer PF. Urethral surgery and stricture disease. In: Droller M, editor. Surgical management of urologic disease. St Louis (MO): Mosby-Yearbook; 1992. p. 394; with permission.)

by urethral stricture formation.[67] Straddle injuries are the most common cause, and the most frequently injured segment is the fixed bulbar portion, found in 85% of anterior urethral injuries. This is in contrast to the mobile penile urethra.[68] Pelvic fractures are the principle cause (80%–90%) of posterior urethral injury because the prostate is tethered to the pelvic bones via the puboprostatic ligaments. In fact, posterior urethral disruptions occur in up to 25% of pelvic ring fractures.[69] High-energy injuries can fracture and distract pelvic bones, creating shearing forces that may lead to stretching (25%), partial disruption (25%), or even complete disruption (50%) at the prostatomembranous junction of the urethra.[70] Recognition and treatment of these injuries are important to decrease the incidence of resultant stricture, impotence, and incontinence.[71] However, given the forces needed to cause significant urethral trauma, these injuries may be easily overlooked when confounded by concomitant life-threatening injuries.[72]

Patients with urethral trauma often complain of hematuria or the inability to void. Others are minimally symptomatic or even asymptomatic, thus necessitating a high index of suspicion in any patient with pelvic fracture, straddle-type injury, or other trauma in the area of the perineum. Physical examination may demonstrate blood at the urethral meatus (37%–93% of posterior urethral injuries, 75% of anterior urethral injuries) or vaginal introitus (80% of women with urethral injuries).[73] Hematuria is neither a sensitive nor specific sign, but urinalysis should be performed in any patient with significant abdominal or pelvic trauma. In addition, it should be noted that the degree of hematuria does not directly correlate with the degree of injury because a severe rupture may result in only scant hematuria on urinalysis.[73] A high-riding prostate may be palpated on digital rectal examination because of the disruption of the prostatic and membranous urethra. The prostate may feel boggy if there is a significant traumatic hematoma. Perineal ecchymoses may exist but are neither sensitive nor specific for urethral injury.[73] If there is any evidence by history taking or physical examination that a urethral injury may exist, urinary catheterization should not be performed until injury is excluded because this may worsen trauma and lead to increased morbidity.

Emergent diagnosis of urethral injury is made by performing an RUG. Typically, the tip of a 16F urinary catheter is introduced into the fossa navicularis, the section of the penile urethra within the glans penis, for the adult patient. The bulb is then inflated with approximately 3 mL of saline, and 20 to 30 mL of contrast medium is then injected through the catheter. Alternatively, the tip of a piston syringe can be introduced into the urethral meatus to introduce contrast. If a urinary catheter has already been placed before consideration of urethral injury, it should remain in place, and contrast material can be injected around the urinary catheter via a 16-guage angiocath. Plain radiographs are then taken of the pelvis to determine if there is contrast extravasation from the urethra, indicating urethral injury.[74] If extravasation does not occur, a urinary catheter may be safely inserted into the bladder.

However, if contrast extravasation does occur, further instrumentation of the urethra should not occur without urologic consultation. If bladder filling occurs with extravasation during an RUG, this typically indicates partial injury, whereas a complete tear does not allow the filling of the bladder with contrast.[71] The classification of urethral injuries is based on urethral location (**Table 3**).

Initial management of urethral injury depends on the type of injury, with the primary goal of not only restoring function but also minimizing the sequelae of impotence, stricture, retention, and incontinence. Partial type I and type V injuries can readily be managed with gentle urinary catheter placement by a urologist. The catheter should be left in place for 2 to 6 weeks to allow healing. A similar method can be used with partial type II or type III tears, with a Foley catheter placed over a guidewire that is

Table 3
Classification of urethral injuries based on anatomic location

Type	Urethral Segment	Description
I	Prostatic	Elongation without disruption
II	Membranous	Disruption above urogenital diaphragm
III	Membranous	Disruption involving the urogenital diaphragm
IV	Prostatic	Disruption involving bladder neck
V	Anterior	Disruption confined to bulbous and/or penile urethra

Adapted from Rosenstein DI, Alsikafi NF. Diagnosis and classification of urethral injuries. Urol Clin North Am 2006;33:74; with permission.

introduced during cystoscopy. A suprapubic catheter is placed when there is complete disruption or when passage of a urinary catheter is not possible, followed by eventual urethral repair. Any open urethral injury should be treated with operative exploration and repair.[75]

EXTERNAL GENITALIA

Trauma to the external genitalia occurs in up to two-thirds of patients who present with GU trauma.[76] Most cases are caused by blunt trauma, but up to 35% of all gunshot wounds to the GU tract involve the external genitalia.[77] Most cases of genital trauma occur in men not only because of anatomic differences but also because of greater rates of exposure to violence in this population as well as participation in contact sports.[78] As with most trauma to the urologic system, most injuries to the genitalia are not life threatening but can lead to significant physical and emotional disabilities, including impotence, urinary retention, and cosmetic disfigurement.[79] It is also important to consider the possibility of sexual abuse in any patient who presents with genital trauma, particularly children.[78]

Penile Trauma

Because of its mobility, blunt injury to the penis is rare, except when it is erect. Penile fracture usually occurs during sexual intercourse (58% of cases), when the erect penis is accidentally thrust against the pubic symphysis or perineum.[80] Technically, a penile fracture is a rupture of the corpus cavernosum through its overlying tunica albuginea, which thins during erection from 2 to 0.5 mm, making it more susceptible to injury.[81] Usually only 1 corpus cavernosum is injured; however, the urethra, which lies within the corpus spongiosum, can be injured in up to 22% of cases.[82] Classically, patients hear a cracking or popping sound, followed by rapid detumescence and severe pain.[80]

On physical examination, the fractured penis is typically swollen and ecchymotic, creating the eggplant deformity, with deviation away from the injury. Blood at the urethral meatus, hematuria, or inability to void can be seen if concomitant urethral injury is present.[80] The diagnosis is mainly a clinical one, but urologists may confirm the diagnosis by performing fluoroscopic cavernosography intraoperatively.[83] Penile ultrasonography and MRI have limited utility in acute injury, mainly because of inaccuracy and cost.[80]

Historically, penile fractures were treated conservatively with splinting, pressure dressings, ice, and analgesics. Recently, however, practice patterns have changed because of the literature suggesting that the complications associated with nonoperative management (abscess formation, penile angulation, missed urethral injury, fibrosis, longer hospital stay) outnumber the risks of immediate operative repair. Therefore, many urologists now take all cases of penile fractures immediately to the operating room for surgical exploration and repair.[84] However, in patients presenting with a penile fracture after more than 24 hours after injury, many experts now recommend delaying surgical repair for 7 to 12 days, provided that there is no coexisting urethral injury.[85,86]

Other examples of traumatic penile emergencies include penile amputation, zipper injury, and strangulation. The amputated penis should be cared for like an amputated digit. The penis should be immediately wrapped in saline-soaked gauze and placed in a bag, which should then be placed on ice until reimplantation is possible. Successful reimplantation rates are directly correlated with a shorter time to implantation, although successful reimplantation can occur up to 16 hours after injury.[87] Intentional or accidental zipper and strangulation injuries should be treated as quickly as possible by releasing the offending object. Rapid treatment decreases the risk of subsequent tissue necrosis and infection.[88] Penetrating injuries to the penis should be treated with operative intervention and exploration as well as the liberal use of antibiotics.[89]

Scrotal Trauma

Injuries to the scrotum are not uncommon and occur most frequently in adolescents and young adults. However, because of the testicular mobility and the protective cremasteric reflex, injuries significant enough to mandate surgical repair are rare. The right testicle lies higher than the left testicle in 60% to 70% of men and is thus more prone to being trapped against the symphysis pubis in blunt trauma.[90] In cases of testicular rupture, the blunt force and trapping of the testicle can lead to rupture of the tunica albuginea, which encapsulates the testicle, resulting in extrusion of the seminiferous tubules.[91]

Patients with testicular rupture typically present with immediate scrotal pain after trauma, which is often accompanied by nausea or vomiting. However, patients may present after a delay, up to days after the injury, if they have a small rupture, which becomes increasingly more painful as time progresses.[92] Examination often reveals a swollen and ecchymotic scrotum, and if the rupture is large enough, the practitioner may not be able to palpate the testicle that has ruptured. Ultrasonography can be used with very high sensitivity to diagnose a rupture, and if confirmed, operative intervention is required.[93] However, if the ultrasonographic result is equivocal, patients should be taken to the operating room for exploration and potential repair if the suspicion for significant injury is high because early repair (within 72 hours) results in a rate of testicular salvage of 90% when compared with delayed repair or conservative management (15%–55% orchiectomy rate).[93] Scrotal ultrasonography can also reveal testicular contusion or hematocele, which are nonsurgical injuries or traumatic torsion or dislocation, which do require surgical intervention but are much less common than testicular rupture.[94]

Female Genital Trauma

Although rare, vulvar trauma can result in life-threatening bleeding or significant disability, including incontinence, urinary retention, and cosmetic disfigurement. Injuries to the vulva may be the only external evidence of associated life-threatening internal injuries, such as vaginal, bladder, or intraperitoneal organ injury. Examination may reveal a vulvar hematoma or blood at the introitus or urethral meatus. Given the short length of the urethra, direct visualization and palpation are necessary to diagnose urethral injury. Therefore, if an injury is noted, performing an examination under anesthesia should be considered to evaluate the degree of injury.

Oftentimes, nonsteroidal antiinflammatory medications (NSAIDs) and ice packs can be used to treat hemodynamically stable women with vulvar injuries, but massive hematomas can occur and must be treated surgically. If a vulvar injury is noted, the practitioner must consider associated bladder, rectum, or bowel injury. As with male genital injuries, the practitioner must also consider sexual abuse as a cause in any woman presenting with genital trauma, regardless of age. Depending on the specific injury pattern, female genital injuries are managed by a gynecologist with or without urologic consultation.[95,96]

SUMMARY

Trauma to the GU tract is relatively common and can occur secondary to blunt or penetrating injury. As they are not always evident on initial examination, injuries involving the kidneys, ureters, bladder, urethra, or genitalia must be considered in any patient presenting with abdominal or pelvic trauma. Although these injuries are rarely life threatening, the emergency practitioner should obtain timely urologic or gynecologic consultation to aid in management.

REFERENCES

1. McAninch JW. Genitourinary trauma. World J Urol 1999;17:95–6.
2. Tezval H, Tezval M, von Klot C, et al. Urinary tract injuries in patients with multiple trauma. World J Urol 2007;25:177–84.
3. McGinty DM, Mendez R. Traumatic ureteral injuries with delayed recognition. Urology 1977;10(2):115–7.
4. Asgari MA, Hosseini SY, Safarinejad MR, et al. Penile fractures. Evaluation, therapeutic approaches and long-term results. J Urol 1996;155:148–9.
5. Dreitlein DA, Suner S, Basler J. Genitourinary trauma. Emerg Med Clin North Am 2001;19:569–90.
6. Kansas BT, Eddy MJ, Mydlo JH, et al. Incidence and management of penetrating renal trauma in patients with multiorgan injury: extended experience at an inner city trauma center. J Urol 2004;172:1355–60.
7. Baverstock R, Simon R, McLoughlin M. Severe blunt renal trauma: a 7-year retrospective review from a provincial trauma centre. Can J Urol 2001;8:1372–6.
8. Dokucu AI, Ozdemir E, Ozturk H, et al. Urogenital injuries in childhood: a strong association of bladder trauma to bowel injuries. Int Urol Nephrol 2006;32(1):3–8.
9. Paparel P, N'Diaye A, Laumon B, et al. The epidemiology of trauma of the genitourinary system after traffic accidents: analysis of a register of over 43,000 victims. BJU Int 2006;97(2):338–41.
10. Ramchandani P, Buckler PM. Imaging of genitourinary trauma. Am J Roentgenol 2009;192:1514–23.
11. Santucci RA, Fisher MB. The literature increasingly supports expectant (conservative) management of renal trauma—a systematic review. J Trauma 2005;59(2):491–501.
12. Gray H. The urinary organs. In: Lewis WH, editor. Anatomy of the human body. 20th edition. Philadelphia: Lea & Febiger; 1918. p. 1215–53.
13. Cass AS. The multiple injured patient with bladder trauma. J Trauma 1984;24:731–4.
14. Volpe MA, Pachter EM, Scalea TM, et al. Is there a difference in outcome when treating traumatic intraperitoneal bladder rupture with or without a suprapubic tube? J Urol 1999;161:1103–5.

15. Hsieh C, Chen R, Fang J, et al. Diagnosis and management of bladder injury by trauma surgeons. Am J Surg 2002;184:143–7.
16. Parry NG, Rozycki GS, Feliciano DV, et al. Traumatic rupture of the urinary bladder: is the suprapubic tube necessary? J Trauma 2003;54:431–6.
17. Carroll PR, McAninch JW. Major bladder trauma: mechanisms of injury and a unified method of diagnosis and repair. J Urol 1984;132:254–7.
18. Cass AS, Luxenberg M. Features of 164 bladder ruptures. J Urol 1987;138:743–5.
19. Corriere JN, Sandler CM. Management of extraperitoneal bladder rupture. Urol Clin North Am 1989;16:275–7.
20. Alli MO, Singh B, Moodley J, et al. Prospective evaluation of combined suprapubic and urethral catheterization to urethral drainage alone for intraperitoneal bladder injuries. J Trauma 2003;55:1152–4.
21. Cass AS. Diagnostic studies in bladder rupture. Urol Clin North Am 1989;16:267–73.
22. Morey AF, Iverson AJ, Swan A, et al. Bladder rupture after blunt trauma: guidelines for diagnostic imaging. J Trauma 2001;51:683–6.
23. Peters PC. Intraperitoneal rupture of the bladder. Urol Clin North Am 1989;16: 279–82.
24. Aihara R, Blansfield JS, Millham FH, et al. Fracture locations influence the likelihood of rectal and lower urinary tract injuries in patients sustaining pelvic fractures. J Trauma 2002;52:205–9.
25. Morey F, Rozanski TS. Genital and lower urinary tract trauma. In: Wein AJ, editor. Campbell-Walsh Urology. 9th edition. Philadelphia: WB Saunders; 2007. p. 2649–55.
26. Iverson AJ, Morey AF. Radiographic evaluation of suspected bladder rupture following blunt trauma: critical review. World J Surg 2001;25:1588–91.
27. Gomez RG, Ceballos L, Coburn M, et al. Consensus statement on bladder injuries. BJU Int 2004;94:27–32.
28. Dobrowolski ZF, Lipczynski W, Drewniak T, et al. External and iatrogenic trauma of the urinary bladder: a survey in Poland. BJU Int 2002;89:755–6.
29. Morey AF, Carroll PR. Evaluation and management of adult bladder trauma. Contemp Urol 1997;9:13–22.
30. Peng MY, Parisky YR, Cornwell EE, et al. CT cystography versus conventional cystography in evaluation of bladder injury. AJR Am J Roentgenol 1999;173: 1269–72.
31. Mee SL, McAnich JW, Federle MP. Computerized tomography in bladder rupture: diagnostic limitations. J Urol 1987;137:207–9.
32. Udekwu PO, Gurkin B, Oller DW. The use of computed tomography in blunt abdominal injuries. Am Surg 1996;62:56–9.
33. Kotkin L, Koch MO. Morbidity associated with nonoperative management of extraperitoneal bladder injuries. J Trauma 1995;38:895–8.
34. Elliott SP, McAninch JW. Extraperitoneal bladder trauma: delayed surgical management can lead to prolonged convalescence. J Trauma 2009;66(1):274–5.
35. McAninch JW, Santucci RA. Renal and ureteral trauma. In: Wein AJ, editor. Campbell-Walsh Urology. Philadelphia: WB Saunders; 2007. p. 1274–8.
36. Presti JC Jr, Carroll PR, McAninch JW. Ureteral and renal pelvic injuries from external trauma: diagnosis and management. J Trauma 1989;29:370–4.
37. Medina D, Lavery R, Ross SE, et al. Ureteral trauma: preoperative studies neither predict injury nor prevent missed injuries. J Am Coll Surg 1998;186:641–4.
38. Amato JJ, Billy LJ, Gruber RP, et al. Vascular injuries. An experimental study of high and low velocity missile wounds. Arch Surg 1970;101:167–74.
39. Evans RA, Smith MJ. Violent injuries to the upper ureter. J Trauma 1976;16:558–61.

40. Campbell EW Jr, Filderman PS, Jacobs SC. Ureteral injury due to blunt and penetrating trauma. Urology 1992;40:216–20.
41. Brandes SB, Chelsky MJ, Buckman RF, et al. Ureteral injuries from penetrating trauma. J Trauma 1994;36:766–9.
42. Mee SL, McAninch JW. Indications for radiographic assessment in suspected renal trauma. Urol Clin North Am 1989;16:187–92.
43. Kawashima A, Sandler CM, Corl FM, et al. Imaging of renal trauma: a comprehensive review. Radiographics 2001;21:557–74.
44. Kawashima A, Sandler CM, Corriere JN Jr, et al. Ureteropelvic junction injuries secondary to blunt abdominal trauma. Radiology 1997;205:487–92.
45. Brown SL, Hoffman DM, Spirnak JP. Limitations of routine spiral computerized tomography in the evaluation of blunt renal trauma. J Urol 1998;160:1979–81.
46. Mulligan JM, Cagiannos I, Collins JP, et al. Ureteropelvic junction disruption secondary to blunt trauma: excretory phase imaging (delayed films) should help prevent a missed diagnosis. J Urol 1998;159:67–70.
47. Gayer G, Zissin R, Apter S, et al. Urinomas caused by ureteral injuries: CT appearance. Abdom Imaging 2002;27:88–92.
48. Tulikangas PK, Gill IS, Falcone T. Laparoscopic repair of ureteral injuries. J Am Assoc Gynecol Laparosc 2001;8:259–62.
49. Elliott SP, McAninch JW. Ureteral injuries from external violence: the 25-year experience at San Francisco General Hospital. J Urol 2003;170:1213–6.
50. Velmahos GC, Degiannis E, Wells M, et al. Penetrating ureteral injuries: the impact of associated injuries on management. Am Surg 1996;62:461–8.
51. Verduyckt FJ, Heesakkers JP, Debruyne FM. Long-term results of ileum interposition for ureteral obstruction. Eur Urol 2002;42:181–7.
52. Bonfig R, Gerharz EW, Riedmiller H. Ileal ureteric replacement in complex reconstruction of the urinary tract. BJU Int 2004;93:575–80.
53. Matlaga BR, Shah OD, Hart LJ, et al. Ileal ureter substitution: a contemporary series. Urology 2003;62(6):998–1001.
54. Hirshberg A, Wall MJ Jr, Mattox KL. Planned reoperation for trauma: a two year experience with 124 consecutive patients. J Trauma 1994;37:365–9.
55. McAninch JW, Carroll PR, Armenakas NA, et al. Renal gunshot wounds: methods of salvage and reconstruction. J Trauma 1993;35:279–83.
56. Hutton JE, Rich NM. Wounding and wound ballistics. In: McAninch JE, editor. Traumatic and reconstructive urology. Philadelphia: WB Saunders; 1996. p. 3–25.
57. Cass AS. Renovascular injuries from external trauma. Urol Clin North Am 1989; 16:213–20.
58. Miller KS, McAninch JW. Radiographic assessment of renal trauma: our 15-year experience. J Urol 1995;154:352–5.
59. Moore EE, Shackford SR, Pachter HL, et al. Organ injury scaling: spleen, liver, and kidney. J Trauma 1989;29:1664–6.
60. American College of Surgeons. Abdominal and pelvic trauma. In: Committee on Trauma, American College of Surgeons, editors. Advanced Traumatic Life Support. 8th edition. Chicago: American College of Surgeons; 2008.
61. Santucci RA, McAninch JW. Diagnosis and management of renal trauma: past, present and future. J Am Coll Surg 2000;191:443–51.
62. Santucci RA, Wessells H, Bartsch G, et al. Evaluation and management of renal injuries: a consensus statement of renal trauma. BJU Int 2004;94:27–32.
63. Matthews LA, Smith EM, Spirnak JP. Nonoperative treatment of major blunt renal lacerations with urinary extravasation. J Urol 1997;157:2056–8.

64. Inoue S, Koizumi J, Iino M, et al. Self-expanding metallic stent for renal artery dissection due to blunt trauma. J Urol 2004;171:347–8.
65. Coburn M. Damage control surgery for urologic trauma: an evolving management strategy. J Urol 2002;160:13.
66. Carter CT, Schafer N. Incidence of urethral disruption in females with traumatic pelvic fractures. Am J Emerg Med 1994;11(3):218–20.
67. Pontes JE, Pierce JM Jr. Anterior urethral injuries: four year of experience at the Detroit General Hospital. J Urol 1978;120:563–4.
68. Mouraviev VB, Santucci RA. Cadaveric anatomy of pelvic fracture urethral distraction injury: most injuries are distal to the external urinary sphincter. J Urol 2005; 173(3):869–72.
69. Watnik NF, Coburn M, Goldberger M. Urologic injuries in pelvic ring disruptions. Clin Orthop Relat Res 1996;329:37–45.
70. Richter ER, Morey AF. Urethral trauma. In: Wessells HB, McAninch JW, editors. Urological emergencies. Totowa (NJ): Humana Press; 2005. p. 57–69.
71. Sandler CM, McCallum RW. Urethral trauma. In: Pollack HM, McClennan BL, Dyer R, et al, editors. Clinical urography. 2nd edition. Philadelphia: WB Saunders Co; 2000. p. 1819–37.
72. Sagalowsky AI, Peters PC. Genitourinary trauma. In: Walsh PC, Retnik AB, Vaughan ED, et al, editors. Campbell's urology. Philadelphia: WB Saunders; 1998. p. 3085–120.
73. Armenakas NA, McAninch JW. Acute anterior urethral injuries: diagnosis and initial management. In: McAninch JW, editor. Traumatic and reconstructive urology. Philadelphia: WB Saunders; 1996. p. 543–50.
74. Walter JR, Webster GD. Surgery for urethral stricture disease. In: Graham SD, Keane TE, editors. Glenn's urologic surgery. Philadelphia: Lippincott Williams & Wilkins; 2009. p. 246–7.
75. Martinez-Pineiro L, Djakovic N, Plas E, et al. EAU guidelines on urethral trauma. Eur Urol 2010;57:791–803.
76. Brandes SB, Buckman RF, Chelsky MJ, et al. External genitalia gunshot wounds: a ten-year experience with fifty-six cases. J Trauma 1995;39:266–71.
77. Phonsombat S, Master VA, McAninch JW. Penetrating external genital trauma: a 30-year single institution experience. J Urol 2008;180:192–5.
78. Adu-Frimpong J. Genitourinary trauma in boys. Clin Pediatr Emerg Med 2009;10: 45–9.
79. Jordan GH, Gilbert DA. Male genital trauma. Clin Plast Surg 1988;15(3):431–2.
80. Nicolaisen GS, Melamud A, William RD, et al. Rupture of the corpus cavernosum: surgical management. J Urol 1983;130:917–9.
81. Seaman EK, Santarosa RP, Walton GR, et al. Immediate repair: key to managing the fractured penis. Contemp Urol 1993;5:13–21.
82. Tsabg T, Demby AM. Penile fracture with urethra injury. J Urol 1992;147:466–8.
83. Dever DP, Saraf PG, Cantanese RP, et al. Penile fracture: operative management and cavernosography. Urology 1983;22:394–6.
84. Karadeniz T, Topsakal M, Ariman H, et al. Penile fracture: differential diagnosis management and outcome. Br J Urol 1996;77:279–81.
85. Naraynsingh V, Ramdas MJ, Thomas D, et al. Delayed repair of a fractured penis: a new technique. Int J Clin Pract 2003;57(5):428–9.
86. Nasser TA, Mostafa T. Delayed surgical repair of a penile fracture under local anesthesia. J Sex Med 2008;5(10):2464–9.
87. Shaw MB, Sadove AM, Rink RC. Reconstruction after penile amputation and emasculation. Ann Plast Surg 2003;50(3):321–4.

88. Nolan JF, Stillwell TJ, Sands JP. Acute management of the zipper-entrapped penis. J Emerg Med 1990;8:305–7.
89. Goldman HB, Dmochowski RR, Cox CE. Penetrating trauma to the penis: functional results. J Urol 1996;155:551–3.
90. Munter DW, Faleski EJ. Blunt scrotal trauma: emergency department evaluation and management. Am J Emerg Med 1989;7:223–34.
91. Mulhall JP, Gabram SG, Jacobs LM. Emergency management of blunt testicular trauma. Acad Emerg Med 1995;2:639–43.
92. Wasko R, Goldstein AG. Traumatic rupture of the testicle. J Urol 1966;95:721–3.
93. Cass AS, Luxenberg M. Testicular injuries. Urology 1991;37:528–30.
94. McAleer IM, Kaplan GW. Pediatric genitourinary trauma. Urol Clin North Am 1995;22:177–88.
95. Goldman HB, Idom CB, Dmochowski RR. Traumatic injuries of the female external genitalia and their association with urological injuries. J Urol 1998;159:956–9.
96. Lynch JM, Gardner MJ, Albanese CT. Blunt urogenital trauma in prepubescent female patients: more than meets the eye. Pediatr Emerg Care 1995;11:372–5.

Urolithiasis in the Emergency Department

Autumn Graham, MD[a,*], Samuel Luber, MD, MPH[b], Allan B. Wolfson, MD[c]

KEYWORDS

• Renal colic • Kidney stone • Urolithiasis • Nephrolithiasis • Ureterolithiasis

Urolithiasis, more commonly referred to as kidney stones, is a frequent emergency department (ED) complaint (**Box 1**). The National Hospital Ambulatory Medical Care Survey (NHAMCS) estimates that kidney stones account for approximately 2 million outpatient visits and $2.1 billion in health care expenditures per year.[1–3] In the year 2000, annual ED visits for kidney stones reached approximately 600,000.[1] It is essential, therefore, for emergency practitioners to develop expertise in the diagnosis and acute management of this disease process.

EPIDEMIOLOGY

Whether from increasing identification or lifestyle changes, the prevalence of kidney stones is increasing in all age groups. It is estimated that approximately 12% of men and 6% of women will experience a symptomatic kidney stone in their lifetime, although this gender gap has narrowed over the last decade.[4–7] The peak incidence is between the ages of 20 and 50 years, and kidney stones remain relatively uncommon in children younger than 10 years. In addition to gender and age variations, Caucasians are almost 3 times as likely as African Americans to develop kidney stones, with Hispanics and Asians at intermediate risk. Epidemiologic studies in the United States have also noted a regional distribution, often referred to as a "stone belt," in the southeastern United States. This regional variation appears to be related to temperature, sunlight, and beverage consumption.[8–10]

[a] Department of Emergency Medicine, Washington Hospital Center, Georgetown University, 3800 Reservoir Road Northwest, Washington, DC 20007, USA
[b] Department of Emergency Medicine, University of Texas Health Sciences Center at Houston, 6431 Fannin Street, JJL 447, Houston, TX 77030, USA
[c] Department of Emergency Medicine, University of Pittsburgh, 230 McKee Place Suite 500, Pittsburgh, PA 15213, USA
* Corresponding author.
E-mail address: autumngraham@gmail.com

Emerg Med Clin N Am 29 (2011) 519–538
doi:10.1016/j.emc.2011.04.007
emed.theclinics.com
0733-8627/11/$ – see front matter

Box 1
Urolithiasis terminology

- Renal Stone Definitions
  - Urolithiasis
    - Calculi in urinary tract, including kidneys, ureters, bladder, and/or urethra
  - Nephrolithiasis
    - Calculi in the kidney
  - Ureterolithiasis
    - Calculi in one or both ureters
  - Kidney stone
    - Common terminology that refers to calculi in the kidneys but often includes calculi in the lower urinary tract as well

ETIOLOGY

While the exact etiology is unknown, distinct phenotypes exist that may influence the specific mechanism of stone development. Most stones are composed of calcium oxalate and less often calcium phosphate, which together account for approximately 80% of all stones. Uric acid (5%), struvite (10%–15%), cystine (1%), and stones of mixed composition account for the remainder.[11] On rare occasions, medications, such as the retroviral protease inhibitor indinavir, have been found to precipitate in the urine and to form medication stones.[12,13]

It is believed that most stones form when dissolved salts in the urine reach a supersaturation point and crystals form. The development of kidney stones begins with the formation of a nucleus around which the stone grows. There are several hypotheses regarding how this process of stone nucleation, retention within the kidney, and growth occurs. One proposed theory links atherosclerotic plaques in the vasa recta arterioles of the renal papillary ducts that erode into the renal tubules and form kidney stones.[11] This theory may explain why urolithiasis is more common in patients with diabetes, hypertension, or obesity.[14–17] Other theories have implicated the lack of urinary inhibitors (urine citrate and magnesium), the presence of nanobacteria that play a role in nucleation, or the presence of Randall plaques, which are areas of salt deposition in the renal papillae that may serve as an anchoring site for stone retention.[11,18,19]

Irrespective of the underlying mechanism, the development of kidney stones is influenced by urine composition. Certain disease processes, genetics, and lifestyle habits affect urine composition, making some patients more susceptible to kidney stones (**Box 2**). In addition to factors that promote crystal formation, the urine contains substances, such as urine citrate and magnesium, which inhibit crystal formation.[11,39,40] With further delineation of the pathophysiology of kidney stones, guidance and interventions directed toward prevention may be developed.

The etiology of renal colic or the pain cycle related to kidney stones has a complex mechanism as well (**Fig. 1**). While there is mechanical injury to the ureteral wall from the passage of kidney stones, the pain associated with urolithiasis is attributed to the obstruction of the urinary tract and the resulting increase in renal pelvic pressures leading to renal capsular distention, stimulation of nocireceptors, and hyperperistalsis of the ureter. With complete obstruction, peak hydrostatic renal pelvic pressures are generally reached within 2 to 5 hours. In the first 90 minutes, there is an increase in renal blood flow from dilation of afferent preglomerular arterioles, causing an increase in urine production and an increase in renal pelvic pressures. Over the next several hours, renal blood flow begins to decrease while intraluminal ureteral pressure continues to increase. By 24 hours, the renal pelvic hydrostatic pressure has dropped because of a reduction in ureteral peristalsis, decreased renal arterial blood flow, decreased urine production on the affected side, and increased lymphatic drainage. Pain generally abates with the decrease in pelvic pressure. However, most stones are only partially obstructing with episodes of complete obstruction as the stone migrates, thus pain may be episodic or prolonged. These complex interactions between the autoregulation of renal blood flow and the renal nervous system are mediated via interactions at the molecular level, involving prostaglandins, thromboxane, angiotensin, and antidiuretic hormone. Knowledge of this process has aided in directing treatment toward these specific factors.[41,42]

CLINICAL PRESENTATION

The classic presentation of urolithiasis is an abrupt, unilateral flank pain that radiates to the groin. The pain is often described as waxing and waning, with maximal intensity lasting 20 to 60 minutes and a dull throbbing flank pain that persists between episodes of colic. As the stone descends in the ureter, the pain may localize to the abdominal area overlying the stone and radiate to the ipsilateral groin. As the stone approaches the ureterovesicular junction, lower-quadrant pain radiating to the tip of the urethra, urinary urgency, urinary frequency, and dysuria are characteristic. One-third of patients report gross hematuria associated with these episodes. Nausea and vomiting are also common, due to the shared splanchnic innervation of the renal capsule and intestines.

Physical examination typically demonstrates a patient who is writhing in distress, trying to find a comfortable position on the stretcher or in the examination room. On abdominal examination, tenderness at the costovertebral angle or lower quadrant may be present, but peritoneal signs should be absent. The skin may be pale, cool, and clammy. However, fever is not common with kidney stones, and if present is suggestive of infection. Although the physical examination is of limited utility in the diagnosis of urolithiasis, it is valuable in ruling out other intra-abdominal pathology such as abdominal aortic aneurysm, diverticulitis, appendicitis, and gynecologic pathology that may mimic renal colic.

EMERGENCY DEPARTMENT EVALUATION

The diagnosis of urolithiasis includes a history and physical examination, evaluating the patient's risk factors, evolution of symptoms, the presence or absence of infection, and the exclusion of renal colic mimics (**Box 3**). The history should also identify factors that may increase the risk of complications related to stone disease, such as previous kidney transplant, immunosuppression, or a solitary functioning kidney.

Confirmatory imaging is not mandatory for all patients with a suspected kidney stone. For instance, in a patient with known urolithiasis, no risk factors for complications, a typical presentation, and ensured follow-up, conservative treatment that focuses on pain control may be a cost-effective and safe ED approach. However, confirmatory imaging should be considered in all patients with a suspected first-time diagnosis of urolithiasis, those with atypical presentations, those with a concern for infection, and patients who are not improving with conservative measures. It is important to recognize that the shared innervation of the genitourinary system with other intra-abdominal organ systems can lead to misdiagnosis. In patients with acute unilateral flank pain, several studies have reported the incidence of urolithiasis on

Box 2
Risk factors for urolithiasis

- Nonmodifiable
  - Family history (2.5× increased risk)
  - Structural Anatomy of Urinary System
    - Calyceal diverticulum
    - Horseshoe kidney
    - Ureterocele
    - Vesicoureteral reflux
    - Ureteral strictures
  - Medical History
    - Gastric bypass
    - Hypertension
    - Diabetes
    - Metabolic syndrome
    - Primary hyperparathyroidism
    - Sarcoidosis
    - Crohn disease
    - Gout
    - Renal tubular acidosis
    - Hyperthyroidism
    - Multiple myeloma
- Modifiable
  - Low fluid intake
  - Low calcium diet
  - High animal protein diet
  - High oxalate intake
  - High sodium diet
  - Hot weather
  - Obesity
  - Decreased exercise
- Medication
  - Medication stones
    - Indinavir
    - Triamterene
    - Acyclovir
  - Promote calcium stones
    - Loop diuretics
    - Acetazolamide
    - Theophylline
    - Glucocorticoids

- Promote uric acid stones
  - Thiazides
  - Salicylates
  - Probenicid
  - Allopurinol

Data from Refs.[12,14–17,19,20–38]

noncontrast computed tomography (CT) to be between 62% and 69%, and the rate of alternative diagnoses between 10% and 45%.[43–47]

Ill-appearing patients in whom there is a suspicion of infection and an obstructing kidney stone must receive an expedited evaluation. Management should include directed resuscitation, early antibiotics, rapid diagnosis, and consultation with urology

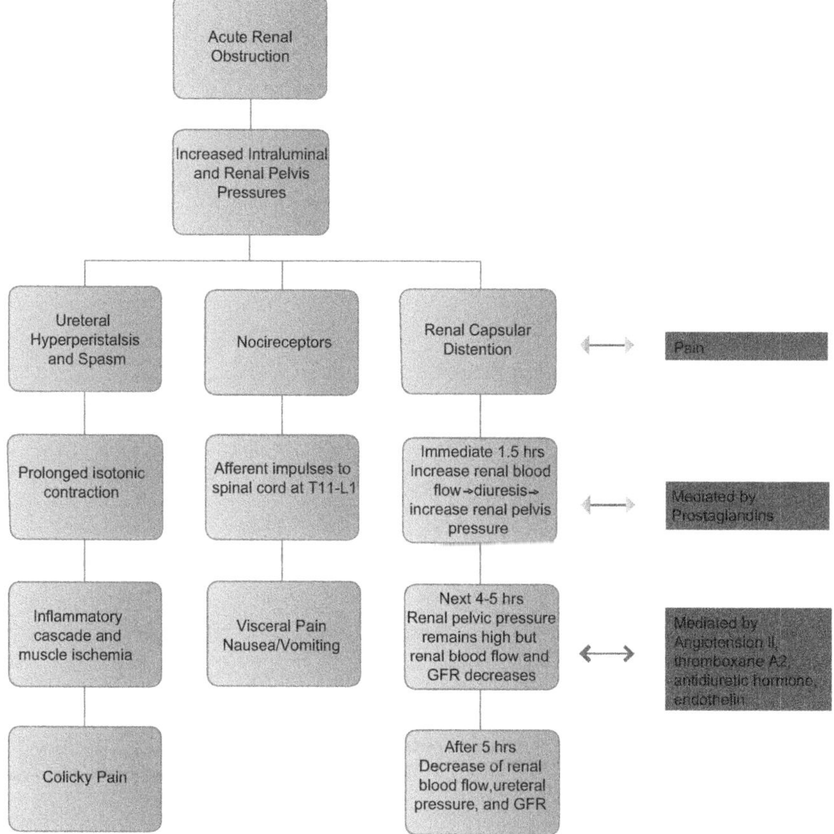

Fig. 1. Mechanisms of pain in renal colic. (*Data from* Shokeir A. Renal colic: new concepts related to pathophysiology, diagnosis, and treatment. Curr Opin Urol 2002;12:263–9; and Travaglini F, Bartoletti R, Gacci M, et al. Pathophysiology of reno-ureteral colic. Urol Int 2004;72(Suppl 1):20–3.)

Box 3
Renal colic mimics

- Gynecologic
  - Hemorrhagic cyst
  - Dermoid cyst
  - Endometrioma
  - Ovarian neoplasm
  - Ovarian torsion
  - Fibroid
  - Ectopic pregnancy
  - Pelvic inflammatory disease
- Gastrointestinal
  - Appendicitis
  - Diverticulitis
  - Biliary disorders
  - Pancreatitis
  - Small bowel obstruction
- Urological
  - Pyelonephritis
  - Urinary tract infection
- Vascular
  - Abdominal aortic aneurysm ± aortic dissection
  - Renal artery thrombosis
  - Renal infarction
  - Mesenteric artery dissection or embolism
  - Intraperitoneal or retroperitoneal hemorrhage
- Musculoskeletal
  - Mechanical low back pain
  - Fractures
- Miscellaneous
  - Herpes zoster infection (shingles)

Data from Rucker CM, Menias CO, Bhalia S. Mimics of renal colic: alternative diagnoses at unenhanced helical CT. Radiographics 2004;24(Suppl 1):11–28.

and/or interventional radiology. An infected, obstructing kidney stone is a urological emergency that requires emergent decompression.

CONFIRMATORY STUDIES

Urinalysis

Urinalysis is a rapid, noninvasive, inexpensive test that is readily and widely available. While it may play a role in the clinical suspicion for urolithiasis, it is neither sensitive nor specific enough to use as a sole diagnostic test. Initial studies that compared microscopic hematuria on urinalysis to intravenous pyelography (IVP) found an 86% to 100% sensitivity in detecting ureterolithiasis in patients with acute flank pain.[48] However, studies that have compared urinalysis and noncontrast CT, the current diagnostic test of choice, found hematuria was present in only about 85% of patients with confirmed kidney stones.[49,50]

Though not an adequate test to screen for urolithiasis, urinalysis does allow the emergency clinician to evaluate for infection. While the presence of leukocyte esterase has been associated with noninfectious inflammation of the ureter, it may also signal infection, as does the presence of nitrites, bacteria, and white blood cells in the urine. On the other hand, the clinician should also not be falsely reassured if the clinical presentation is suggestive of an associated urinary tract infection but the urinalysis does not correlate. It is well recognized that proximal urinary tract infections with an obstructive stone may have a "negative" urinalysis. Unfortunately, there are no studies that correlate the findings on urinalysis with urinary tract infections in association with kidney stones; therefore, emergency medicine clinicians should maintain a high clinical suspicion and consider the clinical presentation when interpreting urinalysis results.

Noncontrast Helical Computed Tomography

Noncontrast helical CT is able to directly visualize or detect secondary signs in the majority of kidney stones, with the exception of indinavir stones.[13] Thus, CT has become the study of choice for confirming the diagnosis of urolithiasis. In multiple investigations, CT has demonstrated specificities nearing 100% and sensitivities of 96% to 98%.[51–54] Furthermore, studies that have directly compared CT to IVP, plain abdominal radiographs, and ultrasonography (US) have shown CT to be superior in the diagnosis of urolithiasis as well as aiding in identifying alternate diagnoses.[55–58]

CT is able to determine the presence of obstruction, as well as the size and the location of kidney stones, which may aid in prognosis. The likelihood of detecting obstruction seems to vary with the duration of symptoms. In a report of 227 patients with acute ureterolithiasis, the following findings were visualized at 2 hours from symptom onset: ureteral dilatation (84%), collecting system dilatation (68%), and perinephric stranding (5%). However, detection of these findings significantly increased at 8 hours after symptom onset: ureteral dilatation (97%), collecting system dilatation (89%), and perinephric stranding (51%).[59]

Even if the stone cannot be directly visualized on CT, secondary signs of stone and stone passage may be found. These signs include hydronephrosis, hydroureter, perirenal stranding, and periureteral stranding. In particular, when CT scans are equivocal because of difficulty in distinguishing stones from phleboliths overlying the course of the ureter, the presence of a "rim" sign due to the circumferential edema from ureteral stones is helpful in making the diagnosis of urolithiasis.[60,61]

There is a growing concern regarding the long-term risk to patients from exposure to ionizing radiation. While CT is superior to other modalities in terms of sensitivity, specificity, and accuracy in the diagnosis of kidney stones, it does expose patients to higher levels of radiation than alternative diagnostic imaging modalities. For instance, whereas CT exposes the patient to 4.5 to 18 mSv of radiation, kidney-ureter-bladder (KUB) plain radiographs and IVP expose the patient to significantly less radiation (0.7 and 3.7 mSv, respectively). In response to these concerns, some institutions have adopted a low-dose CT protocol for kidney stones with reduced radiation dosages ranging from 0.7 to 2 mSv. Sensitivities and specificities of 95% to 97% and 95% to 100%, respectively, have been reported. While comparable with standard CT, low-dose CT may be less accurate in patients with a body mass index greater than 30 kg/m^2 and in those with stones less than 2 mm in size.[62–67]

Another recent advance in CT imaging that may prove beneficial in the diagnosis of urolithiasis is dual-energy computed tomography (DECT). DECT uses both a high-energy source and a low-energy source, which simultaneously conveys two datasets to the image processor. This technology provides a more detailed image of tissue composition, and is being evaluated for a variety of diagnoses. Preliminary studies of DECT suggest that this imaging modality may be able to predict stone composition, which would facilitate treatment decisions. Clinical trials are currently under way to determine whether DECT imaging protocols can be developed that limit patient radiation exposure while maintaining a high detection rate of urolithiasis and stone composition.[68,69]

Ultrasonography

US is the procedure of choice for pregnant women, children, and patients for whom reduced radiation exposure is felt to be a priority. The literature suggests that US has a pooled sensitivity and specificity of 45% and 94%, respectively, for the detection of ureteral calculi,[70] with sensitivities of 85% to 90% and specificities of 90% to 100% for the identification of hydronephrosis.[58,70–76] Therefore, US often cannot visualize the stone itself but can identify the resulting obstruction. Successful US depends on the body habitus of the patient and the skill level of the operator.

The use of US in combination with a KUB radiograph may improve overall accuracy. In one small study, the combination of US and abdominal radiography provided comparable results with those observed with noncontrast helical CT alone. However, more research is needed before drawing conclusions about this diagnostic imaging option.[72]

Abdominal Plain Film

Because 85% to 90% of stones are radiopaque, theoretically the KUB should be able to detect these stones; however, detection is limited by the size of the stone and shadowing from overlying bony structures. In 1985, Roth and colleagues[77] evaluated the utility of plain abdominal radiographs in diagnosing kidney stones in the ED, and found that radiographs only had a sensitivity of 62% and a specificity of 67%. Other retrospective chart reviews have estimated the sensitivity of KUB in the range of 40% to 60%.[78]

In addition to their limited ability to detect urolithiasis, radiographs are also unable to identify urinary tract obstruction or alternative pathology if a kidney stone is not present. KUB may be an appropriate modality to track the progression of stone passage in selected patients. As mentioned earlier, it may also be combined with US in those patients with a known history of a radiopaque stone as a means to reduce the repeated radiation exposure from other imaging modalities.

Intravenous Pyelogram

An IVP in the emergency setting usually consists of a baseline KUB, followed by an injection of intravenous contrast medium and then a series of time-delayed radiographs evaluating the excretion of contrast through the renal system. The IVP has a higher sensitivity and specificity than an abdominal plain radiograph for the detection of kidney stones, and a detection rate as high as 70% to 90%.[56] IVP can only directly visualize radiopaque stones, but can detect filling defects from both radiopaque and radiolucent stones. Of importance, it also provides both structural and functional information, including the site, degree, and nature of obstruction. The drawbacks of IVP include radiation exposure, risk of nephrotoxicity, contrast reaction, and a comparatively long study time, particularly when multiple delayed films are required.

Magnetic Resonance Imaging

Magnetic resonance (MR) urography may be used if there is a specific indication to reduce radiation exposure, such as in pregnant patients.[79] However, its use in the diagnostic workup of urolithiasis is unclear.

ACUTE EMERGENCY DEPARTMENT MANAGEMENT

Most patients with acute renal colic can be managed conservatively with pain control, hydration, and expectant stone passage. Emergent urological consultation in the ED is warranted for patients with urosepsis, renal obstruction with suspicion of a proximal urinary tract infection, acute renal failure, anuria, or intractable pain or vomiting.

Pain Management

Analgesia is the mainstay of treatment for acute renal colic. It is generally accepted that the pain from kidney stones occurs with the passage of a stone into the ureter and the ensuing obstruction. With acute renal obstruction, pain is triggered by the increase in collecting system pressure, ureteral spasm, and renal capsular distention, which is modulated via prostaglandins (see **Fig. 1**). Because of the theoretical benefit of nonsteroidal anti-inflammatory drugs (NSAIDs) via their prostaglandin inhibition and ability to decrease ureteral smooth muscle tone, research has focused on the efficacy of NSAIDs as compared with established opioid analgesics.

A review of the literature would suggest that NSAIDs are at least as effective as opioids in controlling renal colic pain.[80–83] In 2004, a systematic review of 20 trials with 1613 participants found that both NSAIDs and opioids were able to achieve short-term pain relief.[82] However, NSAIDs were associated with fewer side effects, particularly nausea and vomiting, when compared with opioids. The study concluded that given the favorable side-effect profile, the effective analgesia, and the lower requirement for rescue analgesia, NSAIDs were the preferred analgesic for renal colic. This study was limited by the broad spectrum of medications and protocols included in the analysis. Another study that compared morphine (5 mg), ketorolac (15 mg), or a combination of morphine and ketorolac at the same dosages, suggested that it was the combination of NSAIDs and opioids that was most effective. In this study, combination therapy with intravenous morphine and ketorolac was associated with a greater reduction in pain at 40 minutes than with either agent alone, as well as a higher likelihood of complete pain relief at 20 minutes and a lower likelihood of requiring rescue narcotic medication.[83]

In patients with preexisting renal disease or severe dehydration, NSAIDs may interfere with the kidney's autoregulatory response to acute obstruction and cause acute kidney injury (AKI). Thus NSAIDs, particularly ketorolac, should be used cautiously in the elderly, patients with multiple comorbidities, and those with dehydration. As with all NSAIDs, ketorolac inhibits platelets and has been associated with bleeding, predominantly gastrointestinal bleeding. Its use is therefore contraindicated in patients with a recent gastrointestinal bleed, active peptic ulcer disease, or a suspicion of intracranial hemorrhage. A relative contraindication exists for women who are nursing, due to the potential prostaglandin inhibition in neonates. Although most urologists are comfortable with the use of ketorolac for the acute management of renal colic, if emergent surgery or a urological procedure is anticipated, a conversation with the urologist may be helpful in guiding treatment in the ED.

Despite these concerns, in most patients NSAIDs are a safe and effective option for analgesia, and should be considered part of the first-line management of renal colic in addition to opioids. In fact, the literature suggests that a combination approach with opioids and NSAIDs may be the most effective method to manage renal colic in the ED, but further research is needed to clarify the most effective medication, dosage, and route of administration.

Hydration and Diuretics

While some have postulated that high-volume fluid therapy with or without diuretics to increase urine output may facilitate stone passage and decrease the pain associated with renal colic, there is a paucity of literature to support this theory. Many clinicians have concerns that forced hydration will actually worsen hydrostatic pressures and pain in patients with acute ureteral obstruction. In one small study of 43 ED patients, there was no difference in pain scores or the rate of stone passage in patients who received 2 L of saline over 2 hours versus those who received 20 mL of saline per hour.[84,85] Given the lack of randomized controlled studies, and a series of small studies that suggest no benefit, hydration should be aimed at repleting volume in patients who are dehydrated or who have an elevated serum creatinine. Forced diuresis is not recommended.

Medical Expulsion Therapy

Though not considered acute ED care, the use of calcium channel blockers or α-antagonists is becoming common practice. Multiple studies suggest that these agents, thought to relax ureteral smooth muscle, augment the stone expulsion rate when compared with standard therapy.[86–97] In one large meta-analysis, patients treated with a calcium channel blocker (nifedipine) or α-antagonist (tamsulosin) had a 65% greater likelihood of stone passage at the 2- to 6-week follow-up.[93] In a 2007 meta-analysis of medical expulsion therapy (MET), 16 studies with 1235 patients using α-antagonists and 9 studies with 686 patients using the calcium channel blocker nifedipine, suggested that both agents significantly improved spontaneous stone passage of distal ureteral stones compared with standard therapy. α-Antagonists improved the time to stone expulsion by 2 to 6 days compared with controls; the average time to expulsion with α-antagonists was 14 days. Calcium channel blockers also showed improvement over standard therapy and demonstrated a mean passage time of 28 days. Of importance, the meta-analysis noted that adverse effects were reported in 4% of patients receiving α-antagonists and in 15% of patients receiving calcium channel blockers.[98] Most of the side effects in both groups were considered mild, and included nausea, vomiting, dizziness, headache, and asthenia. Transient hypotension was noted in a few cases but did not result in discontinuation of treatment.

Despite the large number of patients included, both meta-analyses were limited by the "methodologic quality within the studies reviewed."[98] A recent small but well-conducted multicenter, randomized, double-blinded trial of tamsulosin use with kidney stones found no statistically significant improvement in the stone passage rate, the time to stone expulsion, or the number of episodes of renal colic.[99] Thus, the efficacy of tamsulosin and MET in improving the spontaneous passage of kidney stones is unclear, and further rigorous research is required to clarify this issue.

Given that this therapy is generally well tolerated and may improve the rate of expulsion of kidney stones, a trial of tamsulosin or nifedipine may be considered at discharge. Based on the literature, tamsulosin seems preferred to nifedipine, due to its reported shorter time to stone passage (14 days vs 28 days) and fewer adverse effects (4% vs 15%). The decision to initiate MET from the ED should also take into consideration the age, comorbidities, and home medications of the patient. For instance, an elderly patient with hypertension who is on a variety of medications may not tolerate MET as well as a 20-year-old healthy patient with no medical conditions, due to a duplication in medication class or the additive effect of home medications.

Other Therapies

Several small studies have found that intranasal desmopressin is effective in controlling the pain associated with renal colic.[100–105] Desmopressin is a synthetic structural analogue of antidiuretic hormone, which decreases free water loss in the kidney and is thought to decrease the hydrostatic pressures in acute obstruction that cause pain. However, given the drug's potential for side effects including hyponatremia, thrombosis, seizure, headache, and hypertension, desmopressin is not an ideal drug for the elderly or for those with significant comorbidities such as coronary disease.[101] At this time desmopressin is not considered first-line management for renal colic, and further studies are needed to determine its efficacy and safety in an emergency setting.

While corticosteroids have been used as part of the acute management of urolithiasis, there are no studies that evaluate their efficacy independent of other therapies. Many of the MET trials included steroids as part of their protocols. When studies of α-blockers versus control were compared with those of α-blockers and corticosteroids versus control, the incremental benefit of steroids was questionable.[93] A similar finding was noted for steroid use with calcium channel blockers. These findings were confirmed in a 2007 meta-analysis that found inconclusive evidence for low-dose steroids promoting stone passage.[98] Although steroids may improve the inflammation associated with urolithiasis, their routine use is currently not recommended.

PROGNOSIS

Stone passage is dependent on the size, shape, and location of the kidney stone. Most stones 4 mm or less in diameter pass spontaneously. For stones larger than 4 mm in diameter, there is a progressive decrease in the spontaneous passage rate as the size of the stone increases (**Table 1**). Shape is also important, and in particular the width of the kidney stone predicts the likelihood of spontaneous passage. In addition, stones that have reached the distal ureter are more likely to pass without intervention. Only about half of the stones in the proximal ureter are expelled spontaneously, while approximately 80% will pass if at the ureterovesicular junction.[106,107]

Recurrence is common. In the absence of preventive measures, the probability of recurrence of symptomatic kidney stones at 5 years is 50%, and 60% by 10 years. Fortunately, the recurrence rate can be decreased by up to 50% in those treated with medication or dietary interventions.[5,6]

Although renal failure and permanent functional injury to the kidney are uncommon with urolithiasis, it is prudent to factor the potential of renal dysfunction into management decisions. Decreases in renal blood flow begin 5 to 18 hours after obstruction, and the degree of reversibility is unclear.[108–110] In one study of 358 patients with ureteral stones, nuclear scintigraphy detected impaired renal function in 27% of asymptomatic patients. Surprisingly, 7% had persistent renal impairment up to 17 months after stone passage.[111] Other studies suggest irreversible damage after 4 weeks of obstruction.[112] Because the patient's symptoms and stone size do not predict loss of renal function and because there is no clear time threshold for irreversible damage, intervention should be considered in any patient with ureteral obstruction unless the ability to closely monitor renal function is available.[113,114]

Table 1
Rate of spontaneous stone passage based on stone size

Size of Stone (mm)	Rate of Spontaneous Passage (%)
1	87
2–4	76
5–7	60
7–9	48
≥9	25

Data from Coll DM, Varanelli MJ, Smith RC. Relationship of spontaneous passage of ureteral calculi to stone size and location as revealed by unenhanced helical CT. AJR Am J Roentgenol 2002;178:101.

In the United States most patients can be treated conservatively with pain management and outpatient urology follow-up for definitive care. Of the 2 million outpatient visits for urolithiasis in 2000, only about 10% were admitted, with an average inpatient hospitalization stay of 2.5 days.[1,2] Admission is indicated for intractable pain and vomiting, single kidney or transplanted kidney with obstruction, concomitant urinary tract infection with obstruction, or hypercalcemic crisis. Admission should also be considered for patients with high-grade obstructions and those with worsening renal function.[114]

DISCHARGE INSTRUCTIONS

Discharge instructions should include outpatient urology follow-up, pain management, and instructions to return to the ED for uncontrolled pain, fever, intractable vomiting, or symptoms persisting for longer than 2 weeks. Capture of the kidney stone by straining the urine can aid urologists in determining the stone composition and directing future treatment. Even if the stone composition is unknown, patients may benefit from increasing fluid intake until urine is a clear color, decreasing the intake of animal protein to less than 52 g/d, and restricting salt intake to less than 50 mmol/d. Decreasing intake of foods such as spinach, rhubarb, chocolate, and nuts will also decrease oxalate excretion and decrease the risk of recurrent stones in susceptible individuals. While counterintuitive given that most stones consist of calcium oxalate, dietary calcium intake should remain high, at greater than 30 mol/d. Low-calcium diets have been associated with an increase in urinary oxalate and increased stone formation.[7] If the type of stone is known, directed treatments may be added to the outpatient regimen.

UROLOGY CONSULTATION

Emergent urological consultation in the ED for decompression and admission is warranted for patients with an obstructing stone with a proximal infection, urosepsis, acute renal failure, anuria, or intractable pain, nausea, or vomiting. Urgent urology follow-up in 1 to 2 days is indicated in well-appearing patients with a nonobstructing kidney stone and associated urinary tract infection, as well as those with a borderline creatinine who are tolerating oral fluids. In these circumstances, a discussion with the urologist before discharge is recommended. Outpatient urology referral in 5 to 7 days is recommended in patients with a stone larger than 10 mm in diameter, those who fail to pass the stone after a trial of conservative management, and those with uncontrolled pain or a history of multiple stones. Even patients with a first-time diagnosis of urolithiasis with spontaneous stone passage may be considered for outpatient urology referral, as some patients may benefit from a metabolic evaluation and determination of stone composition. However, it is not clear whether routine screening is a cost-effective practice for first-time kidney stones.

Current options for treatment of stones that do not pass include shock wave lithotripsy (SWL), ureteroscopic lithotripsy, percutaneous nephrolithotomy, and laparoscopic stone removal. SWL is the treatment of choice in 75% of patients with retained stones, and works best for stones in the renal pelvis and upper ureter. With advances in SWL technology, most patients tolerate the procedure well. Of note, approximately one-third of patients undergoing SWL do develop a transient fever, but fewer than 10% of patients develop obstruction by stone fragments or urinary tract infection. Both SWL and ureteroscopy are considered first-line management options for ureteral stones that require removal, with ureteroscopy yielding higher stone-free rates, but with an increased incidence of complications compared with SWL.[108]

SPECIAL POPULATIONS AND COMPLICATIONS

Infected Kidney Stone

It is well accepted that an upper urinary tract infection in the setting of an obstructed kidney is a urological emergency that requires emergent intervention and decompression. Unfortunately, there are no studies that help characterize which clinical factors are most often associated with this life-threatening complication. Pyonephrosis should be considered in patients with signs or symptoms of sepsis, and in those with systemic leukocytosis, fever, pyuria, or bacteriuria in the setting of an obstructing kidney stone. Patients with immunosuppression, diabetes, or an abnormal genitourinary anatomy are at a higher risk for this complication. Emergent decompression by urology or interventional radiology based on local institutional preference is the treatment of choice. Admission for intravenous hydration and antibiotics is also recommended.

Aerobic gram-negative enteric organisms, including *Escherichia coli* and *Klebsiella*, *Proteus*, *Enterobacter*, and *Citrobacter* species, are typical pathogens. If there is a history of recent hospitalization, antibiotic use, or immunosuppression, enterococcal bacteria and fungal etiologies may also be considered. Initial antibiotic regimens may include ampicillin plus gentamycin or piperacillin. For those with a penicillin allergy, intravenous ofloxacin or ciprofloxacin would be appropriate alternatives, depending on local resistance patterns.

In a well-appearing patient, urinary tract infections associated with a nonobstructing stone can be managed with oral antibiotics and close outpatient follow-up in 24 hours. Prophylactic antibiotics have not been shown to decrease the risk of upper urinary tract infections. While potentially beneficial both before and after urological procedure, prophylactic antibiotics are not recommended in routine emergency management of kidney stones.[98]

Renal Stents

Ureteral stents are used to promote drainage of the upper urinary tract, and are considered a temporizing measure to alleviate obstruction while waiting for kidney stones to pass or for more definitive urological intervention. Ureteral stents may be placed emergently if obstruction is complicated by azotemia, infection, obstruction of a solitary kidney, or pain refractory to analgesia. Complications of renal stents frequently include pain, hematuria, and an increased sense of urinary urgency and frequency. Though rare, serious complications of upward migration, infection, and septic shock are also possible. The position of ureteral stents can be evaluated by KUB or CT imaging.

Pregnancy

Symptomatic kidney stones during pregnancy occur in approximately 1 in every 1500 to 3000 pregnancies.[79,115,116] During pregnancy, increased progesterone levels and decreased bladder capacity from the gravid uterus can cause urine stasis, which promotes stone formation. Most pregnant patients with kidney stones present in the second or third trimester.

Renal and pelvic US is the test of choice when an obstructing calculus is suspected. However, normal physiologic hydronephrosis of pregnancy must be distinguished from abnormal pathologic hydronephrosis secondary to obstruction. Other options to evaluate kidney stones in pregnancy include MR urography, low-dose CT, or a limited intravenous pyelogram.[79,116] All diagnostic decision making should be made in conjunction with the patient, obstetrician, urologist, and radiologist, and take into account patient characteristics as well as stage of pregnancy.

Because most stones will pass spontaneously, treatment is generally the same as for the nonpregnant patient, except for the avoidance of NSAIDs. Cystoscopy with insertion of a ureteral stent or ureteroscopy to remove or fragment the stone may be required in the patient who is septic, has persistent severe pain, or has obstruction of a solitary functioning kidney. Pregnancy significantly increases the risk of stent encrustation, possibly necessitating frequent ureteral stent exchange every 4 to 6 weeks until delivery.

SWL is contraindicated in pregnancy, but ureteroscopic stone removal appears to have a similar safety profile in pregnant and nonpregnant patients. There is limited literature regarding the prognosis and outcomes of pregnant patients with urolithiasis, although there is a possibility that preterm labor may be triggered by stone disease.[79]

PEARLS AND PITFALLS

- CT is the diagnostic test of choice for renal colic, but protocols that limit radiation exposure to the patient are preferred.
- Though still under investigation, MET with tamsulosin is an acceptable part of treatment, but patients should have close follow-up and be warned of potential side effects including transient hypotension, dizziness, nausea, and vomiting.
- An infected, obstructing kidney stone is a urological emergency and requires emergent decompression.
- Mimics of renal colic should be considered in all patients who present with unilateral flank pain.

REFERENCES

1. Pearle MS, Calhoun EA, Curhan GC. Urologic diseases in America project: urolithiasis. J Urol 2005;173:848–57.
2. Litwin MS, Saigal CS, Yano EM, et al. Urologic diseases in American Project: analytical methods and principal findings. J Urol 2005;173:933–7.
3. Saigal CS, Joyce G, Timilsina AR. Direct and indirect costs of nephrolithiasis in an employed population: opportunity for disease management? Kidney Int 2005;68:1808–14.
4. Johnson CM, Wilson DM, O'Fallon WM, et al. Renal stone epidemiology: a 25-year study in Rochester, Minnesota. Kidney Int 1979;16:624.

5. Stamaltelou KK, Francis ME, Jones CA, et al. Time trends in reported prevalence of kidney stones in the United States 1976–1994. Kidney Int 2003;63:1817.
6. Lieske JC, Pena de la Vega LS, Slezak JM, et al. Renal stone epidemiology in Rochester, Minnesota: an update. Kidney Int 2006;69(4):760–4.
7. Parmar MS. Kidney stones. BMJ 2004;328:1420.
8. Scales CD Jr, Curtis LH, Norris RD, et al. Changing gender prevalence of stone disease. J Urol 2007;177:979.
9. Curhan GC, Rimm EB, Willett WC, et al. Regional variation in nephrolithiasis incidence and prevalence among United States men. J Urol 1994;151:838.
10. Soucie JM, Coates RJ, McCellan W, et al. Relation between geographic variability in kidney stone prevalence and risk factors for stones. Am J Epidemiol 1996;143:487.
11. Miller LM, Evan A, Lingeman J. Pathogenesis of renal calculi. Urol Clin North Am 2007;34:295–313.
12. Duffey BG, Pedro RN, Makhlouf A, et al. Roux-en-Y gastric bypass is associated with early increased risk factors for development of calcium oxalate nephrolithiasis. J Am Coll Surg 2008;206:1145.
13. Schwartz BF, Schenkman N, Armenakas NA, et al. Imaging characteristics of indinavir calculi. J Urol 1999;161:1085.
14. Curhan G, Willett W, Rimm E, et al. Family history and risk of kidney stones. J Am Soc Nephrol 1997;8:1568–73.
15. Kopp JB, Miller KD, Mican JA, et al. Crystalluria and urinary tract abnormalities associated with indinavir. Ann Intern Med 1997;127:119.
16. Cappuccio FP, Strazzullo P, Mancini M. Kidney stones and hypertension: population based study of an independent clinical association. BMJ 1990; 300:1234.
17. Taylor EN, Stampfer MJ, Curhan GC. Diabetes mellitus and the risk of nephrolithiasis. Kidney Int 2005;68:1230.
18. Coe FL, Parks JH, Asplin JR. The pathogenesis and treatment of kidney stones. N Engl J Med 1992;327:1141.
19. Borghi L, Schianchi T, Meschi T, et al. Comparison of two diets for the prevention of recurrent stones in idiopathic hypercalciuria. N Engl J Med 2002;346(2):77–84.
20. Kim SC, Coe FL, Tinmouth WW, et al. Stone formation is proportional to papillary surface coverage by Randall's plaque. J Urol 2005;173:117.
21. Ettinger B, Tang A, Citron JT, et al. Potassium magnesium citrate is an effective prophylaxis against recurrent calcium oxalate nephrolithiasis. J Urol 1997; 158(6):2069–73.
22. Ettinger B, Citron JT, Livermore B, et al. Chlorthalidone reduces calcium oxalate calculous recurrence but magnesium hydroxide does not. J Urol 1988;139(4): 679–84.
23. Taylor EN, Stampfer MJ, Curhan GC. Obesity, weight gain, and the risk of kidney stones. JAMA 2005;293(4):455–62.
24. Taylor EN, Stampfer MJ, Curhan GC. Dietary factors and the risk of incident kidney stones in men: new insights after 14 years of follow up. J Am Soc Nephrol 2004;15(12):3225–32.
25. Bataille P, Charransol G, Gregoire I, et al. Effect of calcium restriction on renal excretion of oxalate and the probability of stones in the various pathophysiological groups with calcium stones. J Urol 1983;130(2):218–23.
26. Curan G, Willet W, Speizer F, et al. Comparison of dietary calcium with supplemental calcium and other nutrients as factors affecting the risk for kidney stones in women. Ann Intern Med 1997;126:497–504.

27. Curhan GC, Willett WC, Knight EL, et al. Dietary factors and the risk of incident kidney stones in younger women (Nurses' Health Study II). Arch Intern Med 2004;164:885–91.
28. Borhgi L, Meschi T, Amato F, et al. Urinary volume, water and recurrences in idiopathic calcium nephrolithiasis: a 5 yr randomized prospective study. J Urol 1996;155:839–43.
29. Uribarri J, Oh MS, Carroll HJ. The first kidney stone. Ann Intern Med 1989;111:1006.
30. Hiatt RA, Ettinger B, Caan B, et al. Randomized controlled trial of a low animal protein, high fiber diet in the prevention of recurrent calcium oxalate kidney stones. Am J Epidemiol 1996;144:25.
31. Kocvara R, Plasgura P, Petrik A, et al. A prospective study of nonmedical prophylaxis after a first kidney stone. BJU Int 1999;84:393.
32. Asplin JR, Coe FL. Hyperoxaluria in kidney stone formers treated with modern bariatric surgery. J Urol 2007;177:565.
33. Gillen DL, Coe FL, Worcester EM. Nephrolithiasis and increased blood pressure among females with high body mass index. Am J Kidney Dis 2005;46:263.
34. Gillen DL, Worcester EM, Coe FL. Decreased renal function among adults with a history of nephrolithiasis: a study of NHANES III. Kidney Int 2005;67:685.
35. Rodgers AL, Greyling KG, Noakes TD. Crystalluria in marathon runners. III. Stone-forming subjects. Urol Res 1991;19:189.
36. Daudon M, Traxer O, Conort P, et al. Type 2 diabetes increases the risk for uric acid stones. J Am Soc Nephrol 2006;17:2026.
37. Ekeruo WO, Tan YH, Young MD, et al. Metabolic risk factors and the impact of medical therapy on the management of nephrolithiasis in obese patients. J Urol 2004;172:159.
38. Abate N, Chandalia M, Cabo-Chan AV Jr, et al. The metabolic syndrome and uric acid nephrolithiasis: novel features of renal manifestation of insulin resistance. Kidney Int 2004;65:386.
39. Glowacki LS, Beecroft ML, Cook RJ, et al. The natural history of asymptomatic urolithiasis. J Urol 1992;147:319.
40. Worcester EM, Coe FL. Nephrolithiasis. Prim Care 2008;35(2):369–91, vii.
41. Shokeir A. Renal colic: new concepts related to pathophysiology, diagnosis, and treatment. Curr Opin Urol 2002;12:263–9.
42. Travaglini F, Bartoletti R, Gacci M, et al. Pathophysiology of reno-ureteral colic. Urol Int 2004;72(Suppl 1):20–3.
43. Ha M, MacDonald RD. Impact of CT scan in patients with first episode of suspected nephrolithiasis. J Emerg Med 2004;27:225.
44. Hoppe H, Studer R, Kessler TM, et al. Alternate or additional findings to stone disease on unenhanced computerized tomography for acute flank pain can impact management. J Urol 2006;175(5):1725–30.
45. Ahmad NA, Ather MH, Rees J. Incidental diagnosis of diseases on un-enhanced helical computed tomography performed for ureteric colic. BMC Urol 2003; 17(3):2.
46. Katz DS, Scheer M, Lumerman JH, et al. Alternative or additional diagnoses on unenhanced helical computed tomography for suspected renal colic: experience with 1000 consecutive examinations. Urology 2000;56:53–7.
47. Kirpalani A, Khalili K, Lee S, et al. Renal colic: comparison of use and outcomes of unenhanced helical CT for emergency investigation in 1998 and 2002. Radiology 2005;236(2):554–8.
48. Press SM, Smith AD. Incidence of negative hematuria in patients with acute urinary lithiasis presenting to the emergency room with flank pain. Urology 1995;45:753.

49. Bove P, Kaplan D, Dalrymple N, et al. Reexamining the value of hematuria testing in patients with acute flank pain. J Urol 1999;162:685.
50. Kobayashi T, Nishizawa K, Mitsumori K, et al. Impact of date of onset on the absence of hematuria in patients with acute renal colic. J Urol 2003;170:1093.
51. Smith RC, Verga M, McCarthy S, et al. Diagnosis of acute flank pain: value of unenhanced helical CT. AJR Am J Roentgenol 1996;166:97.
52. Colistro R, Torreggiani WC, Lyburn ID, et al. Unenhanced helical CT in the investigation of acute flank pain. Clin Radiol 2002;57:435.
53. Ulahannan D, Blakeley CJ, Jeyadevan N, et al. Benefits of CT urography in patients presenting to the emergency department with suspected ureteric colic. Emerg Med J 2008;25:569.
54. Dalrymple NC, Verga M, Anderson KR, et al. The value of unenhanced helical computerized tomography in the management of acute flank pain. J Urol 1998;159:735.
55. Smith RC, Rosenfield AT, Choe KA, et al. Acute flank pain: comparison of non-contrast-enhanced CT and intravenous urogram. Radiology 1995;194:789.
56. Worster A, Preyra I, Weaver B, et al. The accuracy of noncontrast helical computed tomography versus intravenous pyelography in the diagnosis of suspected acute urolithiasis: a meta-analysis. Ann Emerg Med 2002;40:280.
57. Pfister SA, Deckart A, Laschke S, et al. Unenhanced helical computed tomography vs intravenous urography in patients with acute flank pain: accuracy and economic impact in a randomized prospective trial. Eur Radiol 2003;13:2513.
58. Sheafor DH, Hertzberg BS, Freed KS, et al. Nonenhanced helical CT and US in the emergency evaluation of patients with renal colic: prospective comparison. Radiology 2000;217:792.
59. Varanelli MJ, Coll DM, Levine JA, et al. Relationship between duration of pain and secondary signs of obstruction of the urinary tract on unenhanced helical CT. AJR Am J Roentgenol 2001;177:325.
60. Heneghan JP, Dalrymple NC, Verga M, et al. Soft-tissue "rim" sign in the diagnosis of ureteral calculi with use of unenhanced helical CT. Radiology 1997;202:709.
61. Smith RC, Verga M, Dalrymple N, et al. Acute ureteral obstruction: value of secondary signs of helical unenhanced CT. AJR Am J Roentgenol 1996;167:1109.
62. Mancini J, Ferrandino M. The impact of new methods of imaging on radiation dosage delivered to patients. Curr Opin Urol 2010;20(2):163–8.
63. McCollough CH, Primak AN, Braun N. Strategies for reducing radiation dose in CT. Radiol Clin North Am 2009;47:27.
64. Mulkens TH, Daniette S, De Wijngaert R. Urinary stone disease: comparison of standard-dose and low-dose with 4D MDCT tube current modulation. AJR Am J Roentgenol 2007;188:553.
65. Poletti PA, Platon A, Rutschmann OT, et al. Low-dose versus standard-dose CT protocol in patients with clinically suspected renal colic. AJR Am J Roentgenol 2007;188(4):927–33.
66. Kluner C, Hein PA, Gralia O, et al. Does ultra-low-dose CT with a radiation dose equivalent to that of KUB suffice to detect renal and ureteral calculi? J Comput Assist Tomogr 2006;30(1):44–50.
67. Kim BS, Hwang IK, Choi YW, et al. Low dose and standard dose unenhanced helical computed tomography for the assessment of acute renal colic: prospective comparative study. Acta Radiol 2005;46(7):756–63.
68. Matlaga BR, Kawamoto S, Fishman E. Dual source computed tomography: a novel technique to determine stone composition. Urology 2008;72:1164.

69. Boll DT, Patil NA, Paulson EK, et al. Renal stone assessment with dual-energy multidetector ct and advanced postprocessing techniques: improved characterization of renal stone composition—pilot study. Radiology 2009;250:813.
70. Sinclair D, Wilson S, Toi A, et al. The evaluation of suspected renal colic: ultrasound scan versus excretory urography. Ann Emerg Med 1989;18:556–9.
71. Erwin B, Carroll B, Sommer F. Renal colic: the role of ultrasound in initial evaluation. Radiology 1984;152:147–50.
72. Patlas M, Farkas A, Fisher D, et al. Ultrasound vs CT for the detection of ureteric stones in patients with renal colic. Br J Radiol 2001;74(886):901–4.
73. Fowler KA, Locken J, Duchesne J, et al. US for detecting renal calculi with non-enhanced CT as a reference standard. Radiology 2002;222(1):109–13.
74. Goertz J, Lotterman S. Can the degree of hydronephrosis on ultrasound predict kidney stone size? Am J Emerg Med 2010;28:813–6.
75. Ray A, Ghiculete D, Pace K, et al. Limitations to ultrasound in the detection and measurement of urinary tract calculi. Urology 2010;76(2):295–300.
76. Catalano O, Nunziata A, Altei F, et al. Suspected ureteral colic: primary helical CT versus selective helical CT after unenhanced radiography and sonography. AJR Am J Roentgenol 2002;178:379.
77. Roth CS, Bowyer BA, Berquist TH. Utility of the plain radiograph for diagnosing ureteral calculi. Ann Emerg Med 1985;14:311–5.
78. Mutgi A, Williams JW, Nettleman M. Renal colic: utility of the plain abdominal roentgenogram. Arch Intern Med 1991;151:1589–92.
79. McAleer S, Loughlin K. Nephrolithiasis and pregnancy. Curr Opin Urol 2004;14:123.
80. Cordell WH, Wright SW, Wolfson AB, et al. Comparison of intravenous ketorolac, meperidine, and both (balanced analgesia) for renal colic. Ann Emerg Med 1996;28:151.
81. Cordell WH, Larson TA, Lingeman JE, et al. Indomethacin suppositories versus intravenously titrated morphine for the treatment of ureteral colic. Ann Emerg Med 1994;23:262.
82. Holdgate A, Pollock T. Systematic review of the relative efficacy of non-steroidal anti-inflammatory drugs and opioids in the treatment of acute renal colic. BMJ 2004;328:1401.
83. Safdar B, Degutis LC, Landry K, et al. Intravenous morphine plus ketorolac is superior to either drug alone for treatment of acute renal colic. Ann Emerg Med 2006;48:173.
84. Springhart WP, Marguet CG, Sur RL, et al. Forced versus minimal intravenous hydration in the management of acute renal colic: a randomized trial. J Endourol 2006;20:713.
85. Cole RS, Fry CH, Shuttleworth KE. The action of the prostaglandins on isolated human ureteric smooth muscle. Br J Urol 1988;61:19.
86. Preminger GM. Editorial comment. The value of intensive medical management of distal ureteral calculi in an effort to facilitate spontaneous stone passage. Urology 2000;56:582.
87. Porpiglia F, Destefanis P, Fiori C, et al. Effectiveness of nifedipine and deflazacort in the management of distal ureter stones. Urology 2000;56:579.
88. Dellabella M, Milanese G, Muzzonigro G. Efficacy of tamsulosin in the medical management of juxtavesical ureteral stones. J Urol 2003;170:2202.
89. Saita A, Bonaccorsi A, Marchese F, et al. Our experience with nifedipine and prednisolone as expulsive therapy for ureteral stones. Urol Int 2004;1(72 Suppl):43.

90. Dellabella M, Milanese G, Muzzonigro G. Medical-expulsive therapy for distal ureterolithiasis: randomized prospective study on role of corticosteroids used in combination with tamsulosin-simplified treatment regimen and health-related quality of life. Urology 2005;66:712.
91. Dellabella M, Milanese G, Muzzonigro G. Randomized trial of the efficacy of tamsulosin, nifedipine and phloroglucinol in medical expulsive therapy for distal ureteral calculi. J Urol 2005;174:167.
92. Porpiglia F, Ghignone G, Fiori C, et al. Nifedipine versus tamsulosin for the management of lower ureteral stones. J Urol 2004;172:568.
93. Hollingsworth JM, Rogers MA, Kaufman SR, et al. Medical therapy to facilitate urinary stone passage: a meta-analysis. Lancet 2006;368:1171.
94. Yilmaz E, Batislam E, Basar MM, et al. The comparison and efficacy of 3 different alpha1-adrenergic blockers for distal ureteral stones. J Urol 2005; 173:2010.
95. Parsons JK, Hergan LA, Sakamoto K, et al. Efficacy of alpha-blockers for the treatment of ureteral stones. J Urol 2007;177:983.
96. Agrawal M, Gupta M, Gupta A, et al. Prospective randomized trial comparing efficacy of alfuzosin and tamsulosin in management of lower ureteral stones. Urology 2009;73:706.
97. Ferre R, Wasielewski J, Strout T, et al. Tamsulosin for ureteral stones in the emergency department: a randomized, controlled trial. Ann Emerg Med 2009;54(3): 432–9.
98. Singh A, Alter H, Littlepage A. A systematic review of medical therapy to facilitate passage of ureteral calculi. Ann Emerg Med 2007;50:552–63.
99. Vincendeau S, Bellissant E, Houlgatte A, et al. Tamsulosin hydrochloride vs placebo for management of distal ureteral stones: a multicentric, randomized, double-blinded trial. Arch Intern Med 2010;170(22):2021–7.
100. Roshani A, Falahatkar S, Khosropanah I, et al. Assessment of clinical efficacy of intranasal desmopressin spray and diclofenac sodium suppository in treatment of renal colic versus diclofenac sodium alone. Urology 2010;75(3):540–2.
101. Welk BK, Teichman JM. Pharmacological management of renal colic in the older patient. Drugs Aging 2007;24(11):891–900.
102. Lopes T, Dias J, Marcelino J, et al. An assessment of the clinical efficacy of intranasal desmopressin spray in the treatment of renal colic. BJU Int 2001;87: 322–5.
103. Moro U, Stefani S, Crisci A, et al. Evaluation of the effects of desmopressin in acute ureteral obstruction. Urol Int 1999;62:8–11.
104. Preminger GM, Tiselius HG, Assimos DG, et al. 2007 guideline for the management of ureteral calculi. J Urol 2007;178:2418.
105. Miller OF, Kane CJ. Time to stone passage for observed ureteral calculi: a guide for patient education. J Urol 1999;162:688.
106. Coll DM, Varanelli MJ, Smith RC. Relationship of spontaneous passage of ureteral calculi to stone size and location as revealed by unenhanced helical CT. AJR Am J Roentgenol 2002;178:101.
107. Parekattil SJ, Kumar U, Hegarty NJ, et al. External validation of outcome prediction model for ureteral/renal calculi. J Urol 2006;175:575.
108. Lingeman J, Matlaga B, Evan A. Surgical management of upper urinary tract calculi. In: Wein AJ, editor. Campbell-Walsh urology, vol. 2. 9th edition. Philadelphia (PA): Saunders Elsevier; 2007. Chapter 43.
109. Moe OW. Kidney stones: pathophysiology and medical management. Lancet 2006;367(9507):333–44.

110. Vieweg J, Teh C, Freed K, et al. Unenhanced helical computerized tomography for the evaluation of patient with acute flank pain. J Urol 1998;52:982–7.
111. Andren-Sandberg A. Permanent impairment of renal function demonstrated by renographic follow up in ureterolithiasis. Scand J Urol Nephrol 1983;17:81–4.
112. Holm Nielson A, Jorgenson T, Mogensen P, et al. The prognostic value of probe renography in ureteric stone obstruction. Br J Urol 1981;53:504–7.
113. Irving SO, Calleja R, Lee F, et al. Is the conservative management of ureteric calculi of >4 mm safe? BJU Int 2000;85:637–40.
114. Stothers L, Lee L. Renal colic in pregnancy. J Urol 1992;148:1383.
115. Boridy I, Maklad N, Sandler C. Suspected urolithiasis in pregnant women: imaging algorithm and literature review. AJR Am J Roentgenol 1996;167:869.
116. Semins M, Trock B, Matlaga B. The safety of ureteroscopy during pregnancy: a systematic review and meta-analysis. J Urol 2009;181:139–42.

Diagnosis and Management of Urinary Tract Infection and Pyelonephritis

David R. Lane, MD[a,*], Sukhjit S. Takhar, MD[b,c]

KEYWORDS

• Urinary • Pyelonephritis • Cystitis

Urinary tract infections (UTIs) are one of the most common bacterial infections encountered in outpatient settings[1,2] In 2005, 1.8 million patients in emergency departments (EDs) were diagnosed with UTI, and nearly 5% of all patients in EDs had a genitourinary (GU) complaint.[3] More than 50% of women experience 1 UTI in their lifetime, and approximately 10% of women have a UTI annually.[4] Familiarity with the most recent literature and clinical practice guidelines, and local patterns of resistance, is crucial for practicing emergency physicians (EPs). Targeted and appropriate therapy can significantly reduce the morbidity and mortality associated with this spectrum of illness, and may also reduce the development of antimicrobial resistance in uropathogens. This article reports the epidemiology and risk factors of UTIs, and clarifies the diagnostic tools and therapeutic measures that best streamline practices and effectively treat patients with UTIs. This article concentrates on the adult woman with upper and lower tract infections, unless otherwise indicated. Treatment options are discussed in light of bacterial resistance in the twenty-first century.

DEFINITIONS

UTIs are divided into 2 major categories: lower tract infections and upper tract infections. Broadly defined, they can be considered an inflammatory response of the

---

The authors have nothing to disclose.

[a] Department of Emergency Medicine, Georgetown University Hospital & Washington Hospital Center, Georgetown University School of Medicine, 3800 Reservoir Road Northwest, Washington, DC 20007, USA

[b] Department of Emergency Medicine, Brigham and Women's Hospital, Neville House, 75 Francis Street, Boston, MA 02115, USA

[c] Harvard Medical School, Boston, MA, USA

* Corresponding author.

E-mail address: david.lane@gunet.georgetown.edu

Emerg Med Clin N Am 29 (2011) 539–552

doi:10.1016/j.emc.2011.04.001

emed.theclinics.com

urinary tract to microorganisms. UTIs range from asymptomatic cases to life-threatening septic shock. They can be community acquired or catheter associated.

Asymptomatic bacteriuria (ABU) is the presence of significant bacteria with or without pyuria on urinalysis without signs or symptoms that are referable to a UTI. The usual cutoff is a single organism isolated in a quantity of at least 100,000 colony forming units (CFU) per milliliter.[5] Screening and treatment is not generally recommended, with the exception of women who are pregnant or men who are going to undergo a transurethral prostate resection.[6,7]

Cystitis, or lower UTI, is an acute bacterial infection of the urinary bladder and urethra, whereas pyelonephritis is an infection of the upper urinary tract structures, including the ureters or kidneys. Differentiation of the 2 is based on history and examination.

Uncomplicated UTI occurs in young, healthy, nonpregnant women with structurally and functionally normal urinary tracts.[8] Complicated UTI is UTI occurring in anyone else: all men, and women who have a structural or functional GU abnormality or an underlying predisposing medical condition that increases the risk of infection and recurrence or that reduces the effectiveness of antimicrobial therapy (**Box 1**). Both cystitis and pyelonephritis can be defined as either uncomplicated or complicated according to these parameters.

EPIDEMIOLOGY AND RISK FACTORS

UTIs are common, particularly in women, with 11% of women reporting a UTI in any given year, and more than 50% of women having at least 1 infection during their lifetime.[4] Other groups at increased risk for UTI, as well as complications of UTI, include infants, pregnant women, the elderly, and individuals with diabetes, human immunodeficiency virus (HIV)/AIDS, spinal cord injuries, indwelling catheters, or urologic abnormalities.[1]

There is much misunderstanding among patients surrounding risk factors for, and prevention of, UTIs. Proven risk factors for UTI in young women are prior episodes of cystitis, recent sexual activity, and use of spermicidal agents during intercourse.[9] The odds of a UTI increase by a factor of 60 during the initial 48 hours after sexual intercourse.[10,11] Commonly recommended treatments to reduce incidence of UTI, such as increased hydration and prompt postcoital voiding or douching, are not supported by evidence.[12] Cranberries, cranberry tablets, and cranberry juice may have a benefit in preventing recurrent UTIs; the evidence is best in sexually active adult

Box 1
Patient characteristics qualifying UTI as complicated

Pregnancy

Diabetes

Male gender

Immunosuppression

- Immunosuppressive agents, acquired immune deficiency syndrome (AIDS), others

Functional genitourinary abnormality

- Indwelling urinary catheter, neurogenic bladder, others

Structural genitourinary abnormality

- Renal stones, fistula from intestinal tract to bladder, polycystic kidney disease, renal transplant, other women. However, it requires daily cranberry juice intake at a dose of 200 to 750 mL, taken in divided doses daily, and the benefit is only modest.[13,14]

Additional risk factors have been shown to have significance in specific subgroups of the population. In postmenopausal women, cystoceles, urinary incontinence, or prior GU surgery are significant risk factors for recurrent cystitis.[15] In elderly women, the risk of UTI increases with age and debility, specifically increasing in those with impaired voiding or poor hygiene, and is also higher in patients with diabetes.[16–19] In men, risk factors for the development of UTI include insertive anal intercourse, lack of circumcision, urinary tract instrumentation, renal stone disease, and prostatic hypertrophy.[20]

MICROBIOLOGY

The bacterial pathogens responsible for UTI have remained consistent for many years. Gram-negative bacilli are the culprit organisms in most cases. However, the response of some pathogens to common antimicrobials has gradually evolved in the past 2 decades. *Escherichia coli* continues to be the primary offender, causing 75% to 90% of episodes of acute uncomplicated cystitis, and most episodes of complicated UTI and pyelonephritis.[4] Gram-positive organisms are less common; however, *Staphylococcus saprophyticus* accounts for 5% to 15% of UTI, mainly in younger women, and is generally confined to cystitis.[21] If *Staphylococcus aureus* is isolated from the urine, a bacteremic source that has seeded the kidney must be considered. Other aerobic gram-negative rods such as *Klebsiella* species and *Proteus mirabilis*, and the gram-positive enterococci are isolated in most of the remaining cases.[4]

CLINICAL PRESENTATION

The typical clinical presentation for cystitis is a well-appearing woman with urinary frequency, dysuria, and urgency. Suprapubic pain and low back pain may also be present. The symptoms of cystitis are sufficiently classic and repetitive that self-diagnosis can be accurate in this disease: if a woman who previously has had cystitis has symptoms suggesting a recurrence, there is an 84% to 92% chance that an infection is present.[22,23]

The probability of cystitis in a woman with dysuria, urinary frequency, or gross hematuria is 50%.[24] The absence of symptoms suggesting vaginitis or cervicitis, such as vaginal irritation, bleeding, or discharge, raises the probability of UTI to more than 90%, whereas the presence of such symptoms reduces the likelihood to about 30%.[24] Further evaluation of women with symptoms of vaginitis or cervicitis should include a pelvic examination with evaluation for potential gonorrhea, chlamydia, bacterial vaginosis, trichomoniasis, and candidiasis.

For older women, increased or new incontinence is a common symptom of cystitis.[25] Elderly patients may present with any number of nonspecific symptoms, including altered mental status or delirium, general malaise, or, in extreme cases, systemic inflammatory response syndrome, sepsis, or septic shock.

As mentioned earlier, differentiation of cystitis from pyelonephritis is based on history and physical examination. Pyelonephritis presents in a spectrum from well appearing to critically ill with severe sepsis. Classic symptoms include flank or abdominal pain, fever and chills, and nausea or vomiting. Up to 25% of patients with pyelonephritis may have bilateral infection and thus present with pain that is not unilateral.[6] Typically patients report preceding symptoms consistent with cystitis, but this is not essential. As in many diseases, diabetics and the elderly have a predilection for presenting atypically. The lack of fever and presence of altered mental status is common in the elderly.[26]

DIAGNOSTIC TOOLS

Urine Collection

Clean-catch midstream collection of urine is a common technique for obtaining urine samples. However, there is evidence showing that the clean-catch technique does not decrease contamination rates and that routine urination into a sterile container may be considered an adequate specimen collection technique.[27–29] For obtaining samples with minimal contamination, straight catheter collection is only bettered by suprapubic aspiration; however, both techniques introduce unnecessary patient discomfort and resource use, as well as the risk of introducing bacteria into the bladder.[5]

Urinalysis

Urine dipstick has largely replaced urine microscopy as the initial diagnostic tool of choice in UTI in the ambulatory setting, because it is less expensive, more convenient, and its accuracy is comparable with urine microscopy.[5,30] On urine dipstick, the 2 tests of interest are leukocyte esterase, a measure of pyuria, and nitrite, a measure of bacteriuria. Dipsticks are the most predictive when the presence of either nitrite or leukocyte esterase is considered positive, yielding a sensitivity of 75% (67%–100%) and specificity of 82% (67%–98%).[31] If both leukocyte esterase and nitrite must be positive, the specificity improves to 98% to 100%, but the sensitivity declines to 35% to 84%.[5] These diagnostic tests in isolation have limitations. Nitrite positivity alone seems to be more specific than leukocyte esterase alone in the diagnosis of UTI (95%–98% vs 59%–96%), but the usefulness of nitrite positivity in isolation is limited because the uropathogens *S saprophyticus*, *Pseudomonas*, or enterococci do not reduce nitrate.[32,33] Leukocyte esterase sensitivity is decreased by high levels of protein or glucose in the urine, and may be falsely positive when there is contamination by bacteria in vaginal fluid, as occurs in vaginitis or cervicitis.[5]

Urine microscopy previously relied on the manual counting of leukocytes for measuring pyuria or Gram stain evaluation for measuring bacteriuria. Automated instruments now perform most microscopic analyses in modern hospital laboratories.[5] For pyuria, typically a count of greater than 10 leukocytes/mm^3 correlates with high bacterial concentrations of ($\geq 10^5$ CFU/mL). The Gram stain is only reliable with high concentrations of bacteria ($\geq 10^5$ CFU/mL). Thus, it is not always positive for patients with uncomplicated UTI, who may be symptomatic with much lower bacterial concentrations (10^2–10^3 CFU/mL). Because of its labor intensity, Gram stain of the urine is often impractical in most laboratory settings, and thus is unavailable in many hospitals.

The difficulty for the EP remains in diagnosing UTI in patients with questionable urinary symptoms based on the presence, for instance, of urinary leukocyte esterase alone. It is prudent to remember that the specificity of this finding in isolation is good, but imperfect. It is important to consider a broad differential, including other potential causes of abdominal or pelvic inflammation or infection. Likewise, consideration of alternate diagnoses in questionable cases is important before administration of antimicrobials. Antibiotic treatment may mask signs and symptoms or otherwise delay definitive diagnosis of alternative conditions.

Urine Culture

Urine culture is not necessary to make the diagnosis in patients with uncomplicated UTI; a positive dipstick or findings on microscopy, combined with suggestive clinical symptoms, is adequate. The urine culture has much more usefulness in patients with complicated UTI, recurrent UTI, or pyelonephritis, because it helps guide treatment in failed antibiotic therapy. It is also advisable to obtain a urine culture in patients with a high pretest likelihood of UTI but a negative urine dipstick or microscopy result. However, the diagnosis of a UTI should be questioned if pyuria is not present.

There is some debate about the definition of a positive culture. Several factors must be considered in dealing with this question. For example, suprapubic aspirates can be considered positive if there is any degree of bacteriuria. The traditional definition used by most laboratories is 100,000 CFU/mL, which provides a test with high specificity and low sensitivity. However, it has been shown that many women with UTI symptoms have bacterial counts of less than 100,000 CFU/mL with uropathogens.[34] If there are greater than or equal to 10^2 CFU/mL in a clean-catch acquired urine culture with a single bacterial isolate, this should be considered a positive test.[35] If there is more than 1 bacterial isolate in the clean-catch acquired urine culture, then a cutoff of greater than or equal to 10^5 CFU/mL is more appropriate.[5] Therefore, a urine culture with fewer than 10^2 CFU/mL should be considered an indeterminate or negative test. Ultimately, the degree of bacteriuria, sampling method, and patient symptoms must be taken into account when interpreting the results of a urine culture.

Imaging

Imaging is largely unnecessary in the evaluation and treatment decisions in uncomplicated UTI, and imaging is not recommended for routine use in the evaluation of pyelonephritis.[36] The usefulness of ED imaging is primarily for patients with pyelonephritis who are septic or who are not responsive to initial antimicrobial therapy. Those with an initial presentation of septic shock from presumed pyelonephritis should have urgent imaging to evaluate for an infected, obstructed ureteral stone. In general, patients who do not have an appropriate clinical response to therapy within 48 to 72 hours should be evaluated for a perinephric abscess.

Computed tomography (CT) imaging of the abdomen and pelvis with intravenous contrast yields the most information in the evaluation of UTI, identifying renal stones, perinephric abscesses, renal enlargement, obstruction, gas, hemorrhage, and masses.[37] Ultrasound may be considered for detecting masses and obstruction in cases where CT is not feasible, and increasing ED availability as well as research into its usefulness in the acute care setting may increase its everyday use.

TREATMENT

Uncomplicated Cystitis

Treatment of uncomplicated cystitis has been the subject of much study in recent years as rates of microorganism resistance to standard antimicrobials have evolved. In addition, greater importance has been placed on the adverse effects of broad-spectrum antimicrobial therapy. Prudent empiric therapy is often based on analysis of local antibiograms. However, a key limitation in this approach is that antibiograms may falsely overestimate resistance for uropathogens because many patients with simple cystitis and typical symptoms of a UTI do not have a culture performed.

Recently, the Infectious Diseases Society of America (IDSA) released updated clinical practice guidelines.[7] The prior IDSA guidelines, released in 1999, recommended treatment with oral trimethoprim-sulfamethoxazole (TMP-SMX) twice daily by mouth for 3 days as initial therapy for uncomplicated cystitis, except in communities with rates of resistance exceeding 10% to 20%, in which case empiric therapy with a fluoroquinolone was recommended.[38] For unclear reasons, physicians' prescribing practices did not regularly match these recommendations, and fluoroquinolones were more regularly used.[4,39,40]

The 2010 IDSA guidelines suggest stronger consideration for the use of oral nitrofurantoin monohydrate/macrocrystals (Macrobid) 100 mg by mouth twice daily for

5 days as a first-line treatment in patients with suspected UTI (**Table 1**).[7] The primary reasons for this recommendation are increasing resistance among uropathogens to TMP-SMX and clinical failure when the isolate is resistant. TMP-SMX is still considered an appropriate choice for therapy if the local resistance rates of uropathogens do not exceed 20%, or if the infecting strain is known to be susceptible; however, availability of these data to practicing physicians is often limited.

Nitrofurantoin previously has been regarded as an antimicrobial for UTI in pregnancy and, because of its longer treatment course, had been avoided by many EPs for uncomplicated UTI. The standard recommendation was a 7-day course to achieve equivalence to the cure rates of the 3-day TMP-SMX. However, recent studies have shown a 5-day course of oral nitrofurantoin to be clinically equivalent to a 3-day course of oral TMP-SMX, allowing shortened treatment with fewer adverse drug events.[41] With increasing antimicrobial resistance to TMP-SMX, the prominence of nitrofurantoin in the treatment of uncomplicated UTI should increase. The overall clinical cure rate with nitrofurantoin is 88% to 93%.[42,43] Nitrofurantoin is less active against aerobic gram-negative rods, and inactive against *Proteus* and *Pseudomonas* species, and thus should be reserved for uncomplicated UTI.

TMP-SMX is still a reasonable choice in regions in which resistance levels are lower than 20%. It is administered as a 3-day, twice-daily oral course. In areas where resistance is in the 10% to 15% range, the cure rates are equivalent to those with nitrofurantoin and ciprofloxacin.[42–44] Studies of duration of treatment have found that efficacy rates for TMP-SMX peak with a 3-day course, whereas complication rates continue to increase with additional days of therapy. Single-dose oral therapy with TMP-SMX was 87% effective with a complication rate of 11%, whereas a 3-day course was 94% effective with an 18% complication rate, and a 7-day course was 95% effective with a 30% complication rate.[45] The 3-day course maximizes efficacy, and minimizes complications.

Alternatives to nitrofurantoin and TMP-SMX include fluoroquinolones, fosfomycin trometamol, pivmecillinam, and β-lactam agents such as amoxicillin-clavulanate, cefdinir, cefaclor, and cefpodoxime-proxetil.

Table 1
Antimicrobial therapy for uncomplicated cystitis

	Antimicrobial	Comment
First line	Nitrofurantoin 100 mg by mouth twice a day for 5 d	Low rate of resistance. Need a 5-d course
	TMP-SMX 1 tablet DS by mouth twice a day for 3 d	Only if local resistance is less than 20%
Alternative	Ciprofloxacin 250 mg by mouth twice a day for 3 d (or ofloxacin or levofloxacin for 3 d)	Concern for resistance has made quinolones second-line agents
	Fosfomycin trometamol 3 g by mouth single dose	Not available in the United States
	β-Lactam agents (cefpodoxime, cephalexin, amoxicillin/clavulanate)	Multiple trials have shown β-lactam antibiotics inferior to TMP-SMX and quinolones. Third-generation oral cephalosporins may be an exception
Not accepted	Amoxicillin, ampicillin	Resistance rates extremely high worldwide

Abbreviations: DS, double strength; TMP-SMX, trimethoprim-sulfamethoxazole.

The most frequently used and most well-studied alternative to TMP-SMX and nitrofurantoin is the fluoroquinolone ciprofloxacin. The 3-day oral course of ciprofloxacin 250 mg twice a day, with its low cost, widespread success, and equivalent cure rates to TMP-SMX, has been widely regarded by many physicians as the alternative of choice and even a first-line agent. A 500-mg extended-release, once-daily oral ciprofloxacin dosing regimen has been shown to be equivalent, thus increasing the ease of use of this drug.[46,47] Other fluoroquinolones including ofloxacin, norfloxacin, and levofloxacin are considered equally effective to ciprofloxacin. However, the concern of increasing uropathogen resistance to fluoroquinolones, as well as increasing resistance among other organisms that will lead to more difficult-to-treat infections at other sites, has led to strong calls for restricting the use of fluoroquinolones to only those cases in which other antimicrobials are not effective.[7,39] Ciprofloxacin, despite its clear efficacy, convenience, low cost, and equivalence to TMP-SMX and nitrofurantoin, should be considered an alternative agent because of increasing fluoroquinolone antimicrobial resistance among a wide spectrum of organisms.

Additional alternatives for uncomplicated UTI, such as fosfomycin trometamol and pivmecillinam, are not widely available in the United States. Fosfomycin trometamol in a single oral dose of 3 g has been compared with the 5-day course of TMP-SMX and the 7-day course of nitrofurantoin, with equivalent or nearly equivalent clinical cure rates.[43,48] It has also been shown to have efficacy against vancomycin-resistant enterococci (VRE), methicillin-resistant *S aureus* (MRSA), and extended-spectrum β-lactamase (ESBL) –producing gram-negative rods, and thus may increase in usefulness as antimicrobial resistance continues to increase.[49] It is recommended as a first-line agent for uncomplicated UTI by the European Association of Urology, with the obvious advantage of single-dose therapy, although it is not widely available in the United States despite its approval for use by the US Food and Drug Administration (FDA). Pivmecillinam is an extended gram-negative spectrum penicillin used specifically for the treatment of UTI. It has lower bacterial and clinical cure rates than the first-line agents, and is not FDA approved or available in the United States.

β-Lactam antimicrobials are generally considered inferior in cure rates to the fluoroquinolones, nitrofurantoin and TMP/SMX, and also have similar challenges with antimicrobial resistance to the fluoroquinolones.[50] However, one recent study compared the oral third-generation cephalosporin cefpodoxime with TMP/SMX and found equivalent cure rates, but the study had limited power because of a small sample size.[51] Further studies are needed to strengthen support for β-lactam antimicrobials in this setting, particularly given the danger of increasing antimicrobial resistance to broad-spectrum cephalosporins by organisms such as ESBL-producing gram-negative bacteria. Empiric therapy with ampicillin and amoxicillin specifically should be avoided because of frequent bacterial resistance and low cure rates. Ampicillin resistance rates for *E coli* are greater than 30% in most parts of the United States and the world.[8]

Phenazopyridine (Pyridium) acts as a urinary anesthetic and its use for 1 or 2 days may relieve symptoms, but controlled trial data are limited. Side effects are rare; however, it may cause hemolysis in patients with known glucose-6-phosphate dehydrogenase deficiency.[4] In addition, phenazopyridine has been associated with the development of methemoglobinemia with prolonged use.

Complicated UTI

There are limited data to rely on for treatment recommendations for complicated UTI. Common measures include sending a urine culture before treatment, starting with broad-spectrum antibiotic coverage and refining the antimicrobial selection after sensitivity results have returned, and treating for 7 to 14 days. The standard approach has been to treat all UTIs in men as complicated; 7 days of antimicrobial therapy with a fluoroquinolone or TMP-SMX should achieve clinical cure in most. Men with presumed prostatitis need a longer course.[52,53] Further information on UTI in men can be found in previously published reviews.[54–57]

Acute Pyelonephritis

Fluoroquinolones remain the standard recommended antimicrobial for acute uncomplicated pyelonephritis, despite concerns of the expected increase of fluoroquinolone resistance (**Table 2**).[7,58–60] For patients not requiring hospitalization, multiple options are available. Oral ciprofloxacin 500 mg twice daily for 7 days, extended-release ciprofloxacin 1000 mg daily for 7 days, and levofloxacin 750 mg for 5 days are all supported in regions where the fluoroquinolone resistance rates are lower than 10%.[7] If fluoroquinolone resistance rates are unknown or higher than 10%, an intravenous (IV) dose of a longer acting β-lactam antibiotic, such as 1 g of ceftriaxone or a dose of 5 to 7 mg/kg gentamicin, is recommended.[7] As well as potential difficulty in determining the inciting allergen, there is an increased risk of an allergic reaction when using 2 distinct antibiotic classes simultaneously in the same patient. Therefore, a clear understanding of the resistance patterns in a particular area is invaluable in making the decision to initiate this additional therapy. Urine culture and sensitivity should be attained, and follow-up should be performed within 72 hours to ensure appropriate antimicrobial treatment.

TMP-SMX twice daily for 14 days or an oral β-lactam twice daily for 10 to 14 days continue to be second-tier options. If susceptibility is not known, a single IV dose of 1 g of ceftriaxone or a single dose of IV aminoglycoside is recommended. Resistance rates for uropathogens causing uncomplicated pyelonephritis were found to be 27% (range 13%–45%) for TMP-SMX, and only 1% to 3% for ciprofloxacin and levofloxacin in a sample of 11 academic EDs.[58] Note that nitrofurantoin is not an

Table 2
Antimicrobial therapy for uncomplicated pyelonephritis

	Antimicrobial	Comment
First line	Ciprofloxacin 500 mg by mouth twice a day for 7 d Ciprofloxacin ER 1000 mg by mouth twice a day for 7 d Levofloxacin 750 mg by mouth twice a day for 5 d	Consider giving an IV dose of the same or similar fluoroquinolone before staring oral dosing If there is a high level of quinolone resistance in the community, consider giving a dose of ceftriaxone 1 g IV, followed by oral fluoroquinolone
Alternative	TMP-SMX by mouth twice a day for 14 d	High rates of resistance. Give an IV dose of ceftriaxone or another long acting agent
	Cefpodoxime 400 mg by mouth twice a day for 10–14 d Amoxicillin/clavulanate 875 mg by mouth twice a day for 10–14 d	Oral third-generation cephalosporins are more effective than first generation, but more expensive
Not acceptable	Nitrofurantoin	Does not achieve acceptable levels in tissue or serum. Only used for uncomplicated cystitis

Abbreviation: IV, intravenous.

acceptable antibiotic for pyelonephritis. It does not achieve appreciable serum levels and therefore should not be used for pyelonephritis, because these patients are often bacteremic.[61,62]

Broader-spectrum antimicrobial therapy covering pseudomonal species should be considered in patients who present with septic shock or in patients with a prior history of resistant organisms. Piperacillin/tazobactam, imipenem, meropenem, ampicillin plus tobramycin, and vancomycin plus gentamicin or tobramycin are options for such patients.

Therapy can be outpatient if patients do not have factors associated with complicated infection or signs of systemic toxicity, can tolerate oral medications, and can be closely followed (**Box 2**).[63] Follow-up on urine culture results is important, particularly in areas that have increasing resistance to fluoroquinolones. Hospitalization is necessary for patients who are unable to tolerate oral medications or who have sepsis, and often recommended for patients who are pregnant or have complicated pyelonephritis. For patients who are hospitalized, parenteral antibiotic recommendations have not changed, and include a fluoroquinolone, an aminoglycoside, an extended-spectrum cephalosporin or penicillin with or without an aminoglycoside, or a carbapenem. For patients who have a history of recurrent UTIs, it is important to review previous culture results. Carbapenems remain the drug of choice for patients with an ESBL-producing organism. After sensitivity results are determined, therapy can be tailored appropriately. Blood cultures are not routinely warranted for uncomplicated pyelonephritis; urine culture is nearly always sufficient. However, blood cultures may be useful when the initial diagnosis of pyelonephritis is uncertain or if an alternative cause for pyuria and fever is identified, such as in endocarditis.[64,65]

Pyelonephritis Complications

Patients typically improve rapidly with appropriate therapy. For patients who do not improve within 48 to 72 hours, further evaluation with CT or ultrasound diagnostic imaging should be strongly considered. Pyonephrosis, renal abscess, and emphysematous pyelonephritis are uncommon, but potentially severe, complications of pyelonephritis, and prompt recognition and therapy can significantly affect morbidity and mortality.

Pyonephrosis is the combination of infection and obstruction (pus under pressure) with a collection of purulent material trapped in the renal collecting system by a stone, a mass, or other obstruction. In addition to antimicrobial therapy and supportive treatment of sepsis, emergent urologic or interventional radiology consultation for percutaneous nephrostomy tube or ureteral stent placement is indicated. Most patients

Box 2
Criteria for discharge of patients with acute pyelonephritis

Stable vital signs

Normal renal function

No urinary obstruction

Adequate pain control

Adequate hydration

Ability to tolerate oral medication

improve rapidly after surgical treatment, and the obstruction can be definitively treated 1 to 2 weeks after resolution of the infection.

Renal abscess includes perirenal or intrarenal abscess, acute focal or multifocal bacterial nephritis, and xanthogranulomatous pyelonephritis (XGP). XGP is an inflammatory disorder of the renal parenchyma with a central area of necrosis and hemorrhage. It is typically unilateral, is caused by long-term urinary tract obstruction, and can spread to surrounding structures. For intrarenal abscess larger than 3 cm or perirenal abscess, percutaneous drainage after medical stabilization and antibiotic therapy is widely recommended in the urology literature.[66] However, many patients with smaller abscesses require drainage as well. The importance of source/nidus control in dealing with a septic or otherwise unstable patient from a urinary source cannot be overstated.

Emphysematous pyelonephritis is a necrotizing infection with gas formation in the renal parenchyma, with a mortality ranging from 20% to 40% even when treated.[67,68] Patients with diabetes represent approximately 95% of reported cases. An infected obstructing renal calculus is the major predisposing risk factor. Patients typically are clinically very ill, requiring aggressive cardiopulmonary stabilization and early broad-spectrum antibiotic therapy, followed by urologic consultation for either percutaneous drainage or immediate nephrectomy.

Pregnancy

Pregnancy changes the therapeutic approach to UTI and pyelonephritis in 2 crucial ways. First, antibiotic therapy is adjusted. Asymptomatic bacteriuria (ABU), defined by isolation of greater than or equal to 10^5 CFU/mL of a single microorganism, should be empirically treated in pregnancy, because progression to pyelonephritis from both ABU and UTI is more likely.[6] Three days of oral nitrofurantoin 100 mg twice daily or a 3-day course of oral cephalexin 500 mg 4 times daily are among the recommended regimens. Pregnant patients with UTI are commonly treated with oral nitrofurantoin 100 mg twice daily for 7 days; other options include oral amoxicillin/clavulanate or oral cephalosporins. Fluoroquinolones and tetracyclines are contraindicated because of their teratogenic effects on the fetus. Aminoglycosides should also be avoided. Trimethoprim should be used with caution during the first trimester, and sulfonamides should be avoided in the third trimester because of the concern of precipitating kernicterus.

Second, management of acute pyelonephritis is more conservative, because pyelonephritis can induce preterm labor, and also approximately 20% of pregnant women with pyelonephritis develop evidence of sepsis.[69] Admission should be considered in most pregnant patients with pyelonephritis, although outpatient therapy has become accepted in well-hydrated and stable patients when rapid follow-up can be ensured. Ceftriaxone 1 g IV every 24 hours is a standard antimicrobial choice. Aztreonam is an option in a pregnant patient with a severe penicillin or cephalosporin allergy. More extensive information regarding UTI in pregnancy is available in recent reviews.[70,71]

SUMMARY

UTIs are the most common bacterial infections treated in the outpatient setting. These infections can range in severity from minimally symptomatic cystitis to severe septic shock, and affect a wide array of patients. Diagnosis of uncomplicated cystitis can be inferred from history and physical, and confirmed by urinalysis. Only in some circumstances is obtaining a urine culture necessary: complicated UTI, recurrent infections, and in those who have failed empiric treatment. CT or ultrasound imaging is limited to patients with severe or nonresponsive pyelonephritis. Appropriate antimicrobial therapy should rapidly improve symptoms in all UTIs. Antimicrobial selection should be guided by local antibiograms, with caution exercised to minimize growing community antibiotic resistance. EPs should consider a 5-day course of nitrofurantoin in uncomplicated cystitis, and a 7-day fluoroquinolone course in uncomplicated pyelonephritis as first-line regimens. Treatment can then be further tailored according to severity of illness, analysis of individualized risk factors, and antimicrobial resistance patterns.

REFERENCES

1. Foxman B. Epidemiology of urinary tract infections: incidence, morbidity, and economic costs. Am J Med 2002;113(Suppl):5S–13S.
2. Foxman B. Epidemiology of urinary tract infections: incidence, morbidity, and economic costs. Dis Mon 2003;49:53–70.
3. Nawar EW, Niska RW, Xu J. National Hospital Ambulatory Medical Care Survey: 2005 emergency department summary. Adv Data 2007;386:1–32.
4. Fihn SD. Acute uncomplicated urinary tract infection in women. N Engl J Med 2003;349:259–66.
5. Wilson ML, Gaido L. Laboratory diagnosis of urinary tract infections in adult patients. Clin Infect Dis 2004;38:1150–8.
6. Sheffield JS, Cunningham FG. Urinary tract infection in women. Obstet Gynecol 2005;106:1085–92.
7. Gupta K, Hooton TM, Naber KG, et al. International clinical practice guidelines for the treatment of acute uncomplicated cystitis and pyelonephritis in women: a 2010 update by the Infectious Diseases Society of America and the European Society for Microbiology and Infectious Diseases. Clin Infect Dis 2011;52(5): e103–20.
8. David RD, DeBlieux PMC, Press R. Rational antibiotic treatment of outpatient genitourinary infections in a changing environment. Am J Med 2005;118(7A): 7S–13S.
9. Scholes D, Hooton TM, Roberts PL, et al. Risk factors for recurrent urinary tract infection in young women. J Infect Dis 2000;182:1177–82.
10. Nicolle LE, Harding GK, Preiksaitis J, et al. The association of urinary tract infection with sexual intercourse. J Infect Dis 1982;46:574–83.
11. Strom BL, Colins M, West SL, et al. Sexual activity, contraceptive use, and other risk factors for symptomatic and asymptomatic bacteriuria: a case-control study. Ann Intern Med 1987;107:816–23.
12. Krieger JN. Urinary tract infections: what's new? J Urol 2002;168(6):2351–8.
13. Raz R, Chazan B, Dan M. Cranberry juice and urinary tract infection. Clin Infect Dis 2004;38:1413–9.
14. Avorn J, Monane M, Gurwitz JH, et al. Reduction of bacteriuria and pyuria after ingestion of cranberry juice. JAMA 1994;274:751–4.
15. Raz R, Gennesin Y, Wasser J, et al. Recurrent urinary tract infection in postmenopausal women. Clin Infect Dis 2000;30:152–6.
16. Sourander LB. Urinary tract infection in the aged – an epidemiological study. Ann Med Intern Fen Suppl 1966;45:7–55.
17. Brocklehurst JC, Dillane JB, Griffith L, et al. The prevalence and symptomatology of urinary infection in an aged population. Gerontol Clin 1968;10:242–53.
18. Powers JS, Billings FT, Behrendt D, et al. Antecedent factors in urinary tract infections among nursing home patients. Southampt Med J 1988;81:734–5.

19. Boyko EJ, Fihn SD, Scholes D, et al. Diabetes and the risk of acute urinary tract infection among postmenopausal women. Diabetes Care 2002;5:1778–83.
20. Wong ES, Stamm WE. Sexual acquisition of urinary tract infection in a man. JAMA 1983;250(22):3087–8.
21. Ronald A. The etiology of urinary tract infection: traditional and emerging pathogens. Am J Med 2002;113(Suppl 1A):14S–9S.
22. Wong ES, McKevitt M, Running K, et al. Management of recurrent urinary tract infections with patient-administered single dose therapy. Ann Intern Med 1985; 102:302–7.
23. Gupta K, Hooton TM, Roberts PL, et al. Patient-initiated treatment of uncomplicated recurrent urinary tract infections in young women. Ann Intern Med 2001; 135:9–16.
24. Bent S, Nallamothu BK, Simel D, et al. Does this woman have an acute uncomplicated urinary tract infection? JAMA 2002;287:2701–10.
25. Nicolle LE. Uncomplicated urinary tract infection in adults including uncomplicated pyelonephritis. Urol Clin North Am 2008;35:1–12.
26. Ramakrishnan K, Scheid DC. Diagnosis and management of acute pyelonephritis in adults. Am Fam Physician 2005;71(5):933–42.
27. Lifshitz E, Kramer L. Outpatient urine culture: does collection technique matter? Arch Int Med 2000;160:2537–40.
28. Leisure MK, Dudley SM, Donowitz LG. Does a clean-catch urine sample reduce bacterial contamination? N Engl J Med 1993;328:289–90.
29. Immergut MA, Gilbert EC, Frensilli FJ, et al. The myth of the clean catch urine specimen. Urology 1981;17(4):339–40.
30. Mayo S, Acevedo D, Quinonenes-Torrelo C, et al. Clinical laboratory automated urinalysis: comparison among automated microscopy, flow cytometry, two test strips analyzers, and manual microscopic examination of the urine sediments. J Clin Lab Anal 2008;22(4):262–70.
31. Hurlbut TA, Littenberg B. The diagnostic accuracy of rapid dipstick tests to predict urinary tract infection. Am J Clin Pathol 1991;96:582–8.
32. Rehmani R. Accuracy of urine dipstick to predict urinary tract infections in an emergency department. J Ayub Med Coll Abbottabad 2004;16(1):4–7.
33. Pappas PG. Laboratory in the diagnosis and management of urinary tract infections. Med Clin North Am 1991;75:313–25.
34. Stamm W, Counts GW, Running KR, et al. Diagnosis of coliform infection in acutely dysuric women. N Engl J Med 1982;307:463–8.
35. Platt R. Quantitative definition of bacteriuria. Am J Med 1983;75(1B):44–52.
36. Sandler CM, Choyke PL, Bluth E, et al. Expert panel on urologic imaging. Acute pyelonephritis. Reston (VA): American College of Radiology (ACR); 2005. p. 1–5.
37. Papanicolaou N, Pfister RC. Acute renal infections. Radiol Clin North Am 1996;34: 965–95.
38. Warren JW, Abrutyn E, Hebel JR, et al. Guidelines for antimicrobial treatment of uncomplicated acute bacterial cystitis and acute pyelonephritis in women. Clin Infect Dis 1999;29:74.
39. Hooton TM, Besser R, Foxman B, et al. Acute uncomplicated cystitis in an era of increasing antibiotic resistance: a proposed approach to empirical therapy. Clin Infect Dis 2004;39:75–80.
40. Taur Y, Smith M. Adherence to the Infectious Diseases Society of America guidelines in the treatment of uncomplicated urinary tract infection. Clin Infect Dis 2007;44:769–74.

41. Gupta K, Hooton TM, Roberts PL, et al. Short-course nitrofurantoin for the treatment of acute uncomplicated cystitis in women. Arch Intern Med 2007;167(20):2207–12.
42. Iravani A, Klimberg I, Briefer C, et al. A trial comparing low-dose, short-course ciprofloxacin and standard 7 day therapy with co-trimoxazole or nitrofurantoin in the treatment of uncomplicated urinary tract infection. J Antimicrob Chemother 1999; 43(Suppl A):67–75.
43. Stein GE. Comparison of single-dose fosfomycin and a 7 day course of nitrofurantoin in female patients with uncomplicated urinary tract infection. Clin Ther 1999;21(11):1864–72.
44. Arredondo-Garcia JL, Figueroa-Damian R, Rosas A, et al. Comparison of short-term treatment regimen of ciprofloxacin versus long-term treatment regimens of trimethoprim/sulfamethoxazole or norfloxacin for uncomplicated lower urinary tract infections: a randomized, multicentre, open-label, prospective study. J Antimicrob Chemother 2004;54(4):840–3.
45. Warren JW, et al. Guidelines for antimicrobial treatment of uncomplicated acute bacterial cystitis and acute pyelonephritis in women. Infectious Diseases Society of America. Clin Infect Dis 1999;29:745–58.
46. Fourcroy JL, et al. Efficacy and safety of a novel once-daily extended-release ciprofloxacin tablet formulation for treatment of uncomplicated urinary tract infection in women. Antimicrob Agents Chemother 2005;49(10):4137–43.
47. Henry DC, et al. Comparison of once-daily extended-release ciprofloxacin and conventional twice-daily ciprofloxacin for the treatment of uncomplicated urinary tract infection in women. Clin Ther 2002;24(12):2088–104.
48. Minassian MA, et al. A comparison between single-dose fosfomycin trometamol and a 5-day course of trimethoprim in the treatment of uncomplicated lower urinary tract infection in women. Int J Antimicrob Agents 1998;10(1):39–47.
49. Popovic M, et al. Fosfomycin: an old, new friend? Eur J Clin Microbiol Infect Dis 2010;29(2):127–42.
50. Hooton TM, Scholes D, Gupta K, et al. Amoxicillin-clavulanate vs ciprofloxacin for the treatment of uncomplicated cystitis in women: a randomized trial. JAMA 2005; 293(8):949–55.
51. Kavatha D, Giamerellou H, Alexiou Z, et al. Cefpodoxime-proxetil versus trimethoprim-sulfamethoxazole for short-term therapy of uncomplicated acute cystitis in women. Antimicrob Agents Chemother 2003;47(3):897–900.
52. Lipsky BA. Prostatitis and urinary tract infection in men: what's new; what's true? Am J Med 1999;106:327–34.
53. Hooton TM. The current management strategies for community-acquired urinary tract infection. Infect Dis Clin North Am 2003;17:303–32.
54. Krieger JN, Ross S, Simonsen J. Urinary tract infections in healthy university men. J Urol 1993;149(5):1045–8.
55. Lipsky B. Urinary tract infection in men. Epidemiology, pathophysiology, diagnosis and treatment. Ann Intern Med 1989;110(2):138–50.
56. Sharp VJ, Takacs EB. Prostatitis: diagnosis and treatment. Am Fam Physician 2010;82(4):397–406.
57. Lipsky BA, Byren I, Hoey CT. Treatment of bacterial prostatitis. Clin Infect Dis 2010;50(12):1641–52.
58. Talan DA, Krishnadasan A, Abrahamian FM, et al. Prevalence and risk factor analysis of trimethoprim-sulfamethoxazole and fluoroquinolone-resistant *Escherichia coli* infection among emergency department patients with pyelonephritis. Clin Infect Dis 2008;47:1150–8.

59. Lautenbach E. Finding the path of least antimicrobial resistance in pyelonephritis. Clin Infect Dis 2008;47:1159–61.
60. Czaja CA, Scholes D, Hooton TM, et al. Population-based epidemiologic analysis of acute pyelonephritis. Clin Infect Dis 2007;45(3):273–80.
61. Halliday A, Jawetz E. Sodium nitrofurantoin administered intravenously. A limited study to define its clinical indication. N Engl J Med 1962;266:427–32.
62. Jawetz E, Hopper J, Smith D. Nitrofurantoin in chronic urinary tract infection. AMA Arch Intern Med 1957;100(4):549–57.
63. Stamm WE, McKevitt M, Counts GW. Acute renal infection in women: treatment with trimethoprim-sulfamethoxazole or ampicillin for two or six weeks: a randomized trial. Ann Intern Med 1987;106:341–5.
64. Schrock J, Reznikova S, Weller S. The effect of an observation unit on the rate of ED admission and discharge for pyelonephritis. Am J Emerg Med 2010;28:682–8.
65. Velasco M, Martinez JA, Moreno-Martinez A, et al. Blood cultures for women with uncomplicated acute pyelonephritis: are they necessary? Clin Infect Dis 2003;37:1127–30.
66. Dembry LM. Renal and perirenal abscesses. Curr Treat Options Infect Dis 2002;4:21–30.
67. Huang JJ, Tseng CC. Emphysematous pyelonephritis: clinicoradiological classification, management, prognosis, and pathogenesis. Arch Intern Med 2000;160(6):797–805.
68. Wan YL, Lo SK, Bullard MJ, et al. Predictors of outcome in emphysematous pyelonephritis. J Urol 1998;159(2):369–73.
69. Hill JB, Sheffield JS, McIntire DD, et al. Acute pyelonephritis in pregnancy. Obstet Gyn 2005;105:18–23.
70. Macejko AM, Schaeffer AJ. Asymptomatic bacteriuria and symptomatic urinary tract infections during pregnancy. Urol Clin North Am 2007;34(1):35–42.
71. Gilstrap LC 3rd, Ramin SM. Urinary tract infections during pregnancy. Obstet Gynecol Clin North Am 2001;28(3):581–90.

Genitourinary Imaging in the Emergency Department

Michael S. Antonis, DO, RDMS[a,b,*], Carolyn A. Phillips, MD, RDMS[b], Michael Blaivas, MD, RDMS[c]

KEYWORDS

• Emergency • Ultrasound • Imaging • Genitourinary

An emergency medical (EM) specialist has a vast array of imaging modalities available to decipher various genitourinary (GU) complaints commonly seen in the emergency department (ED) setting. The widespread availability and rapidly achievable results of CT scan imaging has lead to the virtual disappearance of intravenous pyelography (IVP). In addition, MRI and ultrasonography (US) continue to significantly increase their share of the diagnostic imaging performed in the ED. The use of plain radiographs, such as the kidney-ureter-bladder (KUB) film, continues to be used in various clinical settings. In addition, nuclear medicine imaging has a role in GU imaging in select circumstances. However, the use of point-of-care US by the EM specialist has changed the landscape of ED diagnostic imaging in many ways. This article reviews the various diagnostic imaging modalities in the twenty-first century clinician's armamentarium for assessing GU complaints. In addition, the emergence of point-of-care US examinations by the EM specialist is discussed as a technology that continues to provide essential and timely information.[1]

CUMULATIVE RADIATION EXPOSURE

In recent years, concerns regarding the harmful and additive effects of radiation doses and associated cancer risks to our patients have lead to an increased awareness by

---

The authors have nothing to disclose.

[a] Georgetown University School of Medicine, MedStar Health: Georgetown University Hospital, 3800 Reservoir Road, Washington, DC 20007-2113, USA
[b] Department of Emergency Medicine, MedStar Health: Washington Hospital Center, 110 Irving Street, NW, Washington, DC 20010, USA
[c] Department of Emergency Medicine, Northside Hospital Forsyth, 1200 Northside Forsyth Drive, Cumming, GA 30041, USA
* Corresponding author. Department of Emergency Medicine, MedStar Health: Washington Hospital Center, 110 Irving Street, NW, Washington, DC 20010.
E-mail address: michael.s.antonis@medstar.net

Emerg Med Clin N Am 29 (2011) 553–567
doi:10.1016/j.emc.2011.04.010 emed.theclinics.com

the medical community and the public at large. A few of the proposed and implemented solutions include CT scan software upgrades that decrease radiation exposure and allow for postprocessing three-dimensional (3-D) image reconstruction, as well as tracking of longitudinal lifetime radiation exposure for patients (**Table 1**).

The main disadvantage of CT scans is the more recent recognition of the cumulative lifetime risks associated with ionizing radiation exposure. The *New England Journal of Medicine* reported that among nearly one-million adults aged 18 to 64 observed during a 3-year study period, 68.8% underwent at least one imaging procedure. CT scans and nuclear medicine imaging accounted for 75% of the cumulative radiation dose due to diagnostic testing, and 82% of imaging studies were performed in the outpatient setting. A pelvic CT scan consists of 6 mSv of radiation exposure, compared with 0.02 mSv with chest radiography.[2] Another consideration is that a single radiograph emits ionizing radiation from one direction, as compared with the 360-degree helical orientation of CT scan imaging. Another recent study demonstrated that CT scanning has increased threefold since 1993, with an estimated 29,000 future malignancies related to CT scan imaging performed in the United States in 2007.[3] In this study, the largest contribution (approximately 14,000 malignancies) was attributed to CT scans of the abdomen and pelvis. Studies done on survivors of the Japanese atomic bomb during World War II have been used to extrapolate an increase risk of cancer. The risk of solid malignant tumors has a direct linear relationship to radiation dose.[4] There is much debate regarding the extrapolation of a single large dose (atomic bomb) versus a lifetime cumulative exposure of lower dose radiation, but most investigators are in agreement that clinical judgment and risk-benefit to the patient must be considered when choosing an imaging modality[5,6] Another consideration is that children are much more radiosensitive than adults with a precipitous decline in radiosensitivity with age for most malignancies.[5]

KUB RADIOGRAPHY

The KUB, in conjunction with an IVP, was once the diagnostic test of choice for suspected urinary obstruction. The KUB is a cheap, quick, noninvasive test with relatively low ionizing radiation, but is both insensitive and nonspecific. A plain KUB radiograph has essentially been replaced with the advancement and widespread availability of CT scan imaging. Subtle, nonsensitive, nonspecific findings that can be seen on a KUB include scoliosis of the spine from muscle spasm due to an inflammatory process, calculi, and ileus pattern secondary to retroperitoneal injury or inflammation.

Table 1
Average effective radiation dose from common medical imaging procedures

Type of Examination	Average Effective Dose (mSv)
Posteroanterior chest radiograph	0.02
KUB radiograph	0.7
CT scan of the brain	2
Intravenous urography	3
Adult abdominal CT scan	8
Adult pelvic CT scan	6
CT scan angiogram of chest	15

Data from Mettler FA, Huda W, Yoshizumi TT, et al. Effective doses in radiology and diagnostic nuclear medicine. Radiology 2008;248:254–3.

The KUB currently is making a comeback as a scout film in the management of patients treated conservatively for renal stone disease in conjunction with point-of-care US (**Fig. 1**). Clinicians use the KUB to rule out a large midureteral stone and the bedside US to ensure the absence of hydronephrosis from an obstructing calculus.[7]

Retrograde Urethrography and Retrograde Cystography

The hard physical indications to perform a retrograde urethrogram (RUG) in the trauma setting include: (1) blood at meatus, (2) nonpalpable, high-riding prostate, and (3) urethral trauma (**Fig. 2**).

The RUG is an anatomic rather than a physiologic examination, but is critical in the identification of a possible urethral injury before a urinary catheter insertion to preclude a potentially devastating complication.[8] The complications of a missed urethral tear include stricture, incontinence, infection, and impotence (**Fig. 3**).

A RUG should ideally be performed under fluoroscopy to provide real-time imaging, but plain films are an acceptable alternative. A RUG can be performed in the trauma bay by slowly injecting 10 to 15 cc of iodinated radiographic-contrast material into the proximal urethra. Multiple views (oblique, anterior-posterior, lateral) should be obtained to carefully examine the posterior portion of the urethra on males. If no contrast leak is demonstrated, then a urinary catheter can be advanced to the bladder and a retrograde cystogram may be performed. An additional 100 mL of contrast is infused via gravity into the Foley with the addition of anterior-posterior and lateral radiographs. If there is still no contrast extravasation, then an additional 400 cc of contrast material may be infused. With the urinary catheter clamped, additional radiographs, including an oblique view, can be obtained. Finally, an after void radiograph can be obtained after the clamp is released.

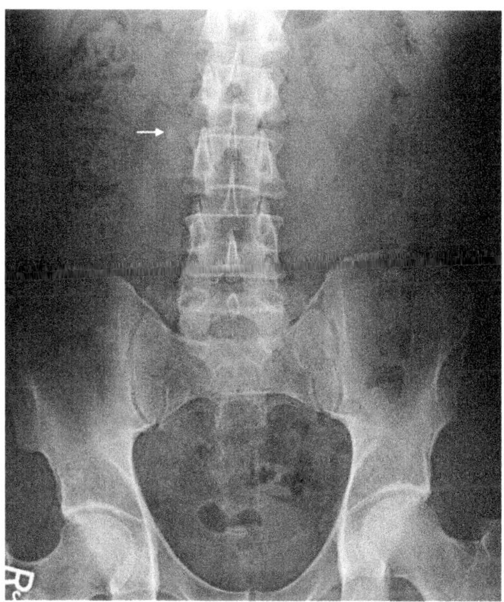

Fig. 1. KUB demonstrating an 8 mm calculus in the lower pole of the right kidney (*arrow*). (*Courtesy of* MedStar Health, Washington, DC; with permission.)

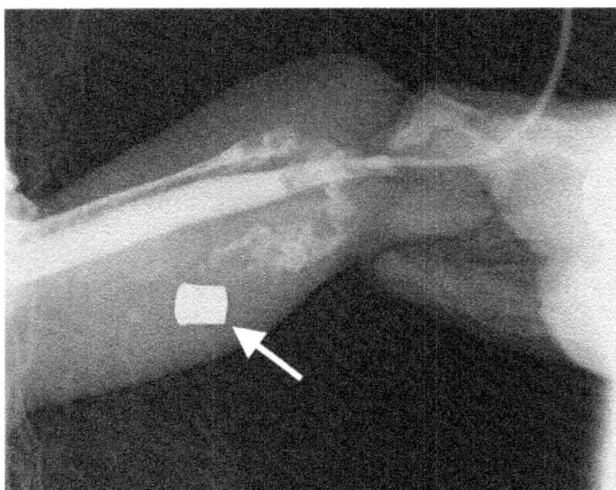

Fig. 2. RUG demonstrating extensive extravasation of contrast from the urethra related to gunshot injury with retained bullet (*arrow*). (*Courtesy of* MedStar Health, Washington, DC; with permission.)

Intravenous Pyelogram

At one time, an IVP (or excretory urogram) was considered the gold standard for the visualization of the entire urinary tract. The advantage of this imaging modality includes the fact that it provides simultaneous functional and anatomic evaluations of the urogenital tract. Disadvantages of the IVP include: (1) potential for subcutaneous contrast extravasation at the injection site, (2) iodinated contrast material reaction or allergy, which is a relative contraindication, (3) comparatively long duration of examination (ideally films are obtained at 1, 5, 15, and 30 minute intervals following the contrast administration and initial imaging), and (4) nephrotoxicity of the contrast agent.

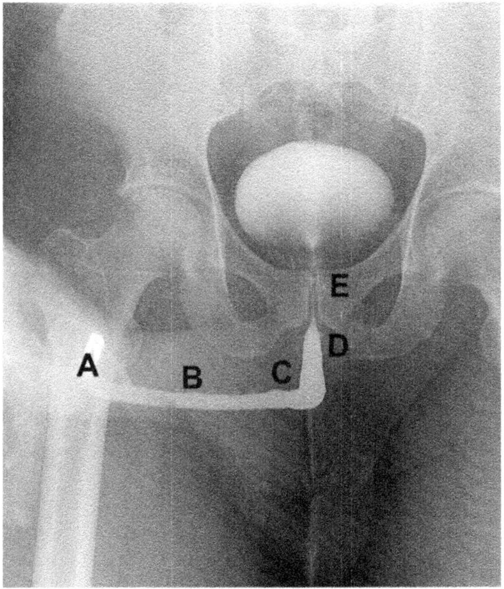

Fig. 3. Normal retrograde urethrogram. Anatomy of the male urethra. (A) Fossa navicularis, (B) pendulous urethra, (C) bulbous urethra, (D) membranous urethra, and (E) prostatic urethra. (*Courtesy of* MedStar Health, Washington, DC; with permission.)

CT Scan

CT scan imaging has become the gold standard for evaluation of the GU track due to the relatively simple and rapid acquisition of high-quality images, often without the need for iodinated contrast administration. Indications for CT scan imaging of the GU track include known or suspected nephrolithiasis, urinary obstruction, pyelonephritis, renal abscess, other infection, or traumatic injury (**Figs. 4** and **5**). CT scans also allow direct visualization of stones, including those radiolucent on KUB. Multiple investigations demonstrate specificities nearing 100% and sensitivities of 96% to 98% with CT scan imaging.[9–12]

One of the biggest advantages of CT scans over other imaging modalities in the evaluation of flank pain is the concurrent assessment for other conditions that may mimic renal colic. Unexpected findings on a nonenhanced abdominal-pelvic CT scan can include ovarian pathology, pelvic inflammatory disease or tuboovarian abscess, appendicitis, abdominal aortic aneurysm, and diverticulitis.

MRI

The use of MRI in the ED has traditionally been reserved for evaluation of neurologic or neurosurgical emergencies. MRI does, however, offer excellent spatial resolution with multiplanar imaging particularly of the soft tissues of the GU tract. Other benefits of this modality include the lack of ionizing radiation, no need for iodinated contrast material, as well as no delays associated with oral preparation of contrast before imaging.

Potential uses of GU MRI outside of the ED include imaging of the nonpregnant female pelvis for issues such as suspected fibroids or other tumors. In the ED, MRI can be useful in the evaluation of abdominal pain in pregnant females, or any patient where radiation or iodinated contrast is contraindicated or undesired and US is nondiagnostic or otherwise not feasible.[13] In the pelvis specifically, MRI does not have much respiratory degradation, which is often an issue in areas such as the thorax because of significant increases in image acquisition time. Other uses of MRI in the GU tract include evaluation for adnexal torsion in females (**Fig. 6**). MRI is more accurate than CT scans in diagnosing torsion owing to its multiplanar imaging capability and increased soft tissue resolution.[14] Despite this, US should typically be the initial diagnostic test of choice due to its ability to rapidly visualize the adnexal structures. The use of MRI for the diagnosis of testicular torsion has been explored, but limitations include speed of imaging and availability.[15,16]

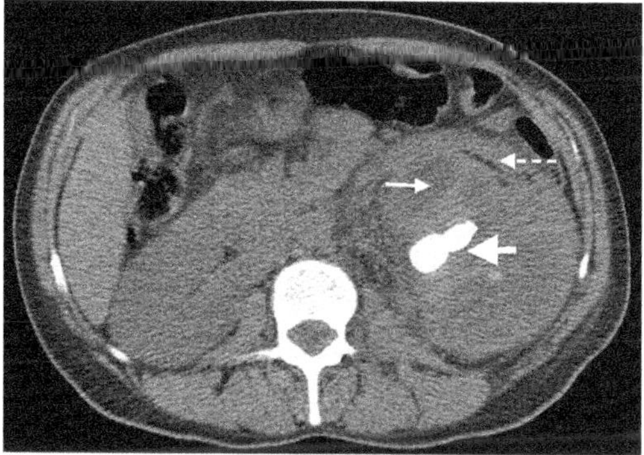

Fig. 4. CT scan image demonstrating an abscess (*small solid arrow*) with surrounding air (*dashed arrow*) with staghorn calculus in the left kidney (*large solid arrow*). (*Courtesy of* MedStar Health, Washington, DC; with permission.)

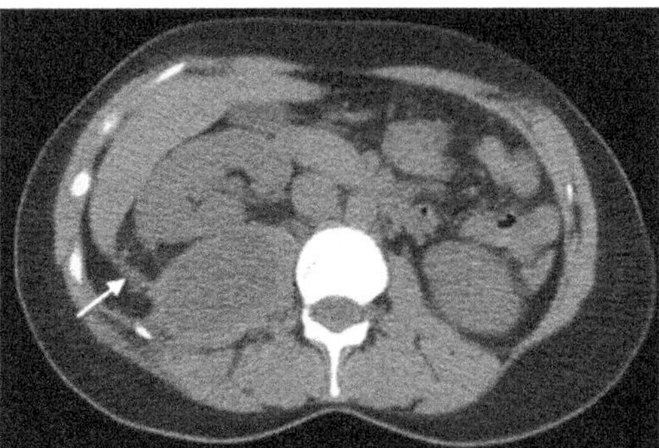

Fig. 5. Noncontrast CT scan demonstrating a right renal abscess and perinephric stranding (*arrow*) in the surrounding perirenal adipose tissue. (*Courtesy of* MedStar Health, Washington, DC; with permission.)

Availability of MRI is a major disadvantage of its use in the ED because of cost of purchase, maintenance, and upkeep of the machines. Also, the MRIs are often located in an area remote from the ED and, because the tests take significantly longer than other imaging modalities, the physician has limited ability to monitor the patient during the examination. Finally, MRI requires the use of a very high-powered electromagnetic field, so patients with metal foreign bodies, including certain pacemakers and defibrillators, are unable to go into the machine without risk of injury to the patient or damage to the magnet. MRI is a very expensive test to have performed and stretches the resources of the department and quite possibility the hospital. MRI has very limited benefit to the ED, and may result in substantial delays in diagnosis of certain emergent conditions.

Nuclear Medicine

The use of nuclear medicine in emergency practice is limited owing to the long duration required for the examinations, and the extended period the patient remains outside the ED. One of the benefits of nuclear medicine testing is that it provides an assessment of function of imaged tissues, including renal function or urinary flow rates, in cases of urinary obstruction. These studies have limited utility on a routine emergency basis.[17]

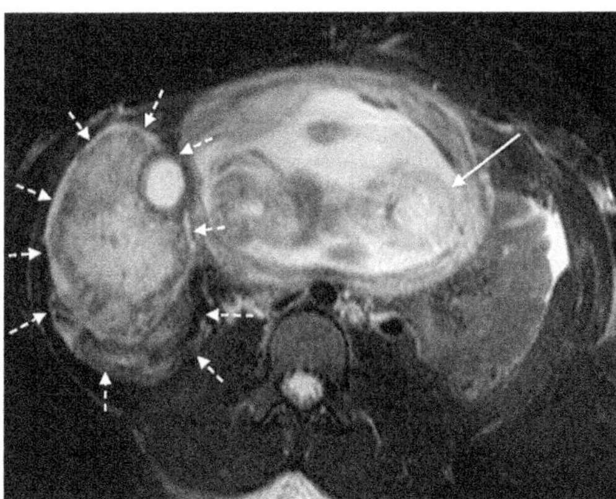

Fig. 6. MRI (T2 series) of pelvis showing a fetus in the uterus (*solid arrow*), and a swollen, ischemic, torsed right ovary (*dotted arrows*). (*Courtesy of* MedStar Health, Washington, DC; with permission.)

For testicular viability, a nuclear scan can assess intratesticular blood flow. Radionuclide scintigraphy and color Doppler US show similar sensitivity, as well as false negative rates, for the diagnosis of testicular torsion.[18] However, due its generally more rapid availability and the ability to perform imaging at the bedside, US remains the gold standard in this evaluation. Similar to MRI, nuclear medicine studies should not prohibitively delay definitive management of potentially emergent conditions.

US: GENERAL PRINCIPLES

The general principles of US allow for a noninvasive examination that provides excellent anatomic detail without ionizing radiation or the need for contrast administration. The US examination requires both cognitive and psychomotor skills that demand extensive training and experience to gain proficiency. US can yield answers to specific clinical questions in organs and structures that are naturally echogenic. US does have limits in regards to patient habitus, location of organ of interest in proximity to air, certain disease states, and operator experience.

The standard US imaging mode used is brightness mode, which converts returning echo signals into a two-dimensional (2-D) grayscale image that appears on the sonogram screen. Doppler mode relies upon "frequency shift" technology that exists with red blood cell movement in a vessel or structure of interest. Spectral Doppler allows a quantitative assessment of blood flow within a specific region of interest. Color Doppler is superimposed on the 2-D image and provides information regarding blood flow directionality and mean velocity of flow. Power Doppler provides improved sensitivity regarding amplitude of motion, but no directionality. Power Doppler is often used specifically in low blood-flow states, such as ovarian or testicular torsion.[19]

The standard of care regarding emergency physician point-of-care US has yet to be fully defined. However, the standard of care typically evolves from the educational objectives and competency requirements of residency training programs. The American College of Emergency Physicians (ACEP) published revised guidelines in 2008 supported by the Society of Academic Emergency Medicine.[20] The guidelines listed 11 core applications of emergency US that include trauma, intrauterine pregnancy, abdominal aortic aneurysm (AAA), cardiac, biliary, urinary tract, deep vein thrombosis, soft-tissue or musculoskeletal, thoracic, ocular, and procedural guidance with new applications including testicular, bowel pathology, and contrast studies.

In 2008, The Council of Residency Directors in Emergency Medicine (CORD) commissioned an Emergency Ultrasound Consensus Committee (EUCC) to establish a standardized minimum US education curriculum for EM residencies.[21] CORD, in conjunction with the Accreditation Council for Graduate Medical Education, further stated that graduating EM residents must demonstrate competency in point-of-care US.

The EUCC's recommendations further specify that residency programs should include training in at least the following core applications: abdominal aorta, cardiac, focused assessment with sonography in trauma (FAST), intrauterine pregnancy (both transabdominal and endocavity scans), and procedural guidance. These five applications were selected due to their crucial role in life-threatening situations. Training in the remaining six core applications is also highly recommended. The requirements of EM residency training are an obvious starting point for accepted standards of practice.

Renal US

US provides excellent anatomic detail without iodinated contrast agents, but historically provided a limited assessment of renal function. The newest generation of US machines allow for the detection of urine entering the bladder as an indirect marker of renal function. Each anatomically normal kidney has an echogenic capsule with surrounding perinephric fat, and a bright, echo-dense central collecting system. Renal US translates easily to the bedside with the ability to use a split screen to compare both kidneys and view the bladder (**Figs. 7** and **8**). The "beans and bladder" view allow detection of the obstruction above or below the level of the bladder in the GU system.

The bedside US has a very limited role for the primary identification of ureteral stones in the middle-third of the ureter. A secondary sign of GU obstruction includes visualization of a large homogenous anechoic area in the collecting system that suggests hydronephrosis or hydroureter (**Fig. 9**). Unilateral renal enlargement may also indicate acute infection, renal vein thrombosis, transplant rejection, or renal abscess.

The reported sensitivity for detection by US ranges from 37% to 64% for urinary calculi, and from 74% to 85% for acute obstruction of the GU tract. These sensitivities can be improved if hydronephrosis or hydroureter are present as secondary signs of obstruction.[7] The sonographic detection of the actual calculi is dependent upon resolution, frequency of the probe used, patient habitus, hydration status, and sonologist experience.

Evaluation of complete (distal) urinary obstruction can be accomplished with US by measurement of ureteral jets (**Fig. 10**). The ureters enter the bladder on both sides, and typically exhibit 1 to 12 antegrade urinary jets per minute on both sides. The detection of ureteral jets essentially excludes the possibility of a total obstruction.[7] The ureteral jets are visualized due to the difference in specific gravity of the urine currently in the bladder and the urine entering from the ureter.

A key role of point-of-care US is to rule out potentially lethal conditions in patients with abdominal or flank pain, such as a leaking or ruptured AAA. With the high morbidity and mortality associated with AAA, US may provide immediate bedside confirmation of its absence if a normal caliber aorta is visualized throughout its length.

Special populations of patients requiring renal US include kidney transplant recipients and pregnant patients with acute flank or abdominal pain. The patient with a transplanted kidney requires a formal evaluation with Doppler examination and measurements of kidney size and arterial and venous flow velocities, which is well beyond the scope of point-of-care ED sonography. The physiologic changes of pregnancy including renal tract dilatation, urinary stasis, hypercalcinuria, and an enlarged uterus may intuitively lead to more symptomatic nephrolithiasis; but, actually, inhibitors of stone formation including magnesium, citrate, and nephrocalcin may assist in the prevention of kidney stone formation.[7] Multiparous women are more affected than

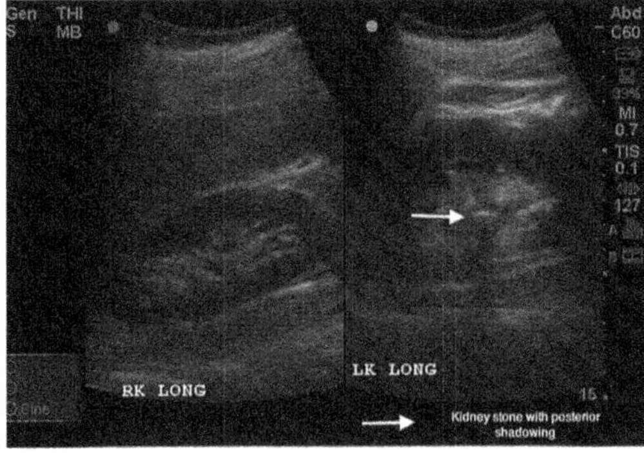

Fig. 7. Split-screen US of right kidney (RK) and left kidney (LK) demonstrating a nonobstructing kidney stone (*arrow*) within the left kidney. (*Courtesy of* MedStar Health, Washington, DC; with permission.)

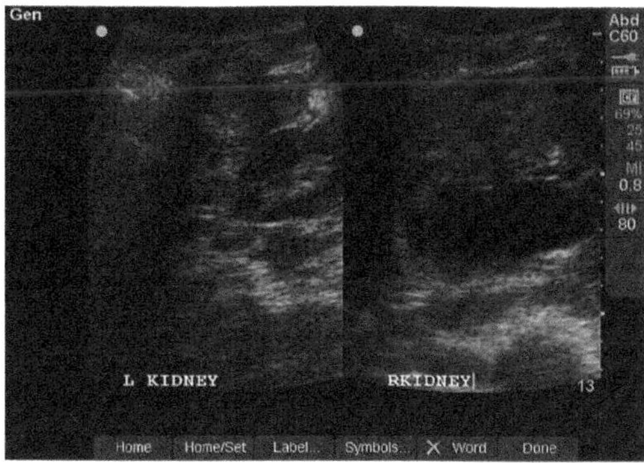

Fig. 8. Split-screen US demonstrating a normal left (L) kidney (left) and a right (R) kidney with severe hydronephrosis with only a small rim of cortex remaining (right). (*Courtesy of* MedStar Health, Washington, DC; with permission.)

primagravida women, with both sides affected with equal frequency even in the second or third trimester. A combination of sound clinical judgment and skilled US assessment can go a long way in sorting through challenging cases in the setting of flank or abdominal pain in pregnancy. Another option may be magnetic resonance urography (MRU), which allows physiologic obstruction that is typical of later-term pregnancy to be distinguished from pathologic obstruction of the ureter.

Scrotal US

Two conditions are of paramount importance to the EM specialist that may clinically present in a similar fashion, yet have significantly different outcomes. Epididymitis (or epididymo-orchitis) and testicular torsion can both cause severe pain, but testicular torsion is a time-dependent diagnosis. Indeed, testicular salvage rates are time sensitive.[22] The blood flow is decreased in torsion (**Fig. 11**), whereas hyperemia results with epididymitis. However, a significant pitfall in this oversimplified approach is a recently detorsed testicle may appear hyperemic. In the authors' experience, a distinct advantage of an emergency sonologist's examination allows for a repeat examination following analgesia and a brief period of observation. A comparison with contralateral

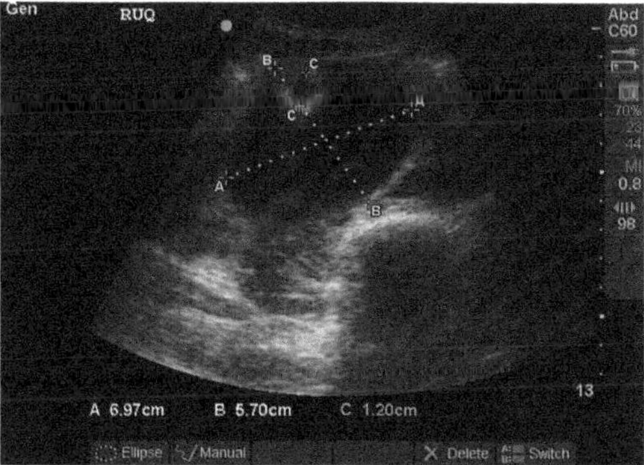

Fig. 9. Right ureter demonstrating severe hydroureter. Caliper measurements (A, B) demonstrate a dilated ureter (7 cm by 5.7 cm). An intraluminal ureteral stent is also seen and measured with the calipers (C). (*Courtesy of* MedStar Health, Washington, DC; with permission.)

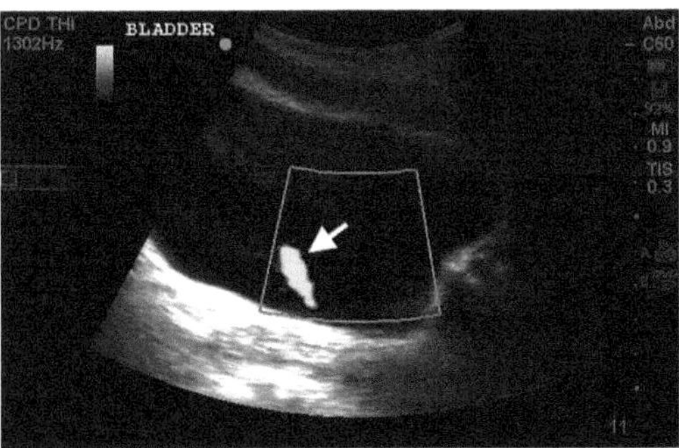

Fig. 10. Ultrasound of bladder with color power Doppler demonstrating a urinary jet (*arrow*). (*Courtesy of* MedStar Health, Washington, DC; with permission.)

testicular blood flow may provide additional supportive diagnostic information with serial point-of-care US examinations.

US remains the bedside diagnostic test of choice for acute scrotal pathology.[23] US has the advantage of better anatomic definition of the scrotal contents. In addition, it may assist in identifying alternate pathologic states, including appendage torsion, incarcerated inguinal hernia, hydrocele, or even Fournier gangrene, which typically presents with air in the perineal soft tissues.[24] The testicular US examination includes grayscale, power Doppler, and spectral Doppler components to assess arterial and venous flow. A high-frequency transducer with power Doppler capability for low-flow states allows for an extremely high degree of accuracy in diagnosing testicular torsion, which carries a large morbidity and professional liability for a failure to diagnose.[25] Emergency physicians with a point-of-care US have shown a 95% sensitivity and 94% specificity in the differentiation of emergent surgical versus other acute scrotal pain causes.[26] The ability of bedside US to diagnose the pathogenesis of acute scrotal pain is unsurpassed by any other imaging modality. Testicular US does have limitations with studies demonstrating a negative predictive value approaching 97%.[27] Surgical exploration remains the only definitive diagnostic modality in assessing for testicular torsion. The EM practitioner must weigh the options of a negative US examination in the setting of a suggestive story versus unnecessary surgery for the patient. An emergent surgical consultation may be prudent in evaluating a patient with an acutely painful scrotum.

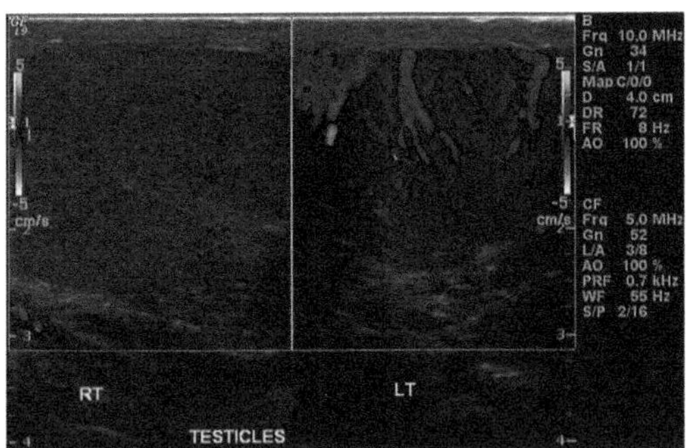

Fig. 11. Testicular US: split-screen, right and left testicular ultrasound demonstrating flow to the left testicle (LT) and absence of flow to the torsed right testicle (RT). (*Courtesy of* MedStar Health, Washington, DC; with permission.)

Ovarian US

US is the definitive imaging modality of choice for pathologic conditions within the ovaries in pregnant and nonpregnant females alike. An ovarian torsion can be partial or complete, acute or chronic, and often intermittent with spontaneous resolution with the diagnosis also hindered by vague complaints. This is further complicated by the fact the ovary more commonly than not has dual arterial supply via the ovarian artery and a branch of the uterine artery. The early diagnosis and resulting surgical intervention of an infarcting ovary allows preservation of the ovary and may serve to avert the potentially life-threatening complications of peritonitis.

Most cases of ovarian torsion are associated with adnexal pathology such as ovarian tumors or cysts. A nonneoplastic ovarian cyst can be found frequently in nonpregnant females. In addition, it may be found commonly in the first trimester or immediately postpartum, as well as with ovarian stimulating agents.[28] The pathology of an ovarian torsion causes initial compromise of the lymphatic and venous system resulting in edema and adnexal enlargement (**Fig. 12**). Until venous or arterial thrombus occurs, reperfusion of the ovary allows reversal of ovarian ischemia. Lack of arterial and venous Doppler flow should enable a confident diagnosis, but false positives do occur, including operator error in setting Doppler flow filters and pelvic depths beyond the penetrating capabilities of the US equipment.[29]

Multiple studies support the use of Doppler examination of ovaries for torsion with a positive predictive value of 94% in the absence of venous flow.[29] The most common grayscale characteristic of torsion is an enlarged ovary or ovarian complex with surrounding fluid. A retrospective study of 60 adolescent and pediatric patients who underwent surgical management for presumed ovarian torsion showed that the findings associated with a high predictive value of torsion included an adnexal mass greater than 5 cm in diameter; patients with this finding were nine times more likely to have torsion.[30] The average size of the adnexal mass in confirmed torsion cases was 8.4 cm compared with 4.4 cm for the group with no operative evidence of torsion. There was a statistically significant association between cyst size and torsion. Pelvic fluid was seen in 64% of all patients with torsion. Interestingly, the presence of arterial and venous flow as determined by color Doppler was noted in 60% of confirmed torsion cases.[30] Ovarian torsion is among the most challenging diagnoses to predict preoperatively in patients with acute pelvic pain. The difficulties result in delays in surgical exploration and a resultant

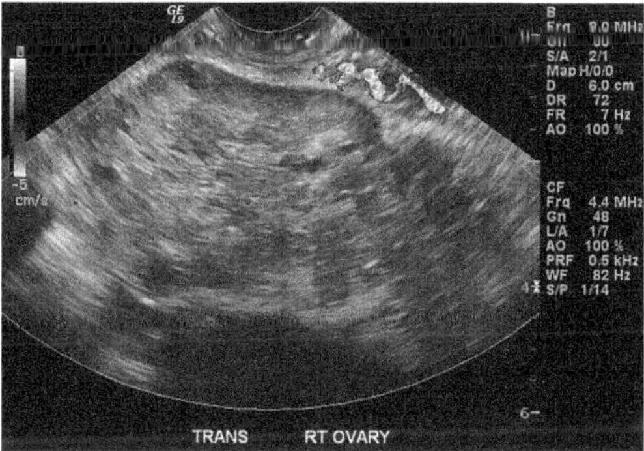

Fig. 12. Pelvic US. Transverse view of right (RT) ovary demonstrating edema surrounding the ovary and lack of color Doppler flow beyond the ovarian pedicle. (*Courtesy of* MedStar Health, Washington, DC; with permission.)

salvage rate of less than 20%.[31] Low yields of the US examination as well as low ovarian salvage rates underscore the importance of serial examinations.

Pediatric US

The point-of-care US usage in the pediatric population has been slow in acceptance, but the transition from adult to pediatric indications and procedures should be intuitive for the EM specialist. The simplest examination that may provide immediate positive feedback from a concerned parent is the use of US to assess bladder volume before urinary catheterization in the febrile infant. Nurses with minimal US training have proven the ability to determine bladder volumes maximizing the chances of successful catheterization without physician involvement.[32] US has many advantages compatible with pediatrics, including noninvasive interrogation, no sedation, no contrast, and, perhaps most importantly, no ionizing radiation. The disadvantages of US in the pediatric setting include, as with adults, the fact that quality is highly operator-dependent and physiology must be inferred from the anatomy. In addition, a complete understanding of developmental anatomy and disease conditions unique to the pediatric population is essential.[8]

US: FUTURE DIRECTIONS

The 2-D US has several disadvantages in comparison to helical imaging techniques including volume calculations based upon estimates and the existence of high inter- and intra-observer variability that severely limits standardization and comparison on follow-up studies. The newer generation live 3-D US has the distinct advantages of improved volume assessment accuracy, improved comprehensive visualization of complex anatomy, and superior standardization at a lower interobserver variability.[33] 3-D GU imaging allows measurement of a volume in many arbitrary planes including the three classical planes (coronal, sagittal, transverse). This capability reduces imaging time, demonstrates complex vasculature, and provides accurate volume assessment for comparison with other imaging modalities.[34] The ability to acquire a complete data map can result in multiple 3-D reconstructions at a computer workstation without the presence of the patient. The rapid dissemination of US technology and proficiency will continue to promote US as the imaging modality of choice in the GU system.

US requires two distinct skill sets for use in the ED. The cognitive component consists of the proper indications for a point-of-care US and the interpretation of the acquired images. The second skill is the psychomotor component of placing the probe on the patient to acquire the appropriate images for interpretation. The paradigm shift of the medical community to clinician-performed point-of-care US has been well documented in the medical literature showing benefit for the indications of trauma, guided procedures, cardiac, abdominal, and pregnancy.[21] Current technology allows contemporaneous image acquisition with a portable US machine by the sonologist. The ability to record and document the obtained images in the electronic medical record in real time has further advanced point-of-care US in the ED setting.

The increasing emphasis on patient safety, quality care, efficiency, less invasive treatment, and nonionizing imaging has allowed further proliferation of US into the realm of the EM specialist. ACEP and CORD each have position statements regarding guidelines for emergency physicians.[20,21] ACEP policy in regards to point-of-care US states "bedside ultrasound evaluation, including examination, interpretation, and equipment, should be immediately available 24 hours a day for emergency patients" and further states, "emergency ultrasound procedures are standard emergency physician skills."[20]

A consideration with the emergence of ED point-of-care US is medical liability for failure to use US when indicated in emergent patient care. A recent review, which searched a comprehensive legal database, demonstrated three documented cases against emergency physicians: one was successfully defended, another was judged for the plaintiff, and a third is pending resolution[35] (with unpublished data from Michael Blaivas, MD, Atlanta, Georgia, 2010). All of these cases resulted in litigation against the ED physician for failure to perform a point-of-care US in a time-sensitive emergent diagnosis, underscoring the role of point-of-care US in modern ED care.[36,37]

SUMMARY

The EM specialist has many imaging options for the evaluation of GU complaints. The advancement in imaging technology has added layers of complexity to the decision-making process. The clinician must weigh the advantages and disadvantages of each imaging modality in the context of hospital resources and capabilities to ensure patient safety and minimize delays in diagnosis. The advent of ED point-of-care US provides a technological advantage to differentiate among many commonly encountered GU conditions.

REFERENCES

1. Moore CL, Copel JA. Point-of-care ultrasonography. N Engl J Med 2011;364: 749–57.
2. Fazel R, Krumholz HM, Wang Y, et al. Exposure to low-dose ionizing radiation from medical imaging procedures. N Engl J Med 2009;361:849–57.
3. Berrington de Gonzalez A, Mahesh M, Kim KP, et al. Projected cancer risks from computed tomographic scans performed in the United States in 2007. Arch Intern Med 2009;169:2071–7.
4. Preston DL, Ron E, Tokuoka S, et al. Solid cancer incidence in atomic bomb survivors: 1958-1998. Radiat Res 2007;1968:1–64.
5. Hall EJ, Brenner DJ. Cancer risks from diagnostic radiology. BJR 2008;81: 362–72.
6. Allen C, Demetriades T. Letters to the editor: radiation risk overestimated. Radiology 2006;240:613–4.
7. Sidhu R, Bhatt S, Dogra VS. Renal colic. Ultrasound Clin 2008;3:159–70.
8. Sty JR, Pan CP. Genitourinary imaging techniques. Pediatr Clin North Am 2006; 53:339–61.
9. Smith RC, Verga M, McCarthy S, et al. Diagnosis of acute flank pain: value of unenhanced helical CT. AJR Am J Roentgenol 1996;166:97.
10. Colistro R, Torreggiani WC, Lyburn ID, et al. Unenhanced helical CT in the investigation of acute flank pain. Clin Radiol 2002;57:435.
11. Ulahannan D, Blakeley CJ, Jeyadevan N, et al. Benefits of CT urography in patients presenting to the emergency department with suspected ureteric colic. Emerg Med J 2008;25:569.
12. Dalrymple NC, Verga M, Anderson KR, et al. The value of unenhanced helical computerized tomography in the management of acute flank pain. J Urol 1998; 159:735.
13. Pedrosa I, Zeikus EA, Levine D, et al. MR imaging of acute right lower quadrant pain in pregnant and non-pregnant patients. RadioGraphics 2007;27:721–53.
14. Scoutt LM, Baltarowich OH, Lev-Toaff AS. Imaging of adnexal torsion. Ultrasound Clin 2007;2:311–25.

15. Terai A, Yoshimura K, Ichioka K, et al. Dynamic contrast-enhanced subtraction magnetic resonance imaging in the diagnostics of testicular torsion. Urol 2006; 67:1278–82.
16. Wanatabe Y, Dohke M, Ohkubo K, et al. Scrotal disorders: evaluation of testicular enhancement patterns at dynamic contrast enhanced subtraction MR imaging. Radiology 2000;217(1):219–27.
17. He W, Fischman AJ. Nuclear imaging in the genitourinary tract: recent advances and future directions. Radiol Clin North Am 2008;46:25–43.
18. Nussbaum AR, Bulas D, Shalaby-Rana E, et al. Color Doppler sonography and scintigraphy of the testis: a prospective, comparative analysis in children with acute scrotal pain. Pediatr Emerg Care 2002;18:67–71.
19. Hecht C, Wilkins J. Physics and image artifacts. In: Ma OJ, Mateer JR, Blaivas M, editors. Emergency ultrasound. 2nd edition. New York: McGraw Hill; 2008. p. 49–63.
20. American College of Emergency Physicians. Policy Statement: Emergency Ultrasound Guidelines—Approved October 2008. Dallas (Texas): American College of Emergency Physicians (ACEP). 2008. Available at: http://www.acep.org/policystatements/. Accessed March 21, 2011.
21. Akhtar S, Theodoro D, Gaspari R, et al. Resident training in emergency ultrasound: consensus recommendations from the 2008 Council of Emergency Medicine Residency Directors Conference. Acad Emerg Med 2009;16(Suppl 2):S32–6.
22. Rampaul MS, Hosking SW. Testicular torsion: most delays occur outside hospital. Ann R Coll Surg Engl 1998;80:169–72.
23. Blaivas M, Sierzenski P. Emergency ultrasonography in the evaluation of the acute scrotum. Acad Emerg Med 2001;8:85–9.
24. Blaivas M, Brannam L. Testicular ultrasound. Emerg Clin North Am 2004;22: 723–48.
25. Dogra V, Bhatt S. Acute painful scrotum. Radiol Clin North Am 2004;42:349–63.
26. Blaivas M, Sierzenski P, Lambert M. Emergency evaluation of patients presenting with acute scrotum using bedside ultrasonography. Acad Emerg Med 2001;8:90–3.
27. Lam WW, Yap T, Jacobsen AS, et al. Colour Doppler ultrasonography replacing surgical exploration for acute scrotum: myth or reality? Pediatr Radiol 2005; 35(6):597–600.
28. Andreotti RF, Shadinger LL, Fleischer AC. The sonographic diagnosis of ovarian torsion: pearls and pitfalls. Ultrasound Clin 2007;2:155–66.
29. Ben-Ami M, Perlitz Y, Haddad S. The effectiveness of spectral and color Doppler in predicting ovarian torsion: a prospective study. Eur J Obstet Gynecol Reprod Biol 2002;104:64–6.
30. Boswell HB, Adigun YE, Sangi-Haghpeykar H, et al. Predictive value of ultrasound in the diagnosis of adnexal torsion in the pediatric and adolescent population. J Pediatr Adolesc Gynecol 2008;21:57–65.
31. Cohen SB, Weisz B, Seidman DS, et al. Accuracy of the preoperative diagnosis in 100 emergency laparoscopies performed due to acute abdomen in nonpregnant woman. J Am Assoc Gynecol Laparosc 2001;8:92–4.
32. Baumann B, McCans K, Stahmer S, et al. Volumetric bladder ultrasound performed by trained nurses increases catheterization success in pediatric patients. Am J Emerg Med 2008;26:18–23.
33. Riccabona M. Pediatric three-dimensional ultrasound: basics and potential clinical value. J Clin Imaging 2005;29:1–5.
34. Riccabona M, Pilhatsch A, Haberlik A, et al. 3-Dimensional ultrasonography based virtual cystoscopy of the pediatric urinary bladder: a preliminary report on feasibility and potential value. J Ultrasound Med 2008;27:1453–9.

35. Blaivas M, Pawl R. Analysis of lawsuits filed against emergency physicians over bedside emergency ultrasound examination performance or interpretation over a 20-year period. Ann Emerg Med 2007;50:S85.
36. Blaivas M, Bunting L, Takla RB. Lawsuit for a misread of ED ultrasound not likely. ED legal letter, 21. Atlanta (GA): AHC Media; 2010. 101–4.
37. Monico EP. The state of emergency ultrasound and standard of care. ED legal letter, 13. Atlanta (GA): AHC Media; 2007. 114–6.

Renal Failure: Emergency Evaluation and Management

Korin B. Hudson, MD[a,*], Richard Sinert, DO[b]

KEYWORDS

- Acute renal failure • Acute kidney injury • Chronic renal failure
- Contrast-induced nephropathy • Emergency

Patients with altered renal function, either acute or chronic, are frequently encountered in the emergency department (ED) and emergency physicians (EPs) often play an important role in the evaluation and management of renal disease. Some of these patients have chief complaints directly related to their failing kidney function, others may show subtle secondary signs, and some may have no signs or symptoms of renal disease. Early recognition, diagnosis, prevention of further iatrogenic injury, and management of renal disease have important implications for long-term morbidity and mortality. This article reviews basic renal physiology, discusses the differential diagnosis and approach to therapy, as well as strategies to prevent further renal injury, for adult patients who present to the ED with renal injury or failure.

PATHOPHYSIOLOGY

Renal function comprises 4 steps: (1) blood flow is delivered to the glomeruli, (2) an ultrafiltrate is formed in the glomeruli and then delivered to the renal tubules, (3) solutes and/or water are reabsorbed/secreted in the renal tubules, and (4) tubular fluid (now urine) exits the tubules, draining to the renal pelvis, the ureters, and the bladder, and urine is then expelled via the urethra. Renal disease can be caused by any process that interferes with any of the structures or steps involved in this process. Furthermore, such insults may be in the setting of an acute kidney injury (AKI), leading to a rapid

The authors have nothing to disclose.

[a] Department of Emergency Medicine, Georgetown University Hospital and Washington Hospital Center, 3800 Reservoir Road North West, Ground Floor, CCC Building, Washington, DC 20007, USA

[b] Department of Emergency Medicine, State University of New York Downstate Medical Center, 450 Clarkson Avenue, Box 1228, Brooklyn, NY 11203, USA

* Corresponding author.

E-mail address: kbh101@gunet.georgetown.edu

Emerg Med Clin N Am 29 (2011) 569–585
doi:10.1016/j.emc.2011.04.005 emed.theclinics.com

decline in renal function, or they may be a result of chronic kidney disease (CKD) and be progressive during months or years (**Table 1**).

Each kidney has approximately 1 million nephrons, each contributing to the total glomerular filtration rate (GFR). The GFR is the volume of fluid filtered per unit time and can be calculated by measuring any chemical whose concentration is at steady state in blood plasma and is freely filtered by the kidney but is neither secreted nor absorbed in the kidney [GFR = (urine concentration × flow)/plasma concentration]. Regardless of the cause, progressive damage to nephrons leads to structural and functional changes within the kidney. Initially, the kidney is able to maintain GFR through hyperfiltration and compensatory hypertrophy of the remaining healthy nephrons, which allows the kidney to maintain normal clearance of plasma solutes. However, if the physiologic insult persists, the damaged nephrons cannot recover and the renal reserve may be exhausted. Renal injury and/or renal failure are usually defined by a decline in GFR, leading ultimately to oliguria, decreased urine output (UOP), or anuria, the absence of urine formation. However, GFR is not a readily measured value and, as such, clinicians and researchers have long searched for ways to accurately and easily measure (or at least estimate) renal function.

Serum creatinine (SCr) is primarily derived from the metabolism of creatine phosphate in muscle tissue and is freely filtered by the glomerulus. The ease of measurement in most laboratories, and in the clinical setting, makes SCr an attractive index for GFR. However, there are several drawbacks to the use of SCr as a surrogate marker for GFR. First, an increase in SCr lags behind falling/declining renal function because it is only when GFR reaches approximately 50% of baseline, and when the renal reserve is no longer able to maintain the level of filtration, that the measured SCr begins to increase. At that point, SCr values approximately double with each 50% decrease in GFR. Therefore, there may be a marked decrease in renal function before the clinician is able to identify a change in SCr. Furthermore, SCr is influenced by many nonrenal factors including body mass, body composition, race, sex, total body volume, muscle metabolism, and diet. These differences in SCr persist even after adjusting for known GFR. There may also be significant day-to-day variations in creatinine excretion, making SCr (particularly any single measurement) an imperfect measure of a patient's true renal function.

Creatinine clearance (CrCl) is also used in some settings as a marker of overall renal function and an estimate of GFR. Most calculations of CrCl depend on measurement of SCr as well as a measurement of urinary creatinine concentrations (UCr) and the measured volume from a 24-hour collection of urine. However, although creatinine is freely filtered by the glomerulus, some creatinine may also be excreted in the proximal tubule, and extrarenal creatinine excretion may be increased in patients with CKD, leading to an overestimation of the true GFR. In addition, certain medications may inhibit creatinine secretion (such as cimetidine and trimethoprim).

Table 1
Key terminology

Acute kidney injury (AKI)	Rapid decline in renal function; formerly termed acute renal failure (ARF)
Chronic kidney disease (CKD)	Progressive/persistent decline in renal function for months or years; previously described as chronic renal failure (CRF)
End-stage renal disease (ESRD)	Minimal/absent renal function, typically requiring renal replacement therapy (RRT) with hemodialysis (HD) or peritoneal dialysis (PD)

Estimations of GFR or CrCl using the Modification of Diet in Renal Disease (MDRD) equation[1] or the Cockcroft-Gault formula[2] are frequently described in the literature and are often used in clinical research. Both make corrections for patient variables such as age and sex. These formulas are available in many medical calculators both online and for handheld electronic devices and the values may be useful in some settings. However, each of these methods assumes that a steady state exists, which is often not the case, particularly in patients with AKI who present to the ED.

Clinical trials are currently underway to evaluate the efficacy of several novel biomarkers to identify the presence of renal disease. Most markers currently being investigated are intended to specifically identify AKI. The goal is to identify a biomarker, or a panel of biomarkers, that would facilitate the early diagnosis of AKI, could differentiate between different types of renal injury, and could provide an accurate prognosis, all with a high degree of specificity and sensitivity. To that end, several biomarkers are currently being evaluated in trials (**Table 2**) including serum measurements of cystatin-C and neutrophil gelatinated–associated lipocalin (NGAL) and urine measurements of interleukin (IL)-18 and kidney injury molecule 1 (KIM-1). The use and availability of these markers in clinical practice is not widespread, and most of the novel biomarkers being studied have not yet been evaluated in patients with CKD or acute exacerbations of chronic renal disease. However, they may represent the future of how clinicians will identify and assess the severity of renal disease.

Therefore, despite the well known limitations outlined earlier, and because measurements of SCr and serum blood urea nitrogen (BUN) are more readily available in clinical practice, EPs more frequently rely on BUN and SCr at the time of presentation and compare them with baseline values (when known) to help guide diagnosis and treatment. Although normal values may vary based on laboratory assay and from facility to facility, creatinine values of 0.7 to 1.2 mg/dL, BUN of 7 to 20 mg/dL, and a BUN/creatinine ratio of 10:1 are generally considered to be normal.

CKD

A thorough discussion of CKD is beyond the scope of this article. However, it is appropriate to recall that approximately 20 million individuals in the United States have CKD,

Table 2
Several novel biomarkers for AKI

Biomarker	Function Evaluated/Affected	Use
Cystatin-C (serum)	Marker of glomerular filtration	Shows good accuracy for early diagnosis of AKI Seems to be particularly useful in patients with sepsis
NGAL (serum)	Marker of renal tubular inflammation	Correlates well with acute changes in SCr
IL-18 (urine)	Marker of renal tubular inflammation	Facilitates the diagnosis of AKI Marked increased in patients with acute tubular necrosis Predicts mortality
KIM-1 (urine)	Marker of injury to the proximal tubule, especially following ischemic insult	May be highly effective at distinguishing acute tubular necrosis from other types of renal injury

Abbreviations: IL-18, interleukin-18; KIM-1, kidney injury molecule 1; NGAL, neutrophil gelatinated–associated lipocalin.

Data from Refs.[44–47]

defined by the National Kidney Foundation as persistent or sustained damage lasting longer than 3 months and resulting in a GFR of less than 60 mL/min/1.73 m^2. Patients with CKD are more likely to be admitted to the hospital and are likely to have longer hospital stays than matched patients who do not have CKD.[3]

The most frequent causes of CKD in the United States include diabetes mellitus, hypertension, human immunodeficiency virus, and autoimmune and inherited diseases (including polycystic kidney disease and sickle cell disease). Of these, diabetes and hypertension are the most frequently encountered comorbidities with one or the other found in more than 75% of US patients with CKD, according to the US Renal Data System.[4] With the proportion of the population with diabetes and hypertension steadily increasing, the incidence of renal failure will continue to increase as well.

EPs frequently encounter patients with CKD, which may complicate their evaluation and treatment of a wide range of emergency conditions, from administration of contrast media to medication dosing, even when patients present with complaints not directly related to their kidney disease. Furthermore, patients with chronic or end-stage kidney disease may frequently present for emergency care for conditions that are directly related to their disease, including fluid overload, electrolyte imbalance, or infection. In addition, several acute insults, including nephrotoxic agents, hypovolemia, and decreased renal perfusion, can cause acute worsening of renal failure in patients who already suffer from CKD. Any of the causes of AKI (discussed later) can be superimposed on chronic renal insufficiency, leading to acute worsening of renal function. The role of EPs is not typically to diagnose CKD or end-stage renal disease (ESRD) but to recognize the presence of the disease process in their patients and limit further renal insults during diagnosis and treatment of emergency conditions.

Although a discussion of renal replacement therapy (RRT), including peritoneal dialysis (PD) and hemodialysis (HD), is worthy of an entire manuscript unto itself, EPs frequently encounter patients who are chronically receiving RRT and should be prepared for complications that arise in this specific patient population. In brief, patients on RRT are at higher risk for infections, bleeding, complications related to volume management, and electrolyte abnormalities. Complications in fluid management and electrolyte management in particular are also problematic when patients fail to get their RRT as scheduled. In addition, infections are the second leading cause of death among patients with ESRD, and the increased mortality caused by sepsis in this patient population is not related to HD or PD access catheters.[5] Furthermore, mortality from sepsis has been found to be at least 100-fold higher in patients on dialysis (both HD and PD) compared with the general population.[5]

It is also important to recall that a percentage of patients with ESRD on RRT proceed to renal transplantation. More than 15,000 renal transplants are performed in the United States every year, a number that is increasing with advances in nonmatched living donor transplantation. It is important for the EP to recall that worsening renal function in the patient having a renal transplant may be caused by any of the insults that can cause AKI (discussed later) and that early identification of the cause and rapid treatment are crucial in the patient with only a single functioning kidney. Furthermore, acute or subacute worsening of renal failure in the patient receiving a transplant may also be a sign of transplant rejection, and the patient's transplant surgeon or nephrologist (depending on local customs) should be consulted early in the course of evaluation and treatment.

AKI

AKI, previously referred to as acute renal failure, is defined by a rapid decline in renal function and filtration. This decline is usually marked by an abrupt decrease in GFR.

Clinically, this may be first evident in an increase in SCr, azotemia (increased BUN), or alterations of other biomarkers as noted earlier. Patients with AKI may or may not present with oliguria or anuria. This abrupt decline usually occurs in hours to days and results in the failure of the kidney to excrete nitrogenous waste or to maintain normal plasma volume or electrolyte balance. Knowledge of a patient's baseline renal function makes it easier to recognize this acute change.

Epidemiology of AKI

Despite significant advances in critical care medicine and technological advances in RRT, the morbidity and mortality associated with AKI remains high. In the United States, as many as 5% to 7% of hospital admissions each year are complicated by AKI, numbering approximately 17 million patients at a cost of nearly $10 billion per year.[6] AKI has long been known to be associated with increased intensive care unit (ICU) and overall hospital length of stay, as well as with increased morbidity and mortality. In a large multinational, multicenter study, Uchino and colleagues[7] report a prevalence of AKI in the ICU population of approximately 6% and, in their study of 30,000 patients, as many as 60% of critically ill patients with AKI died before hospital discharge. Although many of these patients succumbed to non–renal-related conditions (eg, sepsis, hemorrhage), up to 13% of survivors required ongoing RRT at the time of discharge.

More recently, it has become clear that even mild or moderately severe episodes of AKI are associated with an increased risk of longer-term adverse outcomes, including death, even when risks are adjusted for other comorbidities.[8] In their meta-analysis, Coca and colleagues[9] report that, in hospitalized patients, even modest increases in SCr (10%–20% or 0.3–0.4 mg/dL) are associated with a doubling in the risk of short-term mortality, whereas greater changes in SCr (25%–29% or 0.5–0.9 mg/dL) are associated with a threefold to fivefold increase in risk of death.

Defining AKI

Although the term AKI implies a structural injury to the kidney, the term is most often used to describe a decrease in kidney function, often defined by rising SCr or decreased UOP, even in light of the known limitations of these markers. For years, the lack of a clear definition of AKI hampered research and clinical efforts alike, making it difficult to compare results from various therapies or several different clinical trials. However, in recent years, 2 classifications systems have been proposed in an attempt to simplify and coordinate the definition of AKI.

In 2004, the Acute Dialysis Quality Initiative created the RIFLE criteria to define the stages and degree of acute renal dysfunction.[10] These criteria seek to classify patients with renal dysfunction into 5 categories (**Table 3**): risk of renal dysfunction (R); injury to the kidney (I); renal failure (F); loss of kidney function (L); and ESRD (E). Note that only 1 of the conditions (increased creatinine, decreased GFR, or decreased urine output) must be present to meet the classification. This classification system relies on a clinician having prior knowledge of a patient's baseline renal function. If baseline function is not known, the patient's GFR may be estimated using 1 of the formulas discussed earlier, and proportional decrease may be calculated using a baseline of 75 mL/min/ 1.73 m^2 (the lower limit of normal). Uchino and colleagues[11] showed that these criteria for risk, injury, and failure identified 9%, 5%, and 4% respectively of all hospital admissions, and 17%, 12%, and 7% of critical care admissions, and that these criteria are predictive for hospital mortality among patients admitted for all causes.

The second classification system was put forth by the Acute Kidney Injury Network (AKIN) who met in 2005 and agreed on an interim definition that includes an abrupt

Table 3
RIFLE classification for AKI

Classification	Creatinine	GFR	Urine Output
(R) Risk	Increased 1.5×	Decreased ≥25%	<0.5 mL/kg/h × 6 h
(I) Injury	Increased 2×	Decreased ≥50%	<0.5 mL/kg/h × 12 h
(F) Failure	Increased 3× or serum Cr >4 mg/dL with acute increase of 0.5 mg/dL	Decreased ≥75%	<0.3 mL/kg/h × 24 h or anuria for 12 h
(L) Loss	Persistent failure with complete loss of function >4 weeks	—	—
(E) End-Stage	Loss of function >3 mo	—	—

Data from Bellomo R, Ronco C, Kellum JA, et al. Acute renal failure: definition, outcome measures, animal models, fluid therapy and information technology needs: the Second International Consensus Conference of the Acute Dialysis Quality Initiative (ADQI) Group. Crit Care 2004;8:R206.

(within 48 hours) reduction in kidney function currently defined as an absolute increase in serum creatinine of either greater than or equal to 0.3 mg/dL or a percentage increase of greater than or equal to 50% (1.5-fold from baseline) or a reduction of urine output (documented oliguria of <0.5 mL/kg/h for >6h).[12] **Table 4** outlines the stages of AKI using the AKIN definition. This definition assumes that, if the UOP criteria are to be used, urinary outflow obstruction has been ruled out and that adequate fluid resuscitation has occurred when appropriate. The AKIN definition has been shown to predict length of stay, in-hospital mortality, and the need for RRT in critically ill patients.[13]

Types of AKI

The different types of AKI are most frequently described in terms of what part of renal function is affected. The most often used classification divides acute renal failure into prerenal, intrinsic renal, and postrenal causes.

Prerenal azotemia

Prerenal azotemia, or prerenal failure, is the most common type of AKI and is frequently seen in the ED setting. Prerenal azotemia represents an adaptive response to renal hypoperfusion, systemic hypotension, and/or severe volume depletion in the setting of

Table 4
AKIN staging system for the definition of acute kidney injury

Stage	Creatinine	Urine Output
I	Increased SCr ≥0.3 mg/dL OR SCr 150%–200% (1.5-fold to 2-fold) from baseline	<0.5 mg/kg/h for 6 h
II	SCr ≥200%–300% (>2-fold to 3-fold) from baseline	<0.5 mg/kg/h for 12 h
III	SCr ≥300% (>3-fold) from baseline OR absolute SCr ≥4.0 mg/dL with an absolute increase of ≥0.5 mg/dL OR need for RRT	<0.3 mg/kg/h for 24 h OR anuria for 12 h

Data from Mehta RL, Kellum JA, Shah SV, et al. Acute Kidney Injury Network (AKIN): report of an initiative to improve outcomes in acute kidney injury. Crit Care 2007;11:R31.

normal glomerular and tubular function. Conditions that can lead to prerenal failure include hypovolemia from any type of volume loss including decreased fluid intake, hemorrhage, GI fluid losses, and burns. In addition, any condition that leads to systemic hypotension, including conditions that decrease effective arterial blood flow, such as congestive heart failure, liver disease, and sepsis, may also result in decreased renal perfusion and prerenal failure.

This classification also includes decreased renal perfusion caused by renal arterial disease such as renal artery stenosis (atherosclerotic or fibrodysplastic), renal artery emboli (septic, cholesterol, or hematologic), or arteriolar vasoconstriction, which may occur in cases of hypercalcemia, after use of radiocontrast agents, nonsteroidal antiinflammatory drugs (NSAIDs), amphotericin, or vasopressors. Certain medications, such as angiotensin converting enzyme (ACE) inhibitors or angiotensin receptor blockers (ARBs), may contribute to acute prerenal failure in patients who are already in a volume depressed state.

Prerenal azotemia is often reversible if identified and treated early. Fluid management and restoration of adequate renal perfusion are the mainstays of therapy. In cases of hypovolemia, crystalloid replacement remains the recommended emergency intervention. In cases of decreased renal perfusion caused by distributive shock (eg, sepsis, anaphylaxis) the underlying condition should be treated. However, crystalloids should not be withheld while more definitive therapies are initiated. Vasopressors may be required to maintain renal perfusion but are not a substitute for fluid therapy, when indicated. In addition, care should be taken to avoid nephrotoxic medications, contrast agents, or other renal insults in this setting.

If not promptly identified and corrected, the decreased perfusion associated with prerenal disease may lead to ongoing damage and progress to intrinsic renal disease. Decreased renal blood flow eventually leads to tissue ischemia and cell death. Ischemia at the level of the kidney may occur before systemic hypotension is evident. The initial ischemic insult initiates a cascade of events at the cellular level including the production of free radicals and cytokines eventually leading to endothelial activation, leukocyte adhesion, and the initiation of apoptosis. This process causes cellular injury that may persist even after renal blood flow is restored. Damage to tubular cells can allow leakage of glomerular filtrate, which can further depress GFR. Furthermore, damaged cells may slough off and, in effect, clog the tubules, further affecting renal function and decreasing the GFR. Therefore, in cases of AKI that present to the ED, it is crucial to consider prerenal azotemia as a possible cause, treat appropriately, and prevent further insults to provide the patient with the best possible chance of restoring normal renal function.

Postrenal failure

Postrenal failure is best described as obstructive processes affecting the outflow of urine at any point from the renal collecting system to the level of the urethra. Depressed renal function in cases of obstruction occurs because of an increase in tubular pressure that leads to a decrease in the driving forces of filtration. Bilateral obstruction (or distal obstruction at the level of the bladder or urethra) must be present for renal function to be affected, although, in patients with only a single functioning kidney, unilateral obstruction may have the same deleterious effect.

Postrenal or obstructive renal failure is more common in the elderly and in men, most often caused by prostatic disease. However, obstructive uropathy is also common in patients with neurogenic bladder and in patients with in-dwelling urinary catheters, which may themselves become obstructed. In addition, abdominal or pelvic tumors can cause ureteral or urethral obstructions, as can adhesions or scarring from prior abdominal or pelvic surgeries or radiation therapy. Certain medications (eg, methysergide, propranolol, hydralazine) can also cause adhesions or fibrosis. Kidney or bladder stones can cause obstructive disease, including stones caused by uric acid, calcium oxalate (caused by ethylene glycol poisoning), myeloma light chains (in multiple myeloma), or because of certain medications (eg, acyclovir, methotrexate, triamterene, indinavir, or sulfonamides). Bilateral or distal stones/obstructions must be present to lead to decreased renal function in patients with 2 functioning kidneys.

As in other forms of renal disease, obstructive disease often presents acutely, as in acute urine retention, although the disease process may also have a more insidious onset, as in cases of benign prostatic hypertrophy. The role of the EP is to diagnose the obstructive condition and correct it as rapidly as possible. In these cases, patients often complain of acute decrease in UOP in addition to a sense of lower abdominal pain, pressure, or fullness. Often a distended bladder may be appreciated on physical examination. Ultrasound is a fast and noninvasive way to evaluate bladder volume at the bedside. If a full bladder is identified, the obstruction may be considered to be distal to that and a urethral (or suprapubic) catheter may be placed to drain urine and relieve the obstruction. If a more proximal obstruction is suspected, renal ultrasound or noncontrast computed tomography (CT) scan may be useful to evaluate for hydronephrosis or hydroureter and may identify the cause and degree of the obstruction. In cases of proximal obstruction, urostomy or nephrostomy tubes may be required to restore proper urine drainage; this is not typically an ED procedure and consultation with a urologist is often the best way to proceed.

Hyperkalemia may occur as a complication of acute urinary obstruction caused by impaired acidification of urine before and/or after relief of the obstruction, which leads to impaired excretion of hydrogen and potassium ions, leading to a hyperkalemic distal renal tubular acidosis.[14] Given the potentially serious cardiac complications of acute increases in serum potassium, every patient with acute urinary obstruction should be evaluated with a serum electrolyte panel. If a point-of-care electrolyte or chemistry panel is not available, the EP should consider a screening electrocardiogram if hyperkalemia is suspected. In patients with normal underlying kidney function, relief of obstruction and restoration of normal filtration and urine flow are often sufficient to restore normal serum potassium levels.

Longer duration and larger volumes of urinary retention resulting from obstruction may lead to further complications. Urinary tract infections may result from urinary stasis and should be treated per local antiinfective protocols. Postobstructive diuresis is a rare but serious complication following the relief of urinary obstruction that is marked by significant natriuresis and diuresis that may lead to hypotension. This complication may lead to significant volume depletion as well as electrolyte abnormalities including hypokalemia, hyponatremia, and hypomagnesemia. In the past, it was common for an EP to clamp the urinary catheter after output of 1 L, in theory, to prevent overdieresis and hypotension. However, these recommendations were not evidence based and hypotension related to postobstructive dieresis is not caused by overdrainage of urine from the bladder. Treatment of postobstructive dieresis should be initiated with 0.45% saline at a rate approximately equal to the urine output, and electrolytes should be replaced as needed.

Patient disposition in cases of obstructive renal disease depends on many factors. The degree of renal dysfunction (and change from baseline) that is noted at the time of presentation to the ED; patients with significant decrease in renal function should be observed in the hospital to ensure that renal function returns to normal after the obstruction is relieved and to rule out other causes of renal failure. Further, patients with significant electrolyte abnormalities or postobstructive diuresis may require observation or admission while fluids and electrolytes are replaced. In addition, the cause of the obstruction may warrant further inpatient evaluation and further procedures may be required in the acute setting to prevent worsening obstruction.

Intrinsic renal disease

In contrast with prerenal and postrenal causes of AKI, which both occur outside the kidney itself, intrinsic renal disease is a physiologic response to cytotoxic, inflammatory, or ischemic insults to the kidney itself, with both structural and functional damage to the filtration system. This damage includes a range of conditions that affect the function of the kidney, especially those that affect glomerular and tubular function directly. Intrinsic renal disease may be divided into conditions that affect the glomeruli, the interstitium, or the renal tubules.

Glomerular causes of AKI include nephritic syndromes and nephrotic syndromes, either of which may have acute or insidious onset. Acute nephritis refers to an inflammatory process that includes an active urine sediment with proteinuria, red cells, white cells, and granular or cellular casts. The clinical hallmarks of acute nephritic syndrome are hypertension, hematuria, edema, and a history of recent systemic infection.

The other broad category of acute glomerular disease is nephrotic syndrome, which is not associated with acute inflammatory changes and does not include active urine sediment. The hallmarks of nephrotic syndrome are profound proteinuria, and marked edema. Causes of nephrotic syndrome are often described by the histology seen on renal biopsy and include minimal change disease (MCD), focal segmental glomerulosclerosis (FSGS), and membranous nephropathy. The EP should have a suspicion for nephrotic syndrome based on patient presentation and urinalysis, although a 24-hour urine protein measurement remains the gold standard for diagnosis. Further evaluation and treatment should be guided by a nephrologist.

Conditions that primarily affect the renal interstitium include hypersensitivity reactions (illicit drugs, penicillins, nonsteroidal antiinflammatory drugs, and sulfa drugs are most common); autoimmune diseases (eg, systemic lupus erythematosus or Goodpasture syndrome); infiltrative diseases (eg, sarcoid, lymphoma); infectious causes (including bacterial, viral, fungal, or parasitic infections); pigment-induced conditions (secondary to rhabdomyolysis or hemolysis); or acute transplant rejection. Patients with acute interstitial nephritis may present with a wide range of symptoms depending on the cause. However, on presentation, modest renal dysfunction may be evident and patients may have systemic symptoms such as rash or fever. Proteinuria may or may not be present. The diagnostic gold standard for diagnosis of interstitial disease is renal biopsy, and nephrology consultation should be considered early in suspected cases.

Acute tubular necrosis (ATN) is the most commonly encountered form of intrinsic renal disease, especially among hospitalized and critically ill patients. ATN may have many causes, including drug reactions (**Box 1**), cast nephropathy (often associated with multiple myeloma), tumor lysis syndrome following certain chemotherapy regimens, and, less often, acute phosphate nephropathy associated with certain phosphate-containing bowel preparations. ATN may also present in patients who have experienced prolonged hypotension such as after cardiac arrest, severe hemorrhage, sepsis, or drug overdose.

The diagnosis of ATN is not frequently made in the ED. It is a diagnosis of exclusion in the setting of established or presumed AKI once prerenal and obstructive causes have been ruled out. The initial management of ATN focuses on preventing complications, avoiding further renal insults, and providing an environment conducive to renal recovery. Early in the course of ATN, prevention of further renal injury is crucial. This prevention includes a review of all medications and stopping or avoiding medications

Box 1
Examples of drugs/toxins that may cause ATN. Note: this is not a comprehensive list; many drugs/toxins can cause renal impairment

1. Drugs that may cause direct tubular cell damage:
    a. Aminoglycoside antibiotics
    b. Amphotericin B
    c. Cisplatin
    d. Methotrexate
    e. Tacrolimus
    f. Radiocontrast agents
2. Drugs that may cause afferent arteriolar constriction:
    a. Cyclosporine
    b. Tacrolimus
    c. Radiocontrast agents
3. Drugs that may precipitate and obstruct tubular lumens:
    a. Acyclovir
    b. Sulfonamides
4. Endogenous tubular toxins:
    a. Hemoglobin
    b. Myoglobin
5. Other drugs/toxins:
    a. ACE inhibitors
    b. Ethylene glycol
    c. Heavy metals
    d. NSAIDs
    e. Organic solvents

Data from Devarajan P. Acute tubular necrosis. Available at: www.emedicine.com. Accessed February 2, 2011.

that may be nephrotoxic, adjusting dosages where appropriate for medications that are cleared by the kidney, and, when possible, avoiding contrast agents that may cause further renal insult.

In the ED setting, a trial of parenteral hydration with isotonic fluids may correct AKI/ATN that is complicated by prerenal causes. However, overhydration should be avoided, especially in patients with comorbidities that could lead to pulmonary edema or third spacing of fluids. Euvolemia is the ultimate goal and careful measurement of fluid ins and outs should be undertaken.

In addition, electrolyte and acid/base balance should be maintained. Acidosis, hyponatremia, and hyperphosphatemia should be avoided. In addition, evaluation for and treatment of hyperkalemia should occur early in the course of AKI and serum potassium levels should be rechecked frequently. The management of acute hyperkalemia is familiar to EPs, including evaluation of an electrocardiogram for peaked T-waves, QRS widening, or sine-wave patterns, and the administration of intravenous calcium gluconate (or calcium chloride) in addition to insulin, dextrose, and inhaled β-agonists. Routine administration of sodium bicarbonate is controversial. Given as a single therapy, sodium bicarbonate often fails to provide a fast or sustained decrease in serum potassium levels. Therefore, some recommend that its use should be reserved for cases in which acidemia is known or suspected, or when there is another reason to consider its administration (such as tricyclic antidepressant overdose).[15] However, in small studies of patients with chronic renal disease or ESRD, when given in combination with a β_2-agonist or insulin/dextrose, sodium bicarbonate has been shown to decrease plasma potassium levels more that these other therapies alone.[16,17] Potassium-containing fluids, such as Ringer lactate, should also generally be avoided in favor of other non–potassium-containing crystalloid solutions. The oral or rectal administration of potassium-binding resins has long been common in ED practice. However, in the past several years their safety and efficacy have come into question, especially when administered with sorbitol.[18,19]

Early nephrology consultation has been shown to decrease morbidity and mortality associated with AKI regardless of whether or not RRT is ultimately required. In an ICU study by Mehta and colleagues,[20] factors associated with delayed nephrology consultation included patients with lower creatinine levels and patients with preserved UOP. However, even in these patients, the delay in consultation resulted in increased morbidity and mortality. Urgent initiation of RRT may be required in patients with severe AKI, including those with any of the following: significant fluid overload; severe hyperkalemia or rapidly rising plasma potassium levels; significant signs of uremia, including pericardial effusion, pericarditis, or altered mental status; severe metabolic acidosis; or in cases of certain toxins (**Box 2**). In cases where RRT, such as HD, is considered for the elimination of toxins, a medical toxicologist (or poison control center) and a nephrologist should be consulted promptly.[21]

Several pharmacologic therapies have been suggested as treatments for ATN, and many have been used in ED and critical care scenarios for years without adequate data to support their use. In recent years, clinical trials have been performed to evaluate many of the more commonly used modalities.

Box 2
Toxins that may be removed via extracorporeal removal (ECR). Note: this is not a comprehensive list; many drugs may be eliminated during the use of HD

1. Carbamazepine*
2. Lithium
3. Salycilates
4. Theophylline
5. Toxic alcohols:
   a. Ethylene glycol
   b. Isopropanol
   c. Methanol
6. Valproic acid
7. Vancomycin

* Removal may require the use of high-flux dialyzers.

Data from Fertel B, Nelson L, Goldfarb D. Extracorporeal removal techniques for the poisoned patient: a review for the intensivist. J Int Care Med 2010;25:139–48.

Diuretic therapy, specifically the use of loop diuretics, was long considered appropriate for use in patients with ATN. In theory, loop diuretic therapy may protect cells from hypoxic damage by reducing oxygen demand, increasing tubular flow, and maintaining a favorable GFR with increased renal blood flow. However, in an observational study of 552 patients, Mehta and colleagues[22] found that the use of diuretics in critically ill patients with acute renal failure was associated with an increased risk of death and nonrecovery of renal function. Although this observational study was not designed to show causality, Mehta and colleagues[22] conclude that it is "unlikely that diuretics afford any material benefit in this clinical setting." However, Uchino and colleagues[23] report that diuretics did not increase mortality, but neither did their use have a significant positive effect of renal recovery, decrease the need for RRT, or decrease mortality. To date, a large, blinded, randomized controlled trial of loop diuretics in AKI has not been completed.

Mannitol has also been proposed and used as a potential treatment of ATN. Theoretically, mannitol would increase renal blood flow, increasing UOP, flushing intratubular casts, reducing hypoxic cell swelling and cell death, protecting mitochondrial function, and scavenging free radicals. In early studies, some benefit was seen in animal models[24] and in the clinical setting in human subjects,[25] although this effect was found to be most pronounced when mannitol was administered prophylactically or immediately after an ischemic or nephrotoxic insult (ie, when given just before clamping the renal artery during a partial nephrectomy). This type of pretreatment would be impractical or impossible in the emergency or acute care setting. Later human studies failed to show the effectiveness of mannitol to treat toxic or ischemic AKI.[26,27]

For many years, so-called renal dose dopamine was considered a mainstay of treatment of patients with AKI. At doses of 0.4 to 5 μg/kg/min, dopamine activates D1 receptors and is proposed to increase natriuresis, increase renal blood flow, increase GFR, and increase urine output. However, Bellomo and colleagues[28] found that, when patients in the ICU with AKI were randomized to low-dose dopamine or placebo, there was no difference in mortality. In addition, in a large meta-analysis, Kellum and Decker[29] concluded that "the use of low dose dopamine for the treatment or prevention of acute renal failure cannot be justified on the basis of available evidence and should be eliminated from routine clinical use."

Fenoldopam, a selective D1 agonist, was also proposed as a treatment strategy for AKI. Its proposed mechanism is renal vasodilation without stimulation of D2 or β-adrenergic receptors. Some benefit has been shown in animal models[30] and in small clinical trials, with most trials focusing on the prevention of renal failure associated with cardiopulmonary bypass,[31] or in preventing renal failure after percutaneous coronary interventions when given along with IV hydration.[32] A large, randomized clinical trial of fenoldopam for the treatment of AKI has not yet been performed. Given the lack of evidence, and that fenoldopam is delivered as an IV drip requiring continuous blood pressure and cardiac monitoring, it is not currently considered a mainstay of treatment of AKI in the emergency or acute care setting.

The literature provides little firm guidance on the use of other pharmacologic agents in the prevention or treatment of AKI. Larger clinical trials are needed to define the role of vasoactive medications and other drugs in the treatment of AKI, especially those that may be practical and effective in the ED setting.

CONTRAST-INDUCED NEPHROPATHY

The role of IV contrast agents in contributing to, or frankly causing, AKI is a topic that has been of particular interest to EPs in recent years. Originally described extensively in studies of patients who were receiving percutaneous coronary angiography, the discussion of contrast-induced nephropathy (CIN) has now extended to include both inpatient as well as outpatient procedures, including intravenous contrast-enhanced CT scans.

CIN is the sudden and rapid deterioration of renal function that is directly related to the parenteral administration of contrast media with no alternative clinical explanation. CIN is generally defined as a proportional increase in SCr of 25% from baseline or an absolute increase in SCr of 0.5 mg/dL within 48 hours after parenteral contrast administration. CIN is the third most common cause of hospital-acquired renal failure in the inpatient setting.[33] Although causality is often difficult to prove, patients with CIN have been observed to have significantly increased morbidity and mortality.[34]

Nephropathy secondary to contrast administration has been discussed at length in the literature, although most studies have included inpatients and patients undergoing coronary angiography. More recently, the incidence of CIN has been reported to be greater than 10% in patients who undergo contrast-enhanced CT scans in the outpatient setting.[35] Although significant morbidity and mortality are rare, these rates are still unacceptably high for a condition that may be considered completely iatrogenic.

The pathogenesis of CIN is not well understood and no good animal models exist. CIN is believed to occur via a combination of mechanisms including a transient decrease in systemic blood pressure after IV contrast administration caused by vasodilation and decreased peripheral vascular resistance, a transient decrease in the GFR that results from osmotic dieresis, and direct toxic effects in the kidney related to tubular toxicity and free radical formation. CIN is rarely seen in patients with normal preexisting renal function (GFR >60 mg/kg/1.73m^2 and SCr <1.5 mg/dL) and seems to be more prevalent in patients with underlying renal insufficiency, especially among patients with preexisting diabetic renal disease.[36]

A thorough discussion of the various types of contrast media is outside the scope of this article. However, the literature tells us that low-osmolar and iso-osmolar contrast media have much less effect on the kidney than previously used high-osmolar agents.[36,37] Because of their safety profile, these low-osmolar and iso-osmolar agents are much more frequently used in clinical practice and, therefore, most recent studies on CIN focus on the use of these agents.

Several prevention and/or treatment strategies have been suggested. The most rigorously studied modalities include IV hydration with isotonic crystalloid solution, IV hydration with sodium bicarbonate solutions, and administration of *N*-acetylcysteine (NAC). However, there is scant literature available regarding treatment strategies that are both effective and practical for use in the ED setting.

Volume supplementation has been the mainstay of preventative treatment of CIN. Volume supplementation is believed to result in plasma volume expansion, dilution of contrast media, prevention of renal cortical vasoconstriction, and suppression of the renin-angiotensin-aldosterone system, which may downregulate tubuloglomerular feedback, blunting the effect of the contrast agent on GFR.[38] Various protocols have studied infusion rates and duration of treatment, with many recommending as much as 1 mL/kg/h for 12 hours before and after the proposed procedure. Studies evaluating the use of smaller volumes of fluid given as a bolus during the peri- or immediate preprocedure period seem to be less effective than larger volumes infused over 12–24 hours.[39,40] Other abbreviated protocols for emergency procedures recommend 300 mL/h on call to the procedure (generally in the 30–60 minutes preceding), and continuation of IV hydration for a total of 6 hours after the procedure. Although this type of abbreviated hydration strategy seems to be as effective as the standard 24-hour protocol, it is still perhaps impractical in the outpatient or ED setting. However, these hydration protocols do seem to decrease the incidence, and lessen the severity, of CIN.

The use of hydration with sodium bicarbonate–containing solutions has also been proposed as a potential method to decrease the incidence and/or severity of CIN, although the mechanisms are unclear. It is possible that, in addition to the benefits believed to come from volume expansion and hydration alone, the alkalinization of the urine that occurs with sodium bicarbonate administration may reduce the generation of free radicals and prevent oxidative damage, preventing kidney injury. In a meta-analysis by Navaneethan and colleagues,[41] the overall incidence of CIN in patients who received hydration with sodium bicarbonate was lower than in patients who received normal saline alone. Furthermore, they found that hydration with sodium bicarbonate was safe in terms of not worsening preexisting heart failure and not causing increased incidence of pulmonary edema. However, there was no clear difference in the need for RRT, no significant change in hospital length of stay, and no decrease in mortality. To date, a large prospective controlled trial of the use of bicarbonate in the prevention of CIN, focusing on patient-centered outcomes, has not been performed.

Acetylcysteine has been studied for the prevention of CIN as well. It is believed that the antioxidative effects of acetylcysteine may limit the potentially tubulotoxic effects of contrast media. In a meta-analysis that included more than 800 patients, Birck and colleagues[42] suggest that, when compared with periprocedural hydration alone, the use of acetylcysteine plus hydration significantly reduces the relative risk of CIN in patients with preexisting chronic renal insufficiency. However, additional large, prospective, randomized studies with patient-centered outcomes will be helpful in resolving questions surrounding the use of NAC, especially in patients without known preexisting renal disease, and in those receiving common ED diagnostic imaging (CT scans rather than coronary angiography).

Sinert and Doty[43] reviewed the literature in an attempt to discover which methods for preventing CIN might be best used in the ED setting. They point out that one of the most difficult tasks for the EP when reviewing the literature on strategies to prevent CIN is to determine how these strategies may be applied in the outpatient or ED setting, where a 12-hour or 24-hour pretreatment /posttreatment strategy is not practical. Although they found that several published studies include regimens that could be used in the ED setting, many studies had significant limitations, including patients lost to follow up, lack of patient-centered outcomes, and variability in the definition of CIN. Most studies use either a 25% increase in SCr or an absolute increase of 0.5 mg/dL to define CIN, although it is clear that, in some studies, the use of one measure may produce vastly different outcomes and recommendations than the use of the other. Furthermore, neither a percentage increase nor an absolute increase in SCr necessarily portends worse outcomes for patients.

The elderly, diabetics, patients with chronic renal insufficiency, and patients who are already on nephrotoxic medications are at higher risk for poor outcomes following radiocontrast administration. Therefore, it is certainly reasonable for the EP to focus special attention on these groups when considering radiographic testing and the need for IV contrast. If the study is clearly indicated and contrast cannot be avoided, the use of IV hydration to minimize the effect on the kidney is certainly supported by the literature. The use of bicarbonate may also be considered safe and effective. Future trials may provide additional information regarding alternate strategies appropriate for the prevention of CIN in the ED setting.

SUMMARY

EPs encounter many patients who present with either CKD or AKI. It is important that the chronicity is established and, when possible, the etiology be identified. However, in the midst of diagnostic testing, both for renal disease and for other emergency conditions, perhaps the most important role of the EP is to subscribe to the principle of non-maleficence (first, do no harm), and do everything in their power to prevent renal insult or damage by ensuring appropriate hydration and limiting the use of nephrotoxic medications and IV contrast agents in patients who exhibit renal dysfunction. When these agents cannot be avoided, appropriate strategies should be used in an attempt to minimize the risk of further damage. In certain cases, early nephrology consultation and admission for further evaluation and treatment may offer the patient the best opportunity to restore or preserve renal function.

REFERENCES

1. Leavey AS, Bosch JP, Lewis JB, et al. A more accurate method to estimate glomerular filtration rate from serum creatinine: a new prediction equation. Modification of Diet in Renal Disease Study Group. Ann Intern Med 1999;130: 461–570.
2. Cockcroft DW, Gault MH. Prediction of creatinine clearance from serum creatinine. Nephron 1976;16:31–41.
3. Thaemer M, Ray NF, Fehrenbach SN, et al. Relative risk and economic consequences of inpatient care among patients with renal failure. J Am Soc Nephrol 1996;7:751–62.
4. US Renal Data System (USRDS) 2010 annual data report: atlas of chronic kidney disease and end-stage renal disease in the United States. Bethesda (MD): National Institutes of Health, National Institute of Diabetes and Digestive and Kidney Diseases; 2010.
5. Sarnak MJ, Jaber BL. Mortality caused by sepsis in patients with end-stage renal disease compared with the general population. Kidney Int 2000;58:1758–64.
6. Chertow GM, Burdick E, Honour M, et al. Acute kidney injury, mortality, length of stay, and costs in hospitalized patients. J Am Soc Nephrol 2005;16:3365–70.
7. Uchino S, Kellum JA, Bellomo R, et al. Acute renal failure in critically ill patients, a multinational, multicenter study. JAMA 2005;294:813–8.
8. Coca S, Yusuf B, Shlipak M, et al. Long-term risk of mortality and other adverse outcomes after acute kidney injury: a systematic review and meta-analysis. Am J Kidney Dis 2009;6:961–73.
9. Coca S, Peixoto A, Garg A, et al. The prognostic importance of a small acute decrement in kidney function in hospitalized patients: a systematic review and meta-analysis. Am J Kidney Dis 2007;50:712–20.
10. Bellomo R, Ronco C, Kellum JA, et al. Acute renal failure- definition, outcome measures, animal models, fluid therapy and information technology needs: the Second International Consensus Conference of the Acute Dialysis Quality Initiative (ADQI) Group. Crit Care 2004;9(4):R204–12.
11. Uchino S, Bellomo R, Goldsmith D, et al. An assessment of the RIFLE criteria for acute renal failure in hospitalized patients. Crit Care Med 2006;34:1913–7.
12. Mehta RL, Kellum JA, Shah SV, et al. Acute Kidney Injury Network (AKIN): report of an initiative to improve outcomes in acute kidney injury. Crit Care 2007;11:R31.
13. Barrantes F, Tian J, Vazquez R, et al. Acute kidney injury criteria predict outcomes of critically ill patients. Crit Care Med 2008;36:1397–403.
14. Battle D, Arruda J, Kurtzman N. Hyperkalemic distal renal tubular acidosis associated with obstructive uropathy. N Engl J Med 1981;304:373–80.
15. Parham W, Mehdirad A, Biermann K, et al. Hyperkalemia revisited. Tex Heart Inst J 2006;33:40–7.

16. Kim H. Acute therapy for hyperkalemia with the combined regimen of bicarbonate and beta2-adrenergic agonist (salbutamol) in chronic renal failure patients. J Korean Med Sci 1997;12:111–6.
17. Kim H. Combined effect of bicarbonate and insulin with glucose in acute therapy of hyperkalemia in end-stage renal disease patients. Nephron 1996;38:476–82.
18. Kamel K, Wei C. Controversial issues in the treatment of hyperkalemia. Nephrol Dial Transplant 2003;18:2215–8.
19. Sterns R, Rojas M, Bernstein P, et al. Ion-exchange resins for the treatment of hyperkalemia: are they safe and effective? J Am Soc Nephrol 2010;21:733–5.
20. Mehta R, McDonald B, Gabbai F, et al. Nephrology consultation in acute renal failure: does timing matter? Am J Med 2002;113:456–61.
21. Fertel B, Nelson L, Goldfarb D. Extracorporeal removal techniques for the poisoned patient: a review for the intensivist. J Int Care Med 2010;25:139–48.
22. Mehta R, Pascual M, Soroko S, et al. Diuretics, mortality, and non-recovery of renal function in acute renal failure. JAMA 2002;288:2547–53.
23. Uchino S, Doig GS, Bellomo R, et al. Diuretics and mortality in acute renal failure. Crit Care Med 2004;32:1669–77.
24. Burke TJ, Arnold PE, Schrier RW. Prevention of ischemic acute renal failure with impermeant solutes. Am J Physiol 1983;244:F646–9.
25. Wiemar W, Geerglins W, Bijnen AB, et al. A controlled study on the effect of mannitol on immediate renal function after cadaver donor kidney transplantation. Transplantation 1983;35:99–101.
26. Shilliday I, Allison ME. Diuretics in acute renal failure. Ren Fail 1994;16:3–17.
27. Lee RW, Di Giantomasso D, May C, et al. Vasoactive drugs and the kidney. Best Pract Res Clin Anaesthesiol 2004;18:53–73.
28. Bellomo R, Chapman M, Finfer S, et al. Low-dose dopamine in patients with early renal dysfunction: a placebo-controlled randomized trial. Australian and New Zealand Intensive Care Society (ANZICS) Clinical Trials Group. Lancet 2000; 356:2139–43.
29. Kellum J, Decker J. Use of dopamine in acute renal failure: a meta-analysis. Crit Care Med 2001;29(8):1526–31.
30. Halpenny M, Markos F, Snow H, et al. Effects of prophylactic fenoldopam infusion on renal blood flow and renal tubular function during acute hypovolemia in anesthetized dogs. Crit Care Med 2001;29(4):855–60.
31. Halpenny M, Lakshmi S, O'Donnell A, et al. Fenoldopam: renal and splanchnic effects in patients undergoing coronary artery bypass grafting. Anesthesia 2001; 56:953–60.
32. Kini A, Mitre C, Kamran M, et al. Changing trends in incidence and predictors of radiographic contrast nephropathy after percutaneous coronary intervention with use of fenoldopam. Am J Cardiol 2002;89:999–1002.
33. Nash K, Hafeez A, Hou S. Hospital-acquired renal insufficiency. Am J Kidney Dis 2002;39:930–6.
34. Rudnick M, Feldman H. Contrast-induced nephropathy: what are the true clinical consequences? Clin J Am Soc Nephrol 2008;3:263–72.
35. Mitchell A, Jones A, Tumlin J, et al. Incidence of contrast-induced nephropathy after contrast-enhanced computed tomography in the outpatient setting. Clin J Am Soc Nephrol 2010;5:4–9.
36. Katzberg R, Lamba R. Contrast-induced nephropathy after intravenous administration: fact or fiction? Radiol Clin North Am 2009;47:789–800.
37. Barret BJ, Carlisle EJ. Meta-analysis of the relative nephrotoxicity of high and low-osmolality iodinated contrast media. Radiology 1993;188:171–8.

38. Mueller C. Prevention of contrast-induced nephropathy with volume supplementation. Kidney Int 2006;69:S16–9.
39. Bader B, Berger E, Heede M, et al. What is the best hydration regimen to prevent contrast media-induced nephrotoxicity? Clin Nephrol 2004;62:1–7.
40. Krasuski R, Beard B, Geoghagan J, et al. Optimal timing of hydration to erase contrast-associated nephropathy: the OTHER CAN study. J Invasive Cardiol 2003;15:699–702.
41. Navaneethan S, Singh S, Appasamy S, et al. Sodium bicarbonate therapy for prevention of contrast-induced nephropathy: a systematic review and meta-analysis. Am J Kidney Dis 2009;53:617–27.
42. Birck R, Krzossok S, Markowetz F, et al. Acetylcysteine for prevention of contrast nephropathy: meta-analysis. Lancet 2003;362:598–603.
43. Sinert R, Doty C. Prevention of contrast-induced nephropathy in the emergency department. Ann Emerg Med 2007;50:335–44.
44. Molitoris B, Melnikov V, Okusa M, et al. Technology insight: biomarker development in acute kidney injury-what can we anticipate? Nat Clin Pract Nephrol 2008;4:154–65.
45. Wheeler D, Devarajan P, Ma Q, et al. Serum neutrophil gelatinase-associated lipocalin (NGAL) as a marker of acute kidney injury in critically ill children with septic shock. Crit Care Med 2008;36:1297–303.
46. Coca SG, Yalavarthy R, Concato J, et al. Biomarkers for the diagnosis and risk stratification of acute kidney injury: a systematic review. Kidney Int 2008;73:1008–16.
47. Han W, Bailley V, Abichandani R, et al. Kidney injury molecule-1 (KIM-1): a novel biomarker for human renal proximal tubule injury. Kidney Int 2002;62:237–44.

Emergency Department Management of Sexually Transmitted Infections

Joelle Borhart, MD[a,*], Diane M. Birnbaumer, MD[b]

KEYWORDS

- Emergency department • Sexually transmitted infections
- Gonorrhea • Chlamydia • Urethritis • Cervicitis • Genital ulcers

Sexually transmitted infections (STIs) are among the most common infections in the United States. Patients seeking treatment of STIs account for a large number of emergency department (ED) visits per year. Approximately 171,000 adolescents alone present to the ED each year for evaluation of a STI.[1] In addition, ED patients have been shown to have a high rate of asymptomatic STIs.[2] A recent study in Baltimore found that 13.6% of 18- to 31-year-old ED patients seeking medical treatment of any nature tested positive for either gonorrhea or chlamydia.[3]

Despite this large volume of patients, STIs are often missed or treated inappropriately. A 2004 study showed that ED treatment of patients with pelvic inflammatory disease (PID) was fully compliant with the US Centers for Disease Control and Prevention (CDC) recommendations only 27% of the time.[1] A second study found that more than half (58%) of women with gonorrhea or chlamydia infection were discharged from the ED without effective therapy.[4] Due to the high prevalence and incidence of STIs in the United States, it is important that emergency practitioners recognize symptoms consistent with STIs, and treat presumptively. This practice leads to overtreatment of STIs[5,6]; however, when weighed against the public health risk and complications of untreated disease, empiric treatment is recommended. The CDC published their most recent evidence-based treatment guidelines for STIs in 2010, which is an

---

The authors have nothing to disclose.

[a] Department of Emergency Medicine, Georgetown University/Washington Hospital Center, 110 Irving Street NW, Washington, DC 20010, USA

[b] Department of Emergency Medicine, Harbor-University of California, Los Angeles (UCLA) Medical Center, David Geffen School of Medicine at UCLA, 1000 West Carson Street, Building D9, Box 21, Torrance, CA 90509, USA

* Corresponding author.

E-mail address: joelle.borhart@gmail.com

Emerg Med Clin N Am 29 (2011) 587–603
doi:10.1016/j.emc.2011.04.008 emed.theclinics.com
0733-8627/11/$ – see front matter

excellent resource for providers (available from: http://www.cdc.gov/std/treatment/2010/default.htm). A summary of all CDC treatment recommendations for STIs appears in **Table 1**.

EPIDEMIOLOGY

Groups at high risk for STIs include adolescents, men who have sex with men (MSM), pregnant women, and those who exchange sex for money or drugs. Adolescents continue to have the highest rates of STIs, with young people aged 15 to 24 years accounting for almost half of all newly acquired STIs.[7] However, STIs pose a significant public health risk in virtually all demographic groups. It is important for emergency physicians to maintain a high level of awareness and avoid stereotyping patients. It is interesting that elderly patients have recently emerged as a population at increasing risk for STIs,[8] particularly older men who are widowed or using erectile dysfunction drugs such as sildenafil.[9] One recent study found that men older than 40 using erectile dysfunction drugs were 2 to 3 times more likely than nonusers to contract human immunodeficiency virus (HIV).[10,11]

In 2009, more than 1.2 million new cases of chlamydia—the largest number of cases of any STI—were reported to the CDC. The rate of reported chlamydia infection continues to increase, by 2.8% in 2009 compared with the rate in 2008.[12] The CDC estimates that the national prevalence of herpes simplex type 2, the cause of most cases of genital herpes, is 16.2%.[13] More than 300,000 cases of gonorrhea were reported in the United States in 2009, and reported cases of syphilis have been increasing annually since 2001.[12] As many STIs go undiagnosed, reported cases reflect only a fraction of the true disease burden in the United States.

Among reportable STIs (chlamydia, gonorrhea, and syphilis) there are enormous racial disparities, with African Americans being hardest hit. The racial imbalance is especially striking with respect to gonorrhea. In 2008, blacks made up only 12% of the total United States population but accounted for more than 70% of the gonorrhea cases. Syphilis and chlamydia rates were both about 8 times higher in blacks than in whites. Hispanic Americans are also disproportionally affected, with rates at least twice that of whites for all 3 reportable STIs.[12]

EMERGENCY DEPARTMENT APPROACH TO THE PATIENT WITH POSSIBLE STI

In addition to the standard information obtained during a history and physical examination, emergency physicians should elicit specific information when evaluating a patient with a suspected STI. Patients should be asked if they have a new sexual partner, multiple sex partners, unprotected sex, or recently have had sexual contact with someone known to have an STI. It must be noted that monogamous patients may acquire an STI if their partner is active outside the relationship. Symptoms such as genital lesions (ulcers, papules), rashes, genital or eye discharge, joint complaints, or systemic symptoms help narrow the differential diagnosis in a patient with a possible STI. Physical examination should also focus on these areas; patients with rectal complaints should have a rectal examination performed, and all women should have a pelvic examination.[14] All patients should have specific testing for STIs performed, and women should be tested for pregnancy.

STIs PRESENTING WITH URETHRITIS OR CERVICITIS

It is helpful to divide patients into two groups: those presenting with complaints consistent with urethritis or cervicitis, and those with genital ulcers. The primary pathogens responsible for urethritis and cervicitis are *Chlamydia trachomatis* and *Neisseria gonorrhoeae*; *Trichomonas vaginalis*, *Mycoplasma*, and *Ureaplamsa* have also been implicated. Organisms causing genital ulcers include chancroid, herpes genitalis, syphilis, and the lymphogranuloma venereum (LGV) serotype of *C trachomatis*.

Men are considered to have urethritis if they present with at least one of the following: mucopurulent or purulent discharge, a positive leukocyte esterase test on first void urine, at least 10 white blood cells (WBC) per high-power field in urine sediment, or Gram stain of urethral secretions demonstrating at least 5 WBC per oil immersion field. Cervicitis is defined by the presence of purulent, endocervical exudate, or easily induced endocervical bleeding with gentle use of cotton-tipped swab.[15] It is impossible to clinically distinguish infections caused by chlamydia from those caused by gonorrhea, and they often exist as coinfections. Therefore, the CDC recommends presumptive treatment of both chlamydia and gonorrhea for men with urethritis, and for women with cervicitis if the woman is deemed at high risk for either STI (age less than 25 years, new or multiple sexual partners), especially if follow-up cannot be assured. In addition, all patients with cervicitis and urethritis should be referred for HIV, syphilis, and hepatitis B testing, as coinfection is common.[15]

Chlamydia

Patients with *C trachomatis* infection are often asymptomatic, particularly women. When present, symptoms in women may include mucopurulent cervicitis, dysuria, or PID. Men may present with purulent or mucopurulent discharge, dysuria, urethral pruritus, epididymitis, or proctitis. Chlamydia infections of the upper female genital tract can cause long-term sequelae for women, including infertility and increased risk for ectopic pregnancy.[16] About 1% of patients (mostly men) may develop a reactive arthritis with associated urethritis (formerly known as Reiter syndrome).[17–19]

Diagnosis

Culture and nucleic acid hybridization tests can detect *C trachomatis*, though both require urethral or cervical swabs. Nucleic acid amplification tests (NAATs) can be performed on swabs or urine specimens, and have excellent sensitivity and specificity, and therefore are the test of choice for detecting *C trachomatis*.[20]

Treatment

Both azithromycin, 1 g orally as a single dose and doxycycline, 100 mg orally twice a day for 7 days are equally effective in treating chlamydia. Azithromycin is safe in pregnancy, whereas doxycycline is contraindicated.[15] Single-dose therapy is inadequate to treat chlamydial infection of the upper female genital tract (eg, PID).

Gonorrhea

Gonorrhea infection, the second most commonly reported STI in the United States, is caused by the gram-negative diplococcus *N gonorrhoeae*. Like chlamydia, asymptomatic infection is common for women, but some patients will have vaginal discharge, dysuria, or PID. Men frequently present with purulent discharge and dysuria. The discharge associated with gonorrhea classically is more purulent and copious than that of chlamydia. Gonorrheal infections can be spread to the rectum from contaminated vaginal secretions or through anal intercourse, and may cause tenesmus, itching, or a bloody, mucoid discharge.[21]

N gonorrhoeae can disseminate, typically causing septic arthritis, tenosynovitis, and skin lesions described as necrotic pustules on an erythematous base. Patients with joint manifestations of disseminated gonococcal infection (DGI) typically present

Table 1
Sexually transmitted infections: treatment recommendations

STI	Recommended Treatment	Treatment Alternatives
Chlamydia	Azithromycin 1 g orally in a single dose[a] Doxycycline 100 mg orally twice a day for 7 days	Erythromycin base 500 mg orally 4 times a day for 7 days Erythromycin ethylsuccinate 800 mg orally 4 times a day for 7 days Ofloxacin 300 mg orally twice a day for 7 days Levofloxacin 500 mg orally once a day for 7 days
Gonorrhea (uncomplicated)	Ceftriaxone 250 mg IM in a single dose[a]	Cefixime 400 mg orally in single dose Azithromycin 2 g orally in single dose[b]
Gonorrhea (disseminated)	Ceftriaxone 1 g IV every 24 h	Cefotaxime 1 g IV every 8 h Ceftizoxime 1 g IV every 8 h
Trichomonas	Metronidazole 2 g orally in a single dose[a] Tinidazole 2 g orally in a single dose	Metronidazole 500 mg orally twice a day for 7 days
Bacterial vaginosis	Metronidazole 500 mg orally twice a day for 7 days[a] Metronidazole gel, 0.75%, one full applicator (5 g) intravaginally, once a day for 5 days Clindamycin cream, 2%, one full applicator (5 g) intravaginally at bedtime for 7 days	Tinidazole 2 g orally once daily for 2 days Tinidazole 1 g orally daily for 5 days Clindamycin 300 mg orally twice a day for 7 days[a] Clindamycin ovules 100 mg intravaginally at bedtime for 3 days
Vulvovaginal candidiasis	Fluconazole 150 mg orally in a single dose Butoconazole 2% cream (single dose bioadhesive product), 5 g intravaginally for 1 day Nystatin 100,000-unit vaginal tablet, 1 tablet daily for 14 days Terconazole 0.4% cream 5 g intravaginally for 7 days[a] Terconazole 0.8% cream 5 g intravaginally for 3 days Terconazole 80 mg vaginal suppository, one suppository for 3 days	
Genital herpes (first episode)	Valacyclovir 1 g orally twice a day for 7–10 days Famciclovir 250 mg orally 3 times a day for 7–10 days Acyclovir 400 mg orally 3 times a day for 7–10 days[a] Acyclovir 200 mg orally 5 times a day for 7–10 days[a]	

(*continued on next page*)

Table 1
(continued)

STI	Recommended Treatment	Treatment Alternatives
Genital herpes (recurrent)	Acyclovir 400 mg orally 3 times a day for 5 days Acyclovir 800 mg orally twice a day for 5 days Acyclovir 800 mg orally 3 times a day for 2 days Famciclovir 125 mg orally twice a day for 5 days Famciclovir 1000 mg orally twice a day for 1 day Valacyclovir 500 mg orally twice a day for 3 days Valacyclovir 1 g orally once a day for 5 days	
Syphilis	Benzathine penicillin G 2.4 million units IM as a single dose[a] *If penicillin allergic consider desensitization, particularly if patient is pregnant*	Doxycycline 100 mg orally twice a day for 28 days Tetracycline 500 mg orally 4 times a day for 28 days
Chancroid	Azithromycin 1 g orally in a single dose[a] Ceftriaxone 250 mg IM in a single dose[a] Ciprofloxacin 500 mg orally twice a day for 3 days Erythromycin base 500 mg orally 3 times a day for 7 days	
Lymphogranuloma venereum	Doxycycline 100 mg orally twice a day for 21 days	Erythromycin base 500 mg orally 4 times a day for 21 days[a]
Genital warts (external)	Podofilox 0.5% solution or gel applied to visible warts twice a day for 3 days, then nontherapy for 4 days. Repeat up to 4 cycles Imiquimod 5% cream applied to warts once daily at bedtime 3 times a week up to 16 weeks Sinecatechins 15% ointment applied to warts 3 times a day for up to 16 weeks Podophyllin resin 10%–25% Trichloroacetic acid or bichloroacetic acid 80%–90% Cryotherapy	Intralesional interferon Laser surgery

Abbreviations: IM, intramuscular; IV, intravenous.

[a] Recommended treatment in pregnancy.

[b] CDC does not recommend widespread use because of concerns of resistance.

Data from Centers for Disease Control and Prevention. Sexually transmitted diseases treatment guidelines. MMWR Morb Mortal Wkly Rep 2010;59:1–110.

with monoarticular pain, redness, and swelling.[22] Commonly affected joints include the knees, wrists, ankles, and elbows in decreasing order of frequency. Gonorrhea is the most common cause of septic arthritis in sexually active young adults. In DGI, migratory polyarthralgia is characteristic, and skin lesions are seen in 75% of patients.[23] Patients may have fever and appear toxic. Rarely, DGI can cause endocarditis or meningitis.

Diagnosis

In symptomatic men, a Gram stain of urethral discharge showing intracellular gram-negative diplococci is highly specific (>99%) and considered diagnostic for *N gonorrhoeae* infection.[15] The Gram stain has little utility for women.[24] Culture has a high sensitivity (85%–96%)[25] and provides the ability to isolate organisms for antimicrobial sensitivity, but requires special handling conditions. The CDC recommends the use of NAATs on either urine or urethral/cervical swabs when the necessary culture conditions cannot be assured.

Treatment

In April 2007, the CDC announced that only cephalosporins should be used to treat gonococcal infections in the United States because of increasing resistance to fluoroquinolones.[26] Unfortunately, this means that treatment options are very limited, particularly for patients with cephalosporin allergies. As first-line treatment, CDC now recommends a single intramuscular (IM) dose of ceftriaxone, 250 mg; this represents a change from previous CDC guidelines, which had recommended ceftriaxone 125 mg. If ceftriaxone 250 mg IM is not an option, then a single oral dose of cefixime, 400 mg is also acceptable; however, this does not provide as high, nor as sustained, a bactericidal level as 250 mg ceftriaxone.[15,27] A single oral dose of 2 g of azithromycin can be used in patients with documented cephalosporin allergy and who are unable to be desensitized. This regimen is effective against most uncomplicated gonococcal infections, but the CDC discourages widespread use of azithromycin because of concerns for increasing resistance. Hospitalization is recommended for disseminated infections, and recommended initial treatment is ceftriaxone, 1 g intravenously every 24 hours.[28]

Trichomonal Infections

Trichomoniasis is caused by *Trichomonas vaginalis*, a flagellated protozoan. Frequent signs of infection in women include vaginal irritation and foul-smelling, thin discharge.[29,30] The classic yellow-green discharge, which is sometimes described as "foamy" or "frothy," is seen in only 10% of affected women.[31] Men may present with urethritis. Although clinical symptoms are often relatively benign, trichomonal infections are associated with adverse outcomes during pregnancy, such as premature delivery and low birth weight.[32]

Diagnosis

Culture, while a very sensitive and specific test, is rarely performed. A wet mount is often used to look for the microscopic parasites, but the sensitivity is low (51%–70%).[15,33–36] Vaginal pH is commonly elevated (>4.5). The US Food and Drug Administration has recently cleared two point-of-care tests that are performed on vaginal secretions, and tend to be more sensitive than wet mount preparations (sensitivity >83% for both tests).[15]

Treatment

The only recommended class of drugs for the treatment of trichomonal infections is the nitroimidazoles; specifically a single dose of metronidazole 2 g orally, or a single dose of tinidazole 2 g orally. Metronidazole gel is considerably less efficacious.[15] Treatment of pregnant patients is somewhat controversial, especially in the first trimester, but the CDC states that metronidazole 2 g orally may be used at any stage of pregnancy (pregnancy category B). Lactating women may receive either drug, but should avoid breast-feeding for 24 hours after last dose of metronidazole, and for 3 days after the last dose of tinidazole. All patients should avoid consuming alcohol while on nitromidazoles, as they may experience a disulfiram-type reaction including nausea, vomiting, and skin flushing.

Summary of Diseases Characterized by Cervicitis/Urethritis

Chlamydia, gonorrhea, and trichomoniasis are all common STIs, and patients with these infections frequently present to the ED. Although more rapid testing now exists to detect gonorrhea and chlamydia infections, the results are usually not available during the same patient visit. Certain EDs do have access to direct microscopy, and wet mounts of vaginal secretions can be prepared to establish a definitive diagnosis of *Trichomonas* infection in some women. Several studies have examined whether confirmed *Trichomonas* infection be used as a marker for the presence of coinfection with chlamydia, gonorrhea, or both. Older studies found that *Trichomonas* is frequently associated with chlamydia and/or gonorrhea infection.[37,38] However, more recent literature suggests that there is no relationship between *Trichomonas* infection and infection with gonorrhea and/or chlamydia,[39] or perhaps even a negative association.[40] As coinfection with *Trichomonas* and chlamydia and/or gonorrhea is known to occur, and the health consequences of untreated disease can be severe, the authors recommend that emergency physicians have a low threshold for presumptively treating all 3 infections in high-risk patients.

DISEASES CHARACTERIZED BY VAGINAL DISCHARGE

Bacterial vaginosis and vulvovaginal candidiasis are common causes of vaginal discharge and irritation. These infections are not typically transmitted sexually, but are discussed briefly because they are often diagnosed in women being evaluated for STIs. Trichomoniasis also commonly causes vaginal discharge.

Bacterial Vaginosis

Bacterial vaginosis (BV) occurs when the normal, lactobacilli-dominant vaginal flora is replaced with higher concentrations of anaerobic bacteria. As no transmissible agent has been identified, BV is not considered an STI.[41] However, BV is associated with having new or multiple sex partners, and women who have never been sexually active are rarely affected. The majority of women with BV are asymptomatic. Those experiencing symptoms most frequently report a foul vaginal odor often described as "fishy." Vaginal discharge may also be present, and is classically thin and gray-white in color.[15]

Diagnosis

The diagnosis of BV can be made using clinical criteria requiring at least 3 of the following: homogeneous vaginal discharge that smoothly covers the vaginal walls, presence of clue cells on microscopic examination, pH of vaginal fluid greater than 4.5, and a fishy odor of vaginal discharge before or after addition of 10% potassium hydroxide (ie, whiff test). Gram stain may also be used and is considered the gold standard.[15]

Treatment

Treatment recommendations include metronidazole, 500 mg orally twice a day for 7 days, or metronidazole gel, 0.75%, one full applicator (5 g) intravaginally once a day for 5 days, or clindamycin cream, 2%, one full applicator (5 g) intravaginally at bedtime for 7 days. Metronidazole gel is equally efficacious compared with oral metronidazole when treating BV (unlike *Trichomonas* infection). It must be noted that metronidazole 2 g orally (recommended treatment of *Trichomonas* infection) is not effective against BV. To effectively treat for both *Trichomonas* and BV, metronidazole 500 mg orally twice a day for 7 days should be used.[15]

Vulvovaginal Candidiasis

Vulvovaginal candidiasis (VVC) is caused by *Candida albicans* in about 90% of cases. The predominant symptom is pruritus, which may be associated with vulvar burning, edema, excoriations, or fissures. Many women will also have discharge that is thick and white, often described as "cottage-cheese like" or "curdy." The discharge usually does not have an odor.[41]

Diagnosis

The diagnosis of VVC is established by either Gram stain or wet preparation (saline, 10% potassium hydroxide) of vaginal secretions that shows yeast or pseudohyphae. Vaginal culture for *Candida* may also be used. Vaginal pH is typically normal (<4.5).

Treatment

Fluconazole, 150 mg orally as a one-time dose may be used as treatment. A variety of prescription and over-the-counter topical formulations are also effective (see **Table 1**).

Summary of Diseases Causing Vaginal Discharge

There is significant overlap of clinical signs and symptoms among conditions causing vaginal discharge. In a review of studies published between 1966 and 2003, the clinical examination was found to be of limited usefulness in distinguishing between BV, VVC, and trichomoniasis. Several symptoms can support the diagnosis of one condition over another, such as "cheesy" discharge being strongly predictive of VVC. However, symptoms alone were not found to be sufficient in making an accurate diagnosis.[42,43] Microscopy lacks sensitivity in diagnosing all 3 diseases.[15,42]

Vaginal pH has been investigated for its usefulness as a diagnostic tool. One study found that for women with vaginitis symptoms undiagnosed by pelvic examination and wet mount, empiric treatment based on pH reduced symptoms and was cost effective.[44] However, many factors can temporarily alter vaginal pH, such as the presence of semen, making pH unreliable.[41,42] Perhaps most frustrating is that even after a thorough clinical evaluation, approximately 30% of women with vaginal discharge remain undiagnosed.[42]

Vaginal discharge is common, and challenging to diagnose effectively in the ED. Current vaginitis research has several weaknesses, and it is difficult to draw firm conclusions regarding empiric treatment recommendations. One consistent theme in the vaginitis literature is the need for an updated diagnostic approach.[42,45–48] Until then, the authors recommend that emergency physicians consider empirically treating women with fluconazole, metronidazole, or both, based on clinical suspicion. Moreover, women with chlamydia and gonorrhea infections may also present with vaginal discharge. The authors believe that this warrants considering single-dose treatment for both gonorrhea and chlamydia in women with vaginal discharge who are deemed at high risk for these infections.

STIs CAUSING GENITAL ULCERS

The most prevalent disease in the United States causing genital ulcers is genital herpes.[15] Syphilis, chancroid, and LGV also cause genital ulcers, and patients can be infected with more than one of these diseases concurrently.

Symptoms of the 4 infections are similar and may overlap, making a clinical diagnosis challenging. An important distinction is whether the ulcers are painful or painless (**Table 2**). Herpes and chancroid lesions tend to be painful, whereas the primary syphilis lesion and ulcers associated with LGV are typically painless. All 4 diseases can be associated with regional lymphadenopathy. In herpes and syphilis, patients often present with bilateral lymphadenopathy that is tender in herpes but nontender in syphilis. Both chancroid and LGV are typically associated with a unilateral, tender lymphadenopathy.[49] Primary infection with herpes genitalis often causes systemic symptoms such as fever, fatigue, and myalgias.

Because early treatment is important to the successful treatment of genital ulcers and decreases transmission to others, emergency practitioners are encouraged to treat empirically for the most likely diagnosis, based on presentation and epidemiologic data, while waiting for the results of confirmatory diagnostic tests.

Genital Herpes

Herpes simplex virus type 2 (HSV-2) and herpes simplex virus type 1 (HSV-1) are extremely prevalent worldwide, and cause lifelong, incurable infections. HSV-2 is primarily contracted sexually, and in addition to causing most cases of genital herpes can make people at least twice as likely to become infected with HIV.[50] HSV-1 can also cause genital ulcers, but more commonly manifests as orolabial lesions, and is usually transmitted among children via nonsexual contact.[51]

Most HSV-2 infections are unrecognized. When symptoms are present, the clinical manifestations classically include multiple painful vesicles on an erythematous base (**Fig. 1**). Vesicles may be accompanied by fever, malaise, myalgias, and clear watery discharge in cases of first-episode genital herpes. Vesicles typically appear within 7 to 10 days after contact with an infected person, ulcerate and crust over 3 to 5 days after appearance, and heal completely within 3 weeks. Of importance is that individuals may continue to shed virus, thereby remaining infective to others even after the sores have healed.[52]

Some patients, particularly those with primary genital herpes, may develop complications. Up to 10% of patients develop aseptic meningitis, with symptoms and laboratory workup consistent with viral meningitis. Sacral radiculopathy syndrome can also occur, which is characterized by urinary retention and may require temporary urinary catheterization. Resolution typically occurs within 4 to 8 weeks.[52]

Table 2
Classic signs and symptoms of common STIs causing genital ulceration

STI	Lesion(s) Painful?	Inguinal Adenopathy
Genital herpes	Yes	Bilateral, painful
Chancroid	Yes	Unilateral, painful
Primary syphilis	No	Bilateral, painless
Lymphogranuloma venereum	No	Unilateral, painful

Note that these are broad generalizations; significant overlap in signs or symptoms may exist.

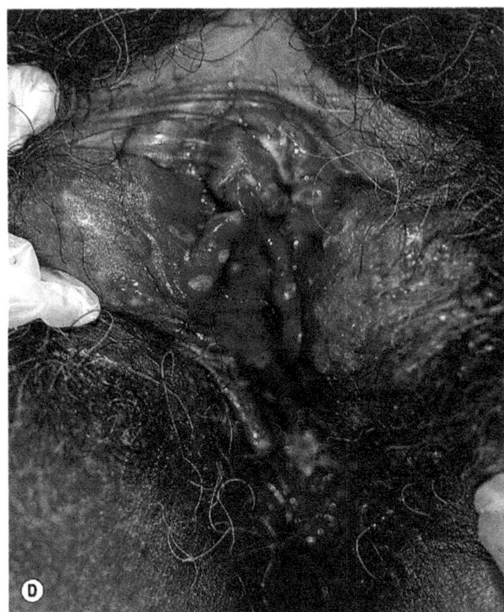

Fig. 1. Genital herpes. (*From* Habif TP. Sexually transmitted viral infections. In: Clinical dermatology: a color guide to diagnosis and therapy. 5th edition. Philadelphia: Mosby Elsevier; 2009. p. 433, with permission.)

Diagnosis

In the ED, diagnosis of genital herpes is often made clinically by recognizing the classic lesions. However, as clinical diagnosis is insensitive and nonspecific, the diagnosis should be confirmed by laboratory testing. Viral culture is the test of choice, though sensitivity is low (70%–80%) and further decreases as lesions heal.[21] The polymerase chain reaction is the test of choice for diagnosing HSV encephalitis and neonatal infections, though potential for genital herpes detection is unclear. Type-specific HSV serologic testing may be considered in some instances.[53]

Treatment

The CDC recommends that all patients receive antiviral therapy for first-episode herpes.[15] Acyclovir, valacyclovir, and famciclovir are the drugs of choice, and show equal efficacy. For severe, disseminated infection, the recommended regimen is acyclovir, 5 to 10 mg/kg intravenously every 8 hours. The majority of patients with a symptomatic first episode of genital herpes will go on to experience recurrence, albeit typically less clinically severe than the initial episode.[54] Episodic treatment of recurrent herpes can be effective if initiated within 1 day of lesion onset, or ideally during the prodrome phase that may precede an outbreak. For patients having more than 6 outbreaks per year, daily suppressive therapy is available, which in addition to consistent condom use can reduce transmission to sexual partners.

Syphilis

Syphilis, caused by the spirochete *Treponema pallidum*, progresses through primary, secondary, and tertiary stages if left untreated. The primary lesion, the chancre, is a painless ulcer with indurated borders that appears at the site of inoculation (**Fig. 2**). It will never appear vesicular. The chancre typically presents as a single lesion,

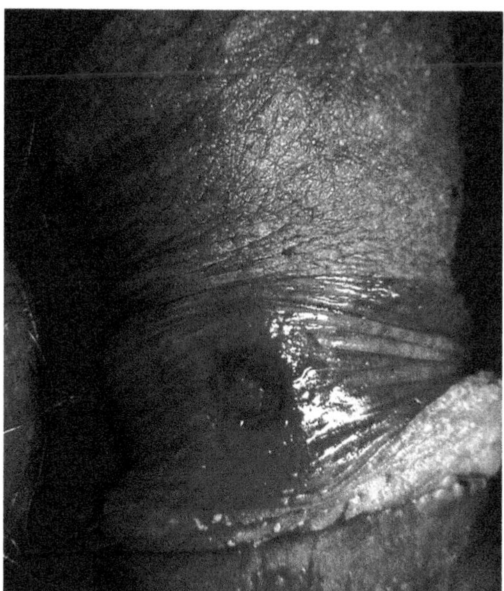

Fig. 2. Primary chancre of syphilis. (*From* Habif TP. Sexually transmitted bacterial infections. In: Clinical dermatology: a color guide to diagnosis and therapy. 5th edition. Philadelphia: Mosby Elsevier; 2009. p. 398; with permission.)

but they can be multiple, especially if the patient is coinfected with HIV.[55] The incubation period is approximately 21 days.[56] The chancre heals spontaneously within 6 weeks, and often goes unnoticed.

Weeks later, systemic systems such as generalized lymphadenopathy, malaise, fever, and rash develop as the patient enters the secondary stage. The rash of secondary syphilis is characteristically macular; lesions most often affect the trunk and flexor surfaces of limbs, and are found on the palms and soles 50% to 80% of the time.[57,58] The rash can mimic many dermatologic conditions, but like the primary chancre will never be vesicular. If untreated, the infection then enters latency. About one-third of these untreated patients will go on to develop tertiary syphilis, which can include cardiac, ophthalmic, and central nervous system manifestations over a period of years.[55–59]

Diagnosis

The definitive method for diagnosing early syphilis is dark-field microscopy of lesion exudate. It is possible to make the diagnosis using 2 types of serologic testing: nontreponemal (VDRL, RPR) and treponemal (FTA-ABS). A positive nontreponemal test must be confirmed with a treponemal test because a variety of conditions can cause a nontreponemal test to be falsely positive. After treatment, nontreponemal tests usually become nonreactive, although some patients have persistently detectable titers for life, also known as the serofast reaction. Treponemal tests remain reactive for life for the majority of patients.[15]

Treatment

For more than 50 years, penicillin G has been the mainstay of treatment for syphilis. The recommended regimen is benzathine penicillin G, 2.4 million units IM in a single dose. Doxycycline is the treatment alternative for patients allergic to penicillin, with the exception of pregnant patients who should be referred for desensitization. Patients should be informed of the possible Jarisch-Herxheimer reaction experienced by up to 60% of patients treated for early syphilis.[58] This reaction is characterized by a transient fever and is associated with malaise, headache, and myalgias occurring within 24 hours of treatment. In general, this reaction is self-limited and of little clinical significance. It can be treated symptomatically with antipyretics.

Chancroid

Chancroid is a rarely reported infection in the United States, with only 28 cases being reported in 2009.[12] *Haemophilus ducreyi* is the causative agent of chancroid, a disease characterized by painful genital ulcers and lymphadenitis. Within a week of infection, a small red papule forms at the site of inoculation. The papule then becomes pustular (as compared with HSV which is vesicular) before rupturing into a painful ulcer with ragged edges. Most patients will have multiple lesions. About half of patients will develop painful, unilateral lymphadenopathy, and if untreated the lymph nodes may necrose and turn into suppurative buboes, which may require incision and drainage.[60,61]

Diagnosis

The organism causing chancroid is fastidious and difficult to culture, making a definitive diagnosis difficult to obtain in the Unites States. Therefore, a probable diagnosis can be reached clinically if other diseases (such as syphilis) can be excluded.

Treatment

Successful treatment has been achieved using azithromycin, 1 g orally in a single dose, or ceftriaxone, 250 mg IM injection in a single dose, or ciprofloxacin, 500 mg orally twice a day for 3 days, or erythromycin base, 500 mg orally 3 times a day for 7 days.

Lymphogranuloma Venereum

LGV is caused by specific serotypes of *C trachomatis* and occurs sporadically in the United States. A recent increase in cases was noted in Europe, with the majority of cases affecting MSM also coinfected with HIV. These patients frequently presented with severe proctitis.[62] LGV infection classically has 3 stages, beginning with a painless ulcer or papule at the site of inoculation, which often goes unnoticed. The second stage is characterized by unilateral, tender, inguinal lymphadenopathy. Most patients will present in the second stage, after the primary lesion has resolved. In the last stage patients may develop scarring, strictures, and fistulas involving the anus, rectum, urethra, vagina, or uterus; this is caused by lymphatic damage from the second stage, and is sometimes confused with inflammatory bowel disease.[63]

Diagnosis

Specific LGV serologic tests are not widely available. The CDC recommends that providers treat empirically for LGV based on the clinical presentation after excluding other etiologies of proctitis, inguinal lymphadenopathy, or genital ulcers.

Treatment

Doxycycline, 100 mg orally twice a day is the treatment of choice. Erythromycin base, 500 mg orally 4 times a day is the treatment alternative for pregnant women. The duration of treatment should be 21 days, regardless of the agent used.

Genital Warts

Genital warts are caused by human papillomavirus (HPV). There are more than 100 different genotypes of HPV, 30 to 40 of which can cause warts in the anogenital area,[64] though types 6 and 11 account for 90% of cases.[65] Other types can cause cervical cancer. It is estimated that 75% of sexually active adults become infected with some form of genital HPV over their lifetime.[66] Like many STIs, most HPV infections are subclinical. Patients may present with multiple, painless flesh-colored papules or cauliflower-like lesions on the vulva or shaft of the penis (**Fig. 3**). Warts can also occur internally on the cervix or anus, even in people who do not have anal intercourse.

Diagnosis

The diagnosis of genital warts is made clinically by observing the characteristic growths. Biopsy can confirm the diagnosis if needed.

Treatment

Many treatment options for genital warts exist, and may be applied by either patient or provider. There is no evidence that one method is superior to others. The goal is to remove warts; treatment does not eliminate HPV infection or infectivity.[15] Patient-applied treatments include podofilox 0.5% solution (applied with cotton swab) or gel (applied with fingers) to warts twice a day for 3 days, then 4 days of no therapy, with the cycle repeated up to 4 times. An alternative treatment is imiquimod 5% cream, applied at bedtime 3 times per week for up to 16 weeks. If using imiquimod cream, the patient should be instructed to wash the treatment area 6 to 10 hours after application. Patients may also apply sinecatechin 15% ointment to warts using fingers 3 times daily until complete clearance of warts, with treatment time not to exceed

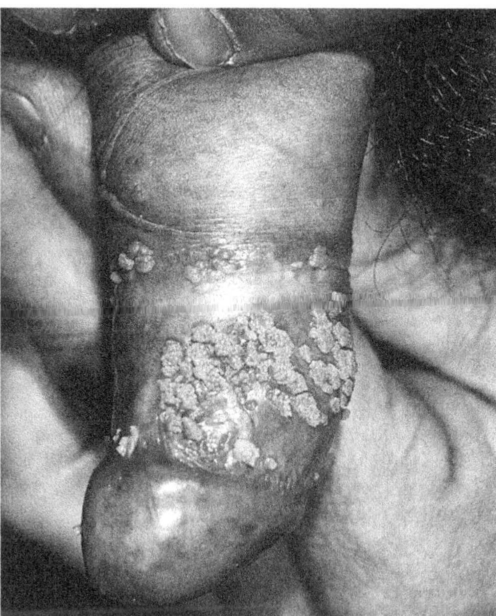

Fig. 3. Genital warts under foreskin. (*From* Habif TP. Sexually transmitted viral infections. In: Clinical dermatology: a color guide to diagnosis and therapy. 5th edition. Philadelphia: Mosby Elsevier; 2009. p. 421; with permission.)

16 weeks. Sinecatechin ointment should not be washed off after use. Provider-applied treatments include cryotherapy, podophyllin resin, trichloroacetic acid, and laser surgery, which are all typically performed in an office setting.[15]

DISPOSITION

With the exception of patients with complications of primary genital herpes infection or those with DGI, the vast majority of patients diagnosed with one of the aforementioned STIs will be able to be discharged home from the ED. If STI testing has not been obtained during the ED visit, the patient should be referred for follow-up testing, including HIV testing. Patients should be instructed to abstain from sexual activity for at least 7 days following initiation of treatment, regardless of treatment duration. Providers should urge their patients with STIs to notify their sexual partner(s) to seek medical evaluation and treatment. Physicians may prescribe antibiotics for the patient's sexual partner in a system known as Expedited Partner Therapy; however, laws regarding this practice vary by state, and physicians should familiarize themselves with the law in the state in which they practice (for more information, see http://www.cdc.gov/std/ept/default.htm). Patients should be educated on prevention of future STIs and the use of condoms, and appropriate follow-up should be arranged.[15,67,68]

SUMMARY

STIs are extremely common in the United States, and patients will continue to use the ED as a primary source of health care. As a result, emergency care providers have a unique opportunity to directly influence this serious public health issue. It is important to maintain a high index of suspicion for such infections, be familiar with signs and symptoms of common STIs, and have a low threshold for initiating empiric treatment in the ED.

REFERENCES

1. Beckmann KR, Melzer-Lange MD, Gorelick MH. Emergency department management of sexually transmitted infections in US adolescents: results from the national hospital ambulatory medical care survey. Ann Emerg Med 2004;43:333–8.
2. Mehta SD, Hall J, Lyss SB, et al. Adult and pediatric emergency department sexually transmitted disease and HIV screening: programmatic overview and outcomes. Acad Emerg Med 2007;14:250–8.
3. Mehta SD, Rothman RE, Kelen GD, et al. Unsuspected gonorrhea and chlamydia in patients of an urban adult emergency department: a critical population for STD control intervention. Sex Transm Dis 2001;28:33–9.
4. Bachmann LH, Pigott D, Desmond R, et al. Prevalence and factors associated with gonorrhea and chlamydia infection in at-risk females presenting to an urban emergency department. Sex Transm Dis 2003;30:335–9.
5. Levitt MA, Johnson S, Engelstad L, et al. Clinical management of chlamydia and gonorrhea infection in a community teaching emergency department: concerns in overtreatment, undertreatment, and follow-up treatment success. J Emerg Med 2003;25:7–11.
6. Todd CS, Haase C, Stoner BP. Emergency department screening for asymptomatic sexually transmitted infections. Am J Public Health 2001;91:461–4.
7. Weinstock H, Berman S, Cates W Jr. Sexually transmitted diseases among American youth: incidence and prevalence estimates, 2000. Perspect Sex Reprod Health 2004;36:6–10.

8. Kuehn BM. Time for "the Talk"—again. Seniors need information on sexual health. JAMA 2008;300:1285–7.
9. Smith KP, Christakis NA. Association between widowhood and risk of diagnosis with a sexually transmitted infection in older adults. Am J Public Health 2009; 99:2055–62.
10. Jena AB, Goldman DP, Kamdar A, et al. Sexually transmitted diseases among users of erectile dysfunction drugs: analysis of claims data. Ann Intern Med 2010;153:1–7.
11. Merchant RC, DePalo DM, Stein MD, et al. Adequacy of testing, empiric treatment, and referral for adult male Emergency Department patients with possible chlamydia and/or gonorrhea urethritis. Int J STD AIDS 2009;20:534–9.
12. Center for Disease Control and Prevention. Sexually transmitted disease surveillance, 2009. Atlanta (GA): CDC; 2009. Available at: http://www.cdc.gov/std/stats09/main.htm. Accessed January 1, 2011.
13. Center for Disease Control and Prevention. Seroprevalence of herpes simplex virus type 2 among persons aged 14–49 years—United States, 2005–2008. MMWR Morb Mortal Wkly Rep 2010;59:456–9.
14. Kravitz J, Promes SB. Sexually transmitted diseases. In: Tintinalli JE, Kelen GD, Stapczynski JS, editors. Emergency medicine: a comprehensive study guide. 6th edition. New York: McGraw-Hill; 2004. p. 909–13.
15. Center for Disease Control and Prevention. Sexually transmitted diseases treatment guidelines. MMWR Morb Mortal Wkly Rep 2010;59:1–110.
16. Paavonen J, Eggert-Kruse W. *Chlamydia trachomatis*: impact on human reproduction. Hum Reprod Update 1999;5:433–47.
17. Brill JR. Diagnosis and treatment of urethritis in men. Am Fam Physician 2010;81: 874–8.
18. Keat A. Extra-genital *Chlamydia trachomatis* infection as sexually-acquired reactive arthritis. J Infect 1992;25:47–9.
19. Miller KE. Diagnosis and treatment of *Chlamydia trachomatis* infection. Am Fam Physician 2006;8:1411–6.
20. Cook RL, Hutchison SL, Ostergaard L, et al. Systemic review: non-invasive testing for *Chlamydia trachomatis* and *Neisseria gonorrhoeae*. Ann Intern Med 2005;142:914–25.
21. Trigg BG, Kerndt PR, Aynalem G. Sexually transmitted infections and pelvic inflammatory disease in women. Med Clin North Am 2008;92:1083–113.
22. Dalla Vestra M, Rettore C, Sartore P, et al. Acute septic arthritis: remember gonorrhea. Rheumatol Int 2008;29:81–5.
23. Rice PA. Gonococcal arthritis (disseminated gonococcal infection). Infect Dis Clin North Am 2005;19:853–61.
24. Stefanski P, Hafner JW, Riley SL, et al. Diagnostic utility of the gram stain in ED patients. Am J Emerg Med 2010;28:13–8.
25. Yealy DM, Greene TJ, Hobbs GD. Underrecognition of cervical *Neisseria gonorrhoeae* and *Chlamydia trachomatis* infections in the emergency department. Acad Emerg Med 1997;4:962–7.
26. Center for Disease Control and Prevention. Update to CDC's 2006 sexually transmitted guidelines, 2006: fluoroquinolones no longer recommended for treatment of gonococcal infections. MMWR Morb Mortal Wkly Rep 2007;56:332–6.
27. Center for Disease Control and Prevention. Availability of cefixime 400 mg tablets-United States. MMWR Morb Mortal Wkly Rep 2008;57:435.
28. Cucurull E, Espinoza LR. Gonococcal arthritis. Rheum Dis Clin North Am 1998;24: 305–22.

29. Sena AC, Miller WC, Hobbs MM, et al. *Trichomonas vaginalis* infection in male sexual partners: implications for diagnosis, treatment, and prevention. Clin Infect Dis 2007;44:13–22.
30. Heine P, McGregor JA. *Trichomonas vaginalis*: a reemerging pathogen. Clin Obstet Gynecol 1993;36:137–44.
31. Schwebke JR. *Trichomonas vaginalis*. In: Mandell GL, Bennett JE, Dolin R, editors. Principles and practices of infectious disease. 7th edition. Philadelphia: Elsevier; 2009. p. 3535–8.
32. Cotch MF, Pastorek JG, Nugent RP, et al. *Trichomonas vaginalis* associated with low birth weight and preterm delivery. The Vaginal Infections and Prematurity Study Group. Sex Transm Dis 1997;24:353–60.
33. Pattullo L, Griffeth S, Ding L, et al. Stepwise diagnosis of *Trichomonas vaginalis* infection in adolescent women. J Clin Microbiol 2009;47:59–63.
34. Helms DJ, Mosure DJ, Secor EM, et al. Management of *Trichomonas vaginalis* in women with suspected metronidazole hypersensitivity. Am J Obstet Gynecol 2008;198:370.e1–7.
35. Krieger JN, Anagonou S. *Trichomonas vaginalis* and trichomoniasis. In: Holmes KK, Sparling PF, Mardh PA, et al, editors. Sexually transmitted diseases. 3rd edition. New York: McGraw-Hill; 1997. p. 587–604.
36. Van Der Pol B, Williams JA, Orr DP, et al. Prevalence, incidence, natural history, and response to treatment of *Trichomonas vaginalis* infection among adolescent women. J Infect Dis 2005;192:2039–44.
37. Reynolds M, Wilson J. Is *Trichomonas vaginalis* still a marker for other sexually transmitted infections in women? Int J STD AIDS 1996;7:131–2.
38. Pabst K, Reichart C, Knud-Hansen C, et al. Disease prevalence among women attending a sexually transmitted disease clinic varies with reason for visit. Sex Transm Dis 1992;19:88–91.
39. Wegner S, Jim Yen M, Witting M. Evidence against the “booty pack”: *Trichomonas* not associated with gonorrhea or chlamydia. J Emerg Med 2009;37:124–6.
40. White MJ, Sadalla JK, Springer SR, et al. Is the presence of *Trichomonas vaginalis* a reliable predictor of coinfection with *Chlamydia trachomatis* and/or *Neisseria gonorrhoeae* in female ED patients? Am J Emerg Med 2005;23:127–30.
41. Eckhert LO, Lentz GM. Infections of the lower genital tract: vulva, vagina, cervix, toxic shock syndrome, HIV infections. In: Katz VL, Lentz GM, Lobo RA, et al, editors. Comprehensive gynecology. 5th edition. Philadelphia: Mosby Elsevier; 2009. p. 569–606.
42. Anderson MR, Klink K, Cohrssen A. Evaluation of vaginal complaints. JAMA 2004;291:1368–79.
43. Johnson E, Berwald N. Diagnostic utility of physical examination, history, and laboratory evaluation in emergency department patients with vaginal complaints. Ann Emerg Med 2008;52:294–7.
44. Carr PL, Rothberg MB, Friedman RH, et al. “Shotgun” versus sequential testing: cost-effectiveness of diagnostic strategies for vaginitis. J Gen Intern Med 2005; 20:793–9.
45. Anderson M, Cohrssen A, Klink K, et al. Are speculum examination and wet mount always necessary for patients with vaginal symptoms? A pilot randomized controlled trial. J Am Board Fam Med 2009;6:617–24.
46. Bornstein J, Lakovsky Y, Lavi I, et al. The classic approach to diagnosis of vulvovaginitis: a critical analysis. Infect Dis Obstet Gynecol 2001;9:105–11.
47. Lowe NK, Neal JL, Ryan-Wenger NA. Accuracy of the clinical diagnosis of vaginitis compared to a DNA probe laboratory standard. Obstet Gynecol 2009;113:89–95.

48. Van Der Pol B. Diagnosing vaginal infections: It's time to join the 21st century. Curr Infect Dis Rep 2010;12:225–30.
49. Stamm WE, Batteiger BE. Lymphogranuloma venereum. In: Mandell GL, Bennett JE, Dolin R, editors. Principles and practices of infectious disease. 7th edition. Philadelphia: Elsevier; 2009. p. 2443–61.
50. Freeman EE, Weiss HA, Glynn JR, et al. Herpes simplex virus 2 infection increases HIV acquisition in men and women: systematic review and meta-analysis of longitudinal studies. AIDS 2006;20:73–83.
51. Stanberry LR, Jorgensen DM, Nahmias AJ. Herpes simplex viruses 1 and 2. In: Evans AS, Kaslow R, editors. Viral infections in humans: epidemiology and control. 4th edition. New York: Plenum Publishers; 1997. p. 419–54.
52. Schiffer JT, Corey L. Herpes simplex virus. In: Mandell GL, Bennett JE, Dolin R, editors. Principles and practice of infectious diseases. 7th edition. Philadelphia: Elsevier; 2009. p. 1943–62.
53. Xu F, Sternberg MR, Kottiri BJ, et al. Trends in herpes simplex virus type 1 and type 2 seroprevalence in the United States. JAMA 2006;296:964–73.
54. Wilson SS, Fakioglu E, Herold BC. Novel approaches in fighting herpes simplex virus infections. Expert Rev Anti Infect Ther 2009;7:559–68.
55. Zetola NM, Engleman J, Jensen TP, et al. Syphilis in the United State: an update for clinicians with an emphasis on HIV coinfection. Mayo Clin Proc 2007;82: 1092–102.
56. Tramont E. *Treponema pallidum* (syphilis). In: Mandell GL, Bennett JE, Dolin R, editors. Principles and practices of infectious disease. 7th edition. Philadelphia: Elsevier; 2009. p. 3035–53.
57. Romano AM, Josef MR, O'Donnell JA, et al. Clinical manifestations of early syphilis by HIV status and gender: results of the syphilis and HIV study. Sex Transm Dis 2001;28:158–65.
58. Hook EW. Syphilis. In: Goldman L, Ausiello D, editors. Cecil medicine. 23rd edition. Philadelphia: Elsevier; 2007. p. 2280–8.
59. Rawstron SA. *Treponema pallidum* (syphilis). In: Long SS, editor. Principles and practice of pediatric infectious diseases. 3rd edition. Philadelphia: Churchill Livingstone; 2008. p. 930–6.
60. Trager JD. Sexually transmitted diseases causing genital lesions in adolescents. Adolesc Med Clin 2004;15:323–52.
61. Lewis DA. Chancroid: clinical manifestations, diagnosis, and management. Sex Transm Infect 2003;79:68–71.
62. Savage EJ, van de Laar MJ, Gallay A, et al. Lymphogranuloma venereum in Europe, 2003–2008. Euro Surveill 2009;14:48.
63. Herring A, Richens J. Lymphogranuloma venereum. Sex Transm Infect 2006;82: iv23–5.
64. Herman BE, Corneli HM. A practical approach to warts in the emergency department. Pediatr Emerg Care 2008;24:246–51.
65. Jansen KU, Shaw AR. Human papillomavirus vaccines and prevention of cervical cancer. Annu Rev Med 2004;55:319–31.
66. Da Ros CT, Schmitt CS. Global epidemiology of sexually transmitted diseases. Asian J Androl 2008;10:110–4.
67. Kane BG, Degutis LC, Sayward HK, et al. Compliance with the Centers for Disease Control and Prevention recommendations for the diagnosis and treatment of sexually transmitted disease. Acad Emerg Med 2004;11:371–7.
68. Holmes KK, Levine R, Weaver M. Effectiveness of condoms in preventing sexually transmitted infections. Bull World Health Organ 2004;82:454–61.

Sexual Assault

Heather K. DeVore, MD[a,b,*], Carolyn J. Sachs, MD, MPH[c,d,e]

KEYWORDS

• Sexual assault • Rape • Violence • Forensic medicine

An estimated 18% of women and 3% of men in the United States are victims of attempted or completed rape sometime in their life. This correlates to 1-year incidence of 876,100 women per year and 111,300 men per year.[1] Discovering the true incidence has been problematic due to widespread underreporting, unclear definitions of sexual assault or rape, and varying survey methodology.[2] The definition of sexual assault refers to any type of physical sexual contact without appropriate legal consent.[3] A physical attack may accompany a sexual assault, but is not required per the definition. Other tactics include intimidation, threats, and victim incapacitation.[4] Rape is generally defined as sexual assault that involves genital, anal, or oral penetration.[5] Persons intoxicated by drugs or alcohol, minors, and persons with mental incapacitations are generally seen as unable to provide consent to sexual contact. State laws differ somewhat on definitions and legal capacity to give consent. Updated information regarding state laws can be accessed at the National Districts Attorneys Association Web site: http://www.ndaa.org/ncpca_state_statutes.html. The aftermath of sexual assault includes a wide range of mental health and general health problems, including functional gastrointestinal disorders, chronic pain, depression, substance abuse disorders, and posttraumatic stress disorders.[6–11] In an attempt to prevent or reduce these or other long-term sequelae, clinicians who treat sexual assault victims have a professional, ethical, and moral responsibility to provide the best psychological, medical, and judicial care possible.

Many jurisdictions are affiliated with a sexual assault nurse examiner (SANE) program. Sexual assault nurse examiners are extensively trained and can provide specialized evaluation and treatment of victims. They generally are part of a larger

The authors have nothing to disclose.

[a] Department of Emergency Medicine, Washington Hospital Center and Georgetown University, 110 Irving Street, Northwest Suite NA1177, Washington, DC 20010, USA
[b] District of Columbia Sexual Assault Nurse Examiner Program, The Lighthouse Center for Healing, 5321 First Place, NE, Washington, DC 20011, USA
[c] Department of Emergency Medicine, University of California, 924 Westwood Boulevard, Suite 300, Los Angeles, CA 09924, USA
[d] Department of Medicine, University of California, 924 Westwood Boulevard, Los Angeles, CA 09924, USA
[e] Forensic Nurse Specialists, Orange County, 3435 Cerritos Avenue, Los Alamitos, CA 90720, USA
* Corresponding author. Department of Emergency Medicine, Washington Hospital Center and Georgetown University, 110 Irving Street, Northwest Suite NA1177, Washington, DC 20010.
E-mail address: Heather.K.DeVore@Medstar.net

Emerg Med Clin N Am 29 (2011) 605–620
doi:10.1016/j.emc.2011.04.012 **emed.theclinics.com**
0733-8627/11/$ – see front matter

sexual assault response team that includes law enforcement individuals, victim advocates, prosecutors, and forensic laboratory personnel. This article is designed to aid clinicians who do not have access to these specialized services as well as to further the knowledge of any provider who interacts with this patient population. Prepared and knowledgeable emergency clinicians can help attenuate the psychological and physical impact of sexual assault through proper care of the victim and careful treatment of evidence. This, in turn, can aid in successful prosecution and conviction of sexual offenders.

Although women encompass the majority, men also present for evaluation and treatment after sexual assault. For simplification purposes only, the female pronoun will be used throughout this article.

CLINICAL PRESENTATION

A sexual assault victim may present directly to the emergency department (ED) or be transported by law enforcement or emergency medical services personnel. Because of pervading myths and stigma associated with sexual assault, most victims do not report the assault to anyone and only 25% present for medical evaluation.[12] Victims may present to the ED complaining only of rectal or genital pain, or requesting treatment for sexually transmitted infection (STI) or emergency contraception. Clinicians should remain vigilant in the setting of such complaints and would be prudent to question the patient further regarding the possibility of sexual assault. Clinicians should also familiarize themselves with local guidelines and protocols, including reporting or not reporting to law enforcement agencies and access to victim advocate support services. Applicable state laws pertaining to sexual assault may be found at the National Center for Victims of Crime: http://www.ncvc.org. Additional web-based resources include: http://www.promotetruth.org and http://www.findlaw.com. In 1994, the US Congress passed the Violence Against Women Act (VAWA 1994) as part of the Violent Crime Control and Law Enforcement Act of 1994, which was amended a second time in 2005, uncoupling the pairing of evidence collection and formal reporting to law enforcement.[13] As such, there is currently no requirement for victims of sexual assault to participate in the criminal justice system, cooperate, or even talk with law enforcement in order for forensic evidence collection to occur. This has important implications for emergency care providers, as a full medical-forensic examination may be requested without involvement of law enforcement personnel.

In all cases, the entire ED staff should follow the guiding principle to provide compassionate and confidential treatment in a timely manner. Staff should offer access to a rape crisis victim advocate and allow friends or family to accompany the patient according to her wishes. The patient has undergone an experience where her right to consent was taken away, and creating an environment where the patient feels like she can regain control is imperative to the healing process.

EVALUATION

As with all patients, the clinician's first priority is to treat any life-threatening or limb-threatening injuries. The vast minority of sexually assaulted patients will not require such immediate intervention; however, in such cases of coexisting severe trauma, reasonable care should be taken to prevent or minimize destruction or alteration of evidence on the patient's body.

Consent

Obtaining consent for evaluation and treatment is considered mandatory and should be acquired through written consent at the beginning, as well as verbal consent throughout each step of the evaluation. The patient has a right to refuse medical-forensic examination and treatment at any point in the process. If there is no institution-specific forensic examination form available, use of a standard ED consent form is recommended, including a brief description of the forensic process. If a patient cannot give consent due to a reversible process, including intoxication from drugs or alcohol or an acute psychological reaction, clinicians should defer the forensic examination until clinical circumstances permit informed consent. When patients cannot give consent due to minor status, developmental disability, or severe trauma or coma, consent should be obtained from someone with legal capacity to give authorization, unless that person is a suspect in the assault. In some cases, law enforcement may provide a court order for an examination. When in doubt, it is prudent to seek consultation from institutional legal and/or ethics council before proceeding with an invasive medical-forensic examination.

History

After obtaining informed consent, the evaluation should begin by obtaining an appropriate history. Document pertinent medical history including underlying medical conditions, current medications, allergies, tetanus immunization status, and hepatitis B immunity status. Pertinent gynecologic history includes last menstrual period, history of tubal ligation or hysterectomy, contraceptive history, recent anal-genital injuries, or procedures that may alter the expected normal genital appearance, any other preexisting injuries, and last voluntary sexual contact or intercourse. This information will assist in determining appropriate medical treatment and documentation. The assault history need not be an exhaustive account of the details of the encounter, as any discrepancy noted between the medical and police reports regarding minute details may later prove to be confusing in court. It should include enough information to determine from where and what type of forensic specimens should be collected. The time and date of the assault should be documented to determine appropriateness for evidence collection and medication administration. When looking for corroborating evidence, important descriptive information may include the location of the assault, such as grass or leaves if the assault occurred in a park, or physical violence such as punching, kicking, biting, or pinching that may correlate with injuries discovered on examination. Likewise, it is important to document whether the patient thinks they inflicted injury upon the assailant. For example, a history of scratching may lead the examiner to collect fingernail swabs or scrapings. The number of assailants is important to the forensic lab when they encounter DNA evidence. Document any sexual acts, including fondling of breasts or genitalia, vaginal, oral, or anal penetration or attempted penetration, ejaculation on or in the body, and the use of contraception or lubricants. Whether ejaculation occurred and its location can help guide the examiner to possible evidence sites. Postassault history should include bathing, urinating, eating or drinking, gargling, defecating, douching, and changing undergarments or outer clothing. These actions can alter the recovery of seminal specimens and other evidence. Consider obtaining blood and urine specimens and testing for alcohol or other drugs, when the history suggests lapses of consciousness, impairment in consciousness, or intoxication. Drug-facilitated sexual assault (DFSA) is discussed in more detail below.

General Physical Examination

The physical examination has several different purposes, including recognizing and treating injuries or other medical needs, collecting forensic specimens, and documenting observational findings for others when investigating details of the assault. Throughout the examination, the clinician should again explain the process, answer any questions, and remind the patient that she is in control and can stop or refuse any part of the examination. Allow a support person or victim advocate to remain in the room if the patient desires. It is useful to know local guidelines on the time duration that can transpire from assault to evidence collection, as jurisdictions differ in the maximum time where an evidence kit may be collected. This time frame generally ranges from 72 to 120 hours. Prioritize the sequence of evidence collection based on history and type of assault, obtaining the most important evidence (ie, DNA) first. Evidence collection should stop if the patient becomes too distressed or unable to cooperate, and may resume only with patient consent. The clinician should wear a cap and mask, and maintain gloved hands throughout the collection process, changing gloves often to avoid cross-contamination of DNA evidence or specimens. Chain of custody of evidence begins once a sexual assault examination kit is opened by the examiner, and it is the responsibility of the examiner to maintain physical custody until relinquished to law enforcement or a forensic laboratory.

If available, examiners may choose to look for injury using magnification provided with a simple magnification lens, colposcope, or digital camera—ideally equipped with a macro lens. Reported rates of genital injury increase substantially with the use of magnification.[14,15] It should be emphasized that a completely normal genital examination can still be consistent with forced sexual assault and, likewise, some injuries can be seen after consensual sexual activity.[16,17]

Forensic laboratories often request victim DNA samples such as blood, buccal mucosal cells, scalp hairs, pubic hairs, or skin swabs for comparison testing. The need for such samples will be determined by local protocol. Other tests may include whole blood samples and the patient's first available voided urine when DFSA is suspected. All specimens must be maintained with a chain of custody to ensure admissibility of the results in a court of law.

The physical examination begins with noting and documenting the general demeanor and appearance of the patient. If the patient is wearing the same clothing as the time of the assault, collect the relevant clothes as potential evidence. The patient should disrobe by standing on and then dropping clothes onto a clean sheet or paper cloth. With gloved hands, place each item of clothing in a separate paper bag and itemize each article. The sheet or paper should be bundled together with any material or debris collected, and then sealed in an envelope or bag. Use only paper bags for evidence collection, as plastic restricts air circulation and may lead to fungal or bacterial growth, destroying biologic evidence.

After the patient has put on a hospital gown or other suitable covering, examine her body for signs of trauma and foreign materials as directed by the history of the assault. Uncover one part of the body at a time to retain some modesty throughout the examination. Important focus areas include the mouth, neck, back, thighs, breasts, wrists, and ankles. Document any areas of tenderness, even if an injury is not clearly visualized. Injuries may include scratches, lacerations, incisions, abrasions, contusions, suction injuries, and bite marks. Leaves, grass, sand, carpet fibers, and other foreign material may be found in the hair or on the skin during the full body examination. Retain these as evidence by sealing them in an envelope, dating and signing the envelope seal, and noting their location on the body. All swabs must be air-dried, labeled appropriately, and then sealed in an envelope. Labels should include patient information, date and time of specimen collection, examiner name or initials, and site of collection.

Document areas of significant trauma further with radiographs as indicated by the type and extent of the injury. Document all injuries using words, diagrams, or photography, if available. When using photography, three images should be taken of each injury or group of injuries. The first should be taken from a distance to easily observe the body part where the injury is located. The second image should be a close-up of the injury. The third should be a close-up with a ruler next to, but not covering, the injury. These photographs may serve as evidence or may simply refresh the examiner's memory at the time of trial or other legal proceedings. One study found that documentation of bodily injuries associated with a sexual assault improves the likelihood of a successful prosecution.[18]

Dried semen stains may be visible on the hair or skin of the patient under regular room lighting and may fluoresce when inspected in a dark room using short-wave light such as an ultraviolet light source: a Wood lamp or, preferably, a forensic alternate light source.[19] Semen is not the only substance that fluoresces and it generally stops fluorescing within a day or two of the assault, so it is recommended to collect specimens of all dried secretions as soon as feasible.[20] Using a swab moistened with sterile water, scrub the area and allow the swab to dry thoroughly. Preserve the dried swab in a labeled box or envelope, noting the location on the body, then sign and seal the box or envelope.

If there is suggested involvement of scratching or other physical struggle in the assault history, obtain fingernail clippings or scrapings with a toothpick run under the fingernails, collecting the resulting material on a clean piece of paper and then sign and seal it inside a labeled envelope.

Oropharyngeal Examination

The lips and oral cavity should be examined for signs of trauma. Injuries from forced oral copulation may include lacerations of the labial or lingual frenulum, mucosal abrasions, and contusions. Examine the posterior pharyngeal wall and soft palate for petechiae, which may heal quickly and therefore may not be visible on examination hours or days later. Use moistened swabs to collect dried secretions around the outer lips. Use clean sterile swabs and move between the buccal mucosa and teeth throughout the oral cavity, including both upper and lower gingival surfaces. Dry all swabs and then place in a box or envelope, signing and sealing the envelope. Spermatozoa have been found in oral swab specimens up to 12 hours after an assault, despite tooth brushing or oral intake.[21]

Genital Examination

Before the genital examination, explain the procedure and reobtain verbal consent from the patient. While in the lithotomy position, inspect the patient's inner thighs and perineum for signs of trauma and dried secretions. Injuries and tenderness should be described thoroughly and documented using appropriate anatomic terms (**Figs. 1** and **2**).

Many jurisdictions recommend routine swabbing of the outer genitalia and inner thighs given the high likelihood of evidence being present in these locations. Place a clean piece of paper beneath the patient's buttocks and comb through the pubic hair onto the paper. Any foreign material, including loose pubic hair, should be collected on the paper. The paper, including the comb, should be folded and sealed in a labeled envelope. If suspected dried semen is discovered on pubic hair, the

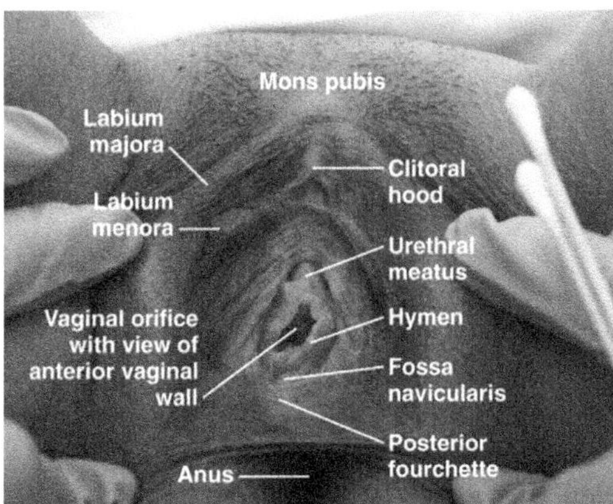

Fig. 1. Female anatomy with appropriate anatomic terms. (*From* Sachs C. Care for the sexual assault victim. In: Roberts JE, Hedges JR, editors. Clinical procedures in emergency medicine, vol. 5. Philadelphia (PA): Saunders, an imprint of Elsevier Inc.; 2009; with permission.)

matted hairs should be trimmed and collected. Forensic laboratories often request 20 to 25 victim pubic hair specimens for DNA comparison testing. Although pulled victim hair specimens provide the best reference sample, this is generally considered insensitive, is quite painful and usually does not alter the course of the investigation. Instead, it is recommended to clip the hair as close to the root as possible to provide the lab a reference sample. In the rare instance that pulled hairs are required for lab evaluation, a patient can provide them later. Significant hair transfer occurs in less than 5% of assaults.[22]

The genital examination of the sexual assault patient differs from the standard pelvic examination. First, carefully inspect the vulva and vaginal introitus for signs of trauma.

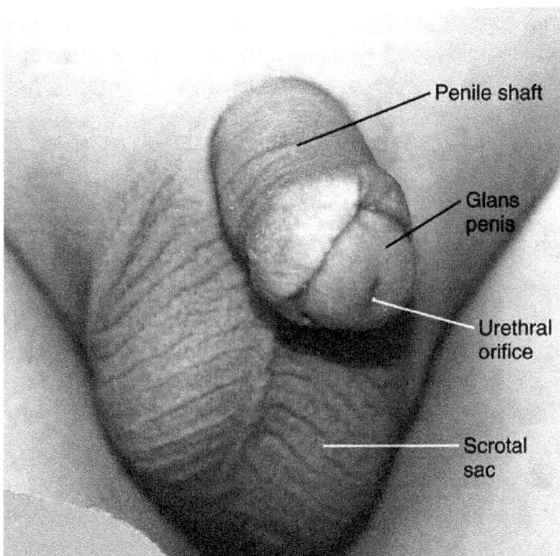

Fig. 2. Male anatomy with appropriate anatomic terms. (*From* Sachs C. Care for the sexual assault victim. In: Roberts JE, Hedges JR, editors. Clinical procedures in emergency medicine, vol. 5. Philadelphia (PA): Saunders, an imprint of Elsevier Inc.; 2009. Figures 58-2, 58-3A, 50-3B; with permission.)

Using both hands, separate the labia laterally in each direction to visualize the posterior fourchette and vaginal introitus. Then use gentle inferior labial traction toward the examiner to visualize the hymen. A mature adult female hymen often becomes fragmented, atrophied, and difficult to identify. In younger women and adolescents, the hymen is often redundant and folded. Use sterile water-moistened swabs to facilitate thorough inspection of the hymen. Alternatively, a 14-French Foley catheter may be inserted through the hymen orifice and then inflated for hymen examination. Prepubertal adolescents lack a fully estrogenized hymen; contact with this area is often painful and should therefore be minimized or avoided altogether. Hymen injuries are most commonly seen in sexually inexperienced adolescents. The most common site of vaginal injuries to occur is the posterior fourchette.[23]

It can be helpful to highlight a genital injury with the use of toluidine blue dye, a nuclear stain proven safe for mucosal application.[24] Toluidine will uptake in injured deepithelialized areas with exposed nucleated cells, but not intact epithelialized areas. Thus, injuries will appear blue. Apply a small amount of toluidine to the entire perineum and wipe off the excess with a lubricant-moistened cotton ball or gauze. Some examiners use diluted acetic acid to remove the excess toluidine, although acetic acid may produce pain when it contacts injured surfaces. Care should be taken to avoid lubricant or toluidine entering into the vaginal canal where it could contaminate other specimens, although toluidine is not generally thought to corrupt DNA evidence.[25,26] Next, using a speculum lubricated only with warm water, gently insert the speculum into the vaginal canal. The vaginal walls should be inspected for injury. Any secretions that have pooled in the posterior fornix should be collected with sterile swabs that are then dried and sealed in a box or envelope labeled vaginal specimens. Alternatively, some forensic labs request vaginal washings that can be obtained by instilling 5 mL of nonbacteriostatic sterile saline solution into the vaginal vault followed by aspiration. Cervical specimens should next be obtained by swabbing the cervix with sterile swabs and then drying and sealing them in the same fashion. Collection of cervical swabs becomes particularly important if more than 48 hours has elapsed from the time of the assault or if there is a history of recent consensual intercourse. Forensic laboratories have recovered sperm from vaginal specimens up to 9 days and cervical specimens up to 12 days following sexual contact.[27] Examiners may choose to create a wet mount of the swabs to look for motile sperm. However, most programs have abolished this step due to lack of formal training and access to microscopes. A bimanual examination is not a routine part of the sexual assault examination and should only be performed if indicated for medical evaluation and treatment.

Anorectal Examination

Because of a reluctance of some victims to admit to anal penetration or a loss of exact recall of the assault, an anal examination should be performed in most cases to look for injury. With consent from the patient, visually inspect the anus by spreading all skin folds. Collect anal specimens by inserting sterile swabs approximately 2 cm into the anal orifice, gently move them in a circular motion, and remove. Air dry, create slides if requested, and package as evidence. Anoscopy is not a routine part of all sexual assault examinations, but is indicated when looking for internal anal or rectal injuries after attempted anal penetration or in a patient who has experienced a lapse of consciousness during the assault period. Anoscopy is especially important in male victims.[28] Anal injuries should be documented geographically using a clock to describe location, with 12 o'clock located closest to the perineum. Extensive anal or rectal injuries may need to be thoroughly examined under anesthesia with consultation from a surgeon.

Sexual Assault-Specific Diagnostic Testing

The US Centers for Disease Control and Prevention (CDC) guidelines recommend testing for gonorrhea and *Chlamydia* at the time of the assault examination.[29] However, most SANE programs do not routinely perform these tests as they can only detect before-assault infection, provide no useful information for the forensic laboratory, and patients are typically empirically treated for these infections anyway.[30] Baseline serologic testing for HIV and hepatitis B (if not previously vaccinated) is routinely recommended in assaults involving penile-vaginal or penile-anal penetration, as the efficacy of after-exposure prophylactic treatment remains variable. Additionally, assault-related seroconversion may qualify an individual for benefits from a crime victims' compensation fund. Syphilis serology should be obtained if antibiotic prophylaxis is not given empirically. Baseline pregnancy testing should be performed on all female victims of childbearing age, as this will affect emergency contraception and STI treatment options. See below for additional information regarding management of possible STI and emergency contraception.

MANAGEMENT

There are four concepts that comprise the routine medical management of a sexual assault patient. These include psychosocial support, medical treatment of injuries or other conditions, pregnancy prevention, and empiric treatment of STIs.

Psychosocial Support

Psychosocial support is important throughout the entire ED visit and should guide all interactions with the patient, maintaining sensitivity and strict patient confidentiality throughout the process. Social workers or rape crisis victim advocates can provide emotional support and confirm that the patient comprehends the entire process. Resources should be given to the patient at the end of the visit for follow up counseling and support.

Medical Treatment

Medical or surgical treatment of associated injuries should follow standard procedure with immediate consultation by urology, gynecology, general surgery, or other consulting specialty services as indicated to manage significant trauma or uncontrolled hemorrhage. During the initial medical evaluation and stabilization, all reasonable attempts should be made to preserve potential evidence if possible. This includes avoiding cutting through holes found in clothing, collecting clothing and other material in paper bags and leaving it with the patient until chain of custody can be confirmed, and not washing away potential DNA evidence. Additionally, if time allows, urinary catheterization and vaginal speculum insertion should be performed after collection of DNA evidence and documentation of injury. It is important to remember that the management of serious coexisting injuries or other acute medical conditions takes precedence over preservation of forensic evidence.

Pregnancy Prevention

In the United States, an estimated 4.7% victims, or 22,000 women per year, become pregnant after a sexual assault.[31,32] Pregnancy prevention, or emergency contraception, should be offered to patients up to 5 days after a penile-vaginal assault.[33,34] Any nonpregnant female of childbearing age who does not have anatomic contraception (ie, intrauterine device, bilateral tubal ligation, or hysterectomy) is eligible for treatment. Single-dose levonorgestrel, 1.5 mg orally, is the preferred treatment as it has better efficacy and causes fewer side effects than other regimens.[35] In the rare case where levonorgestrel is unavailable, another option is a combination of ethinyl estradiol and a progestin, known as the Yuzpe regimen.[34] If the patient vomits within 1 hour of ingesting the medication, the dose should be repeated. No studies to date show untoward effects on a fetus should pregnancy occur despite emergency contraception.[36] Further information and guidance provided by the Association of Reproductive Health Professionals can be accessed at http://www.not-2-late.com.

STI Treatment

The risk of contracting an STI after an assault varies according to geographic location, population, and assault characteristics. Prophylactic treatment should be offered to patients who have suffered any oral-genital or genital-genital assault. Due to potential long-term sequelae, treatment for gonorrhea, *Chlamydia*, and syphilis at the time of the initial examination is standard practice.[37] The treatment of *Trichomonas* and bacterial vaginosis at the time of the initial examination is considered optional, and may in fact be relatively contraindicated in the setting of recent alcohol ingestion by the patient.[30] Complete guidelines for STI prophylaxis following sexual assault are available on the CDC Web site, http://www.cdc.gov/std/treatment/2010/sexual-assault.htm.[37] Of note, fluoroquinolones are no longer recommended as first-line therapy due to widespread gonococcal resistance. To ensure patient compliance, single-dose treatments are preferred whenever feasible.

The hepatitis B vaccination series should be initiated in nonimmunized or incompletely immunized patients.[37] The first dose ideally should be given within 24 hours after the assault with recommendations given to the patient for repeat doses in 1 month and again in 6 months. Hepatitis B immune globulin (HBIG) is indicated only for incompletely vaccinated or unvaccinated patients after a high-risk exposure involving a known hepatitis B-positive assailant. Due to cost or resource restraints, some programs must refer patients for delayed administration of the hepatitis B vaccine or HBIG, which is thought to maintain its effectiveness for up to 72 hours after assault.[37]

The risk of transmission of HIV due to a sexual assault is thought to be higher than consensual receptive vaginal or anal intercourse because of the possible tissue injury sustained during the assault. From studies performed in no-assault circumstances, the risk of transmission of HIV from one episode of unprotected receptive vaginal intercourse with an HIV-positive individual is 0.1% to 0.2%, or approximately 1 in 1000. The risk associated with consensual receptive anal intercourse is 0.8% to 3%, or 8 to 32 in 1000.[38] Postexposure prophylaxis guidelines are extrapolated from research and protocols from occupational exposures such as needlestick injuries. In 2005, the US Department of Health and Human Services Working Group on Nonoccupational Postexposure Prophylaxis (nPEP) recommended administering 28 days of prophylactic anti-retroviral therapy only for HIV-negative patients who present less than 72 hours after vaginal, anal, or oral penetration by a known HIV-positive assailant.[39] Other assault scenarios were not addressed, and many providers are left to make decisions on a case-by-case basis (**Table 1**).

Assistance with nPEP decisions is available to providers by calling the National HIV Telephone Consultation Service (1-800-933-3413). Risks and side effects of antiretroviral therapy must be discussed with the patient before initiation, as well as emphasizing the importance of adhering to the regimen for a full 28-day period. Studies find that approximately 50% of patients fail to complete the prescribed regimen due to poor follow-up or inability to tolerate side effects.[40–42] Repeat HIV antibody, hepatitis B, hepatitis C, and syphilis testing is recommended at 1 to 2 months and again at 4 to 6 months after assault.[39] Consider prescribing an antiemetic medication along with

Table 1
General guidelines to offering HIV nPEP

>72 hours elapsed since assault	YES	Do not offer nPEP but recommend or refer for baseline and follow-up HIV antibody testing
	NO	Continue risk analysis
Victim <12 years old	Yes	Consult pediatric HIV specialist
	No	Continue risk analysis
Known HIV-negative assailant	Yes	Do not offer nPEP
	No	Continue risk analysis
Assault carries measurable risk of transmission (blood exposure, receptive anal penetration, receptive vaginal penetration)	Yes	Consider offering nPEP, especially if there is a break in skin or known STI present, or HIV-positive assailant
	No	HIV nPEP may not be warranted
Assault carries possible risk of transmission (oral penetration with ejaculation, biting, or other mucous membrane involvement; unknown acts occurred)	Yes	Consider offering nPEP if there was an exposure to potentially infectious fluids, break in skin, known STI present, and known HIV-positive assailant
	No	HIV nPEP may not be warranted
Assault with no risk of transmission (kissing, object or digital penetration, blood or ejaculation on intact skin, condom use)	Yes	HIV nPEP may not be warranted
Other risk factors present in assault (presence of blood, known STI in victim or assailant, significant trauma, ejaculation, multiple penetrations)	—	Consider offering nPEP on a case-by-case basis

Data from Centers for Disease Control and Prevention, Smith DK, Grohskopf LA, et al. Antiretroviral postexposure prophylaxis after sexual, injection-drug use, or other nonoccupational exposure to HIV in the United States: recommendations from the U.S. Department of Health and Human Services. MMWR Recomm Rep 2005;54(RR-2):1–20.

nPEP as nausea is a common side effect associated with prophylactic medications and emergency contraception. **Table 2** provides an overview of prophylactic medications that should be considered based on assault history and patient specifics.

DISPOSITION

Sexual assault can precipitate a psychological crisis for the patient that can result in a lack of understanding and information overload. Patients may expect immediate answers and results from the collected evidence and need to be informed that it may not be examined unless law enforcement pursues prosecution of an assailant. Patients may not understand the potential sequelae of STIs and the purpose and side-effects of prophylactic medications should be underscored. Short-term, as well as long-term, psychological consequences, including "flashbacks," should be discussed and reassured as a typical response following an assault. However, patients should be given comprehensive return precautions if serious or concerning side effects or symptoms develop, including suicidal thoughts. Sexual assault victims often develop a posttraumatic stress disorder called rape trauma syndrome, manifest by sleep disturbances, feelings of guilt, memory impairment, avoidance of activities, and blunted emotions.[43] Early intervention can help reduce this response and speed the healing process.

In most cases, the sexual assault victim may be discharged from the ED in the company of relatives or friends. On occasion, hospitalization is necessary for

Table 2
After-assault prophylactic medications

Gonorrhea	cefixime 400 mg po	—
	spectinomycin 2 gm IM	For use in pregnant cephalosporin-allergic patients
Gonorrhea and incubating syphilis	ceftriaxone 250 mg IM	—
	cefpodoxime 400 mg po	May be slightly less effective than ceftriaxone
	cefuroxime 1000 mg po	—
Chlamydia	azithromycin 1 gm po	—
	doxycycline 100 mg po bid × 7 days	—
	erythromycin 500 mg po qid × 7 days	Safe in pregnancy
Trichomonas	metronidazole 2 gm po	Optional treatment, usually deferred. Avoid if alcohol ingested in last 24 hours. Warn patient about a disulfiram reaction
Bacterial vaginosis	metronidazole 2 gm po	Optional, usually deferred. Avoid if alcohol ingested in last 24 hours
Hepatitis B	hepatitis B vaccine, recombinant 1 mL IM, repeat in 1 and 6 months	—
	hepatitis B immune globulin 0.06 mL/kg IM	For high-risk exposures with an assailant known to have acute hepatitis B (for nonimmunized or incompletely immunized patients only)
Pregnancy prevention	single-dose levonorgestrel 1.5 mg po	—
	ethinyl estradiol and norgestrel 2 tabs (0.05 mg ethinyl estradiol/0.5 mg norgestrel) po at time of examination; repeat 2 tabs again in 12 hours	Use only if levonorgestrel is unavailable
HIV postexposure prophylaxis	efavirenz + lamivudine or emtricitabine + zidovudine or tenofovir	Refer to local ID guidelines for occupational postexposure prophylaxis regimens
	zidovudine + lamivudine + lopinavir-ritonavir	—
	zidovudine + lamivudine or emtricitabine	—

Abbreviations: ID, infectious disease; IM, intramuscular dose.

Data from Centers for Disease Control and Prevention, Smith DK, Grohskopf LA, et al. Antiretroviral postexposure prophylaxis after sexual, injection-drug use, or other nonoccupational exposure to HIV in the United States: recommendations from the U.S. Department of Health and Human Services. MMWR Recomm Rep 2005;54(RR-2):1–20; and Linden JA, Oldeg P, Mehta SD, et al. HIV postexposure prophylaxis in sexual assault: current practice and patient adherence to treatment recommendations in a large urban teaching hospital. Acad Emerg Med 2005;12:640–6.

significant injuries requiring continued observation or urgent intervention; exacerbation of preexisting or new medical conditions; or suicidal, homicidal, or psychotic reactions. Follow-up care should be arranged before final discharge with appropriate referrals provided in written form. Local sexual assault crisis agencies may provide follow-up psychological support and services. Medical follow-up should occur with a primary care provider or gynecologist at 4 weeks for retesting of pregnancy and STIs. Adherence counseling and infectious disease follow-up should be arranged for patients initiated on nPEP. Any physical injury or other medical condition requires standard referrals and return precautions. Despite access and offering of services, most sexual assault victims fail to return for follow-up.[44,45] Law enforcement contact information should be given to the patient to determine the status of a report or to make an initial report if previously declined by the patient.

SPECIAL CIRCUMSTANCES

Intimate Partner Violence

Often times, sexual assault patients are also victims of intimate partner violence.[46] Health care providers must be sensitive to this association and screen patients for associated physical and psychological abuse as well as address their safety. Social work or victim advocates may be helpful in providing emergency shelter and other resources. Rarely, a patient may need to be hospitalized to ensure their safety until legal processes and protections are in place.

Male Examinations

The male forensic evaluation includes all of the same history and examination techniques as the female evaluation except for gynecologic history and vaginal specimens. Most males are victims of forced anal or oral penetration. Penile specimens from the glans, shaft, corona, and scrotum may be obtained if there is oral or anal contact with the assailant. HIV risk is increased with anal penetration and should be assessed accordingly. Male victims deserve the same amount of respect and privacy as female victims and should be given appropriate referrals to psychological resources and support.

Pediatric Examinations

Trained pediatric sexual assault experts are best equipped to handle victims of pediatric sexual assault or abuse. However, in departments lacking timely response or availability of a pediatric sexual assault expert, it becomes the provider's responsibility to inspect, document, and possibly collect forensic specimens. In very young female children, the frog-leg position using gentle labial or gluteal separation and traction is the best way to visualize the genitalia and potential injuries. The knee-to-chest position is best for visualizing the hymenal perimeter in prepubertal girls, as well as the anus in both genders. Clear findings of sexual abuse include local areas of hymenal absence in knee-chest position, hymenal transection, or anal laceration. Suspicious or suggestive findings include an extremely narrow hymen (<1 mm), acute abrasions or lacerations of the labia or vagina external to the hymen, and excessive anal dilation (>15 mm without stool in rectum). Nonspecific findings may include redness, increased vascularity, and labial adhesions.[17] The aid of a microscopic lens and photography is helpful in documenting findings that can be later evaluated by an expert. Testing for STIs is routine practice, as presence of such infection may indicate or confirm ongoing abuse.

Suspect Examinations

Suspect examinations and evidence collection are becoming more commonly requested by law enforcement. As such, it is prudent to become familiar with local and state protocols regarding consent and procedure. Some jurisdictions permit suspect examinations without consent, whereas others require a search warrant from the court. Law enforcement should always be in attendance during any suspect examination for the safety of the examiner and staff. The suspect and victim should never see each other during the evaluation period and care should be taken to examine them in different areas of the ED or hospital by different examiners if possible to prevent cross contamination of DNA evidence. Suspect examinations require the same level of professionalism as displayed during victim examinations. It is certainly not within the realm of the examiner's professional duties and responsibilities to pass judgment on the suspect or the victim.

DFSA

Alcohol or other drugs play an important role in many sexual assaults. Half of all sexual assaults involve drugs or alcohol, whether voluntarily ingested by the victim, surreptitiously given by the assailant, or ingested under force or coercion.[47] The drugs most commonly associated with sexual assault include alcohol, marijuana, cocaine and benzodiazepines.[48] The publicized "date rape" drugs, including benzodiazepines and gamma hydroxybutyrate (GHB), are only found in about 5% of cases.[49,50] In DFSAs, the victim may present complaining of an impaired or lapse of consciousness with short segments of memory of a sexual act, genital pain, or may have no memory but are concerned that they may have been a victim of a possible sexual assault due to misplaced or missing undergarments or other concerns. Clinicians should use appropriate prudence in these cases and should consider performing a comprehensive medical-forensic evaluation (with consultation by a SANE, if available). Thoroughly evaluate for injury and collect evidence from all potential oral or genital contact sites including neck, breasts, mouth, vagina or penis, and anus. Toxicology specimens, including serum ethanol, with exact times of collection documented may be warranted depending on particular circumstances. In general, at least 100 mL of urine should be collected in a standard urine collection cup within 96 hours of ingestion.[48] A first-void urine specimen provides the highest concentration of drug levels and is ideal to collect. Blood specimens should be collected within 24 hour of the suspected drugging. It is recommended to collect 10 to 30 mL of blood in gray-top (sodium fluoride, potassium oxalate) tubes.[48] If an extremely intoxicated or unconscious patient presents with surrounding circumstances suspicious for sexual assault (ie, undergarments or clothing missing), care should be taken to collect blood and urine as soon as possible for DFSA testing in addition to the standard physical forensic examination. Most forensic laboratories will offer a "date rape" panel that tests a variety of commonly used drugs. Law enforcement and SANE programs routinely interact with forensic laboratories and are a good resource for assistance in submitting specimens. It is important to get a thorough and accurate list of medications and drugs voluntarily ingested by the patient to help the forensic lab and law enforcement pursue an accurate investigation. One recent study showed that only 40% of victims were forthcoming with their voluntary illegal drug use.[50] As with all specimens, a chain of evidence should be maintained and properly documented to qualify the results to be used in criminal justice proceedings.

SUMMARY

The care of the sexual assault patient begins with presentation to the ED and continues beyond disposition and discharge. A multifactorial, multidisciplinary approach will produce the most efficient and inclusive evaluation and management. Care should be taken to address a patient's psychosocial, medical, and forensic needs. This includes using victim advocacy services, treating associated injuries and medical conditions, collecting forensic evidence while maintaining proper chain of custody, and aptly administering emergency contraception, empiric treatment for STIs, and pertinent postexposure prophylaxis. With the proper knowledge and preparation, appropriate and victim-centered care in the ED can provide the first step toward successful long-term healing after sexual assault.

REFERENCES

1. Rennison CM. Criminal victimization 2000: changes 1999–2000 with trends 1993–2000 National Crime Victimization Survey 2001. NCJ 187007 2001 Bureau of Justice Statistics. Washington DC: United States Government Printing Office; 2001. p. 1.
2. Fanflick PL. Victim responses to sexual assault: counterintuitive or simply adaptive? National District Attorneys' Association. American Prosecutors' Research Institute. Available at: http://www.ndaa.org. Accessed October 22, 2010.
3. Groth S. Evaluation and Management of the sexually assaulted or sexually abused patient. Dallas (TX): American College of Emergency Physicians; 1999. Available at: www.acep.org. Accessed October 22, 2010.
4. Merriam-Webster's Dictionary of Law. Merriam-Webster, Incorporated; 1996. Available at: http://dictionary.lp.findlaw.com/dictionary.html. Accessed October 22, 2010.
5. Tjaden P, Thoennes N. A prevalence, incidence, and consequences of violence against women; Findings from the National Violence Against Women Survey, Research in Brief. Washington, DC: National Institute of Justice, U.S. Department of Justice; 1998. p. 2, 5.
6. Kilpatrick DJ, Acierno R. Mental health needs of crime victims: epidemiology and outcomes. J Trauma Stress 2003;16:119–32.
7. Kilpatrick DJ, Acierno R, Resnick HS, et al. A two-year longitudinal analysis of the relationships between violent assault and substance use in women. J Consult Clin Psychol 1997;65:834–47.
8. Paras ML, Murad MH, Chen LP, et al. Sexual abuse and lifetime diagnosis of somatic disorders; a systematic review and meta-analysis. JAMA 2009;302: 550–61.
9. Conoscenti LM, McNally RJ. Health complaints in acknowledged and unacknowledged rape victims. J Anxiety Disord 2006;20:372–9.
10. Chandler HK, Ciccone DS, Raphael KG. Localization of pain and self-reported rape in a female community sample. Pain Med 2006;7:344–52.
11. Eberhard-Gran M, Schei B, Eskild A. Somatic symptoms and diseases are more common in women exposed to violence. J Gen Intern Med 2007;22:1668–73.
12. Resnick HS, Holmes MM, Kilpatrick DG, et al. Predictors of post-rape medical care in a national sample of women. Am J Prev Med 2000;19:214–9.
13. United States Department of Justice. Frequently asked questions: anonymous reporting and forensic examinations. Available at: http://www.ovw.usdoj.gov/ovw-fs.htm#fs-faq. Accessed February 16, 2011.
14. Sugar NF, Fine DN, Eckert LO. Physical injury after sexual assault; findings of a large case series. Am J Obstet Gynecol 2004;190:71–6.
15. Read KM, Jufera JA, Jackson MC, et al. Population-based study of police-reported sexual assault in Baltimore, Maryland. Am J Emerg Med 2005;23:273–8.
16. Riggs N, Houry D, Long G, et al. Analysis of 1,076 cases of sexual assault. Ann Emerg Med 2000;35:358.

17. Adams JA, Knudson S. Genital findings in adolescent girls referred for suspected sexual abuse. Arch Pediatr Adolesc Med 1996;150:850–7.
18. Rambow B, Adkinson C, Frost TH, et al. Female sexual assault; medical and legal implications. Ann Emerg Med 1992;21:727–31.
19. Nelson DG, Santucci KA. An alternate light source to detect semen. Acad Emerg Med 2002;9:1045–8.
20. Wawryk J, Odell M. Fluorescent identification of biological and other stains on skin by the use of alternative light sources. J Clin Forensic Med 2005;12:296–301.
21. Enos WF, Beyer JC. Spermatozoa in the anal canal and rectum and in the oral cavity in female rape victims. J Forensic Sci 1978;23:231.
22. Mann MJ. Hair transfers in sexual assault: a six-year case study. J Forensic Sci 1990;35:951.
23. Slaughter L, Brown CR, Crowley S, et al. Patterns of genital injury in female sexual assault victims. Obstet Gynecol 1997;176:609.
24. Redman RS, Krasnow SH, Sniffen RA. Evaluation of the carcinogenic potential for toluidine blue O in the hamster cheek pouch. Oral Surg Oral Med Oral Pathol 1992;74:473.
25. Hochmeister MN, Whelan M, Borer UV, et al. Effects of toluidine blue and destaining reagents used in sexual assault examinations on the ability to obtain DNA profiles from postcoital vaginal swabs. J Forensic Sci 1997;42:316.
26. Lauber AA, Souma ML. Use of toluidine blue for documentation of traumatic intercourse. Obstet Gynecol 1982;60:644–8.
27. Morrison AI. Persistence of spermatozoa in the vagina and cervix. Br J Vener Dis 1972;48:141–3.
28. Ernst AA, Green E, Ferguson MT, et al. The utility of anoscopy and colposcopy in the evaluation of male sexual assault victims. Ann Emerg Med 2000;36:432.
29. Sexually Transmitted Diseases Treatment Guidelines, 2010. Sexual Assault and STDs. Centers for Disease Control and Prevention. Available at: http://www.cdc.gov/std/treatment/2010/sexual-assault.htm. Accessed March 30, 2010.
30. Ciancone AC, Wilson C, Collette R, et al. Sexual assault nurse examiner programs in the United States. Ann Emerg Med 2000;35:353.
31. Holmes MM, Resnick HS, Kilpatrick DG, et al. Rape-related pregnancy: estimates and descriptive characteristics from a national sample of women. Am J Obstet Gynecol 1996;175:320.
32. Stewart FH, Trussell J. Prevention of pregnancy resulting from rape. Am J Prev Med 2000;19:228.
33. Ellertson C, Evans M, Ferden S, et al. Extending the time limit for starting the Yuzpe regimen of emergency contraception to 120 hours. Obstet Gynecol 2003;101: 1168–71.
34. Trussell J, Rodriguez G, Ellertson C. Updated estimates of the effectiveness of the Yuzpe regimen of emergency contraception. Contraception 1999;59:147–52.
35. von Hertzen H, Piaggio G, Ding J, et al. Low dose mifepristone and two regimens of levonorgestrel for emergency contraception: a WHO multicentre randomized trial. Lancet 2002;360:1803–10.
36. Korba VD, Heil CG Jr. Eight years of fertility control with norgestrel-ethinyl estradiol (Ovral): An updated clinical review. Fertil Steril 1975;26:973.
37. Workowski KA, Berman S, Centers for Disease Control and Prevention. Sexually transmitted disease treatment guidelines, 2010. MMWR Recomm Rep 2010; 59(No. RR-12):90–5.
38. Royce RA, Sena A, Cates W, et al. Sexual transmission of HIV. N Engl J Med 1997; 336:1072.

39. Centers for Disease Control and Prevention, Smith DK, Grohskopf LA, et al. Antiretroviral postexposure prophylaxis after sexual, injection-drug use, or other nonoccupational exposure to HIV in the United States: recommendations from the U.S. Department of Health and Human Services. MMWR Recomm Rep 2005;54(RR-2): 1–20.
40. Linden JA, Oldeg P, Mehta SD, et al. HIV postexposure prophylaxis in sexual assault: current practice and patient adherence to treatment recommendations in a large urban teaching hospital. Acad Emerg Med 2005;12:640–6.
41. Wiebe ER, Comay SE, McGregor M, et al. Offering HIV prophylaxis to people who have been sexually assaulted: 16 months' experience in a sexual assault service. CMAJ 2000;162:641–5.
42. Myles JE, Hirozawa A, Katz MK, et al. Postexposure prophylaxis for HIV after sexual assault [letter]. JAMA 2000;284:1516–8.
43. Burgess AW, Holmstrom LL. Rape trauma syndrome. Am J Psychiatry 1974;131: 981–6.
44. Ackerman DR, Sugar NF, Fine DN, et al. Sexual assault victims: factors associated with follow-up care. Am J Obstet Gynecol 2006;194:1653–9.
45. Boykins AD, Mynatt S. Assault history and follow-up contact of women survivors of recent sexual assault. Issues Ment Health Nurs 2007;28:867–81.
46. Coker AL, Smith PH, McKeown RE, et al. Frequency and correlates of intimate partner violence by type: physical, sexual and psychological battering. Am J Public Health 2000;90(4):553–9.
47. Abbey A, Zawacki T, Buck PO, et al. Alcohol and sexual assault. Alcohol Res Health 2001;25:43.
48. LeBeau MA, Andollo W, Hearn WL, et al. Recommendations for toxicological investigations of drug-facilitated sexual assaults. J Forensic Sci 1999;44:227–30.
49. Slaughter L. Involvement of drugs in sexual assault. J Reprod Med 2000;45:425.
50. Negrusz A, Juhascik M, Gaensslen RE. Estimate of the incidence of drug-facilitated sexual assault in the U.S. Document 212000. Federal Grant 2000-RB-CX-K003. U.S. Department of Justice. Available at: http://www.ncjrs.gov/pdffiles1/nij/grants/212000.pdf. Accessed April 21, 2011.

Genitourinary Emergencies in the Nonpregnant Woman

Gillian Schmitz, MD[a,*], Carrie Tibbles, MD[b,c]

KEYWORDS

- Pelvic pain • Pelvic inflammatory disease • Ovarian cysts
- Ovarian torsion • Abnormal vaginal bleeding • Bartholin cyst
- Emergency contraception

Lower abdominal and pelvic pains are common symptoms in women who present to the emergency department (ED). Pregnancy should always be ruled out in any woman of child-bearing age. This article reviews diagnostic techniques, therapeutic interventions, as well as new concepts and management principles for common diagnoses in nonpregnant women including pelvic inflammatory disease, ovarian cysts and masses, ovarian torsion, abnormal vaginal bleeding, Bartholin cysts, and emergency contraception.

PELVIC INFLAMMATORY DISEASE

Background

Pelvic inflammatory disease (PID) encompasses an ascending pelvic infection from the cervix and its sequelae, which may include tubo-ovarian abscesses, endometritis, and salpingitis. PID may result in acute or chronic pelvic pain, infertility from scarring of the fallopian tubes, and may increase the rate of ectopic pregnancy.[1] Infection with *Chlamydia trachomatis* remains the most common bacterial sexually transmitted disease (STD) in the United States.[2] Estimates regarding the number of cases are likely underrepresented because most patients remain asymptomatic.[3] The incidence of PID has been reported to be as high as 2% in women of reproductive age and the annual costs of the acute infection and its sequelae in the United States have been estimated at approximately US$ 2 billion.[4]

[a] Department of Emergency Medicine, Georgetown University, Washington Hospital Center, 110 Irving Street NW, Washington, DC 20010, USA
[b] Department of Graduate Medical Education, Beth Israel Deaconess Medical Center, 330 Brookline Avenue, Boston, MA 02215, USA
[c] Harvard Affiliated Emergency Medicine Residency, Beth Israel Deaconess Medical Center, 330 Brookline Avenue, Boston, MA 02215, USA
* Corresponding author.
E-mail address: gillianmd@gmail.com

Emerg Med Clin N Am 29 (2011) 621–635
doi:10.1016/j.emc.2011.04.002
emed.theclinics.com
0733-8627/11/$ – see front matter

Neisseria gonorrhoeae and *Chlamydia trachomatis* have been isolated in many cases of PID; however, laparoscopic cultures suggest mixed infection in 30% to 40% of cases.[5] Studies of adolescent patients demonstrated that patients diagnosed with PID are at risk for subsequent development of STD and recurrent PID infection. Of 110 adolescent women treated for PID as outpatients, 34% had an additional diagnosis of an STD within 2 years and 44% of those patients developed a second episode of PID.[6] Risk factors for PID include multiple sexual partners, history of other STDs, younger age, sexual abuse, and frequent vaginal douching.[7]

Diagnosis

History and physical examination findings

The signs and symptoms of PID are variable. Although lower abdominal pain is the most frequent complaint, patients may also have vaginal discharge, bleeding, dysuria, dyspareunia, fever or malaise, or they may be completely asymptomatic.[4,8] Classic findings on physical examination include lower abdominal tenderness, cervical motion tenderness, and uterine or adnexal tenderness. However, these diagnostic criteria are based on empirical data. Expert opinion as well as the sensitivity and specificity of the findings of pelvic examinations have been questioned in several studies. None of the signs and symptoms (abnormal vaginal discharge, fever >38°C, vomiting, menstrual irregularity, marked tenderness of pelvic organs on bimanual examination) have both high sensitivity and specificity.[9] Increased erythrocyte sedimentation rate (ESR), fever, and adnexal tenderness were found to have a positive association with PID but even these 3 variables correctly classified only 65% of patients with laparoscopically diagnosed PID.[8] Furthermore, the interexaminer reliability of bimanual pelvic examinations performed by emergency physicians in the ED setting has been poor.[10] Compared with the traditional digital bimanual examination, sonographic bimanual examination improved confidence in many aspects of the pelvic examination of nonpregnant women regardless of body mass index (BMI), and it may be a useful adjunct to the physical examination.[11] A clinical prediction rule has been developed to help differentiate PID from appendicitis in women of child-bearing age. Factors favoring PID included (1) no migration of pain, (2) bilateral abdominal tenderness, and (3) absence of nausea and vomiting.[12] When all 3 factors were present, this prediction rule was found to have a sensitivity of 99% in differentiating appendicitis from PID. However, it does not necessarily rule in PID in the undifferentiated patient with pelvic or abdominal pain. This prediction rule requires further prospective validation.

The evidence suggests that positive findings on physical examination are useful when present, but the absence of signs or symptoms does not rule out PID and the results of physical examinations are highly variable between examiners.

Imaging

Although laparoscopy is considered the gold standard in the diagnosis of PID, ultrasound is the imaging modality of choice for the evaluation of pelvic pain in the ED.[13] In a study of emergency medicine (EM) residents and attendings, the use of bedside ultrasound helped to diagnose tubo-ovarian abscesses in cases where only 45% of patients reported cervical motion tenderness or adnexal tenderness. This further demonstrates the limitations of physical examination and clinical criteria for the diagnosis of PID. Findings on ultrasonograms of patients with tubo-ovarian abscesses included complex adnexal mass (70%), echogenic fluid in the cul-de-sac (25%), and pyosalpinx (15%).[14]

Magnetic resonance imaging (MRI) has been shown to be a valuable alternative but is often limited in the ED setting because of limited availability, the expense involved, and the long duration of the imaging process.[15] The role of computed tomography (CT) in the evaluation of pelvic pain may be useful in cases where the ultrasonographic findings are equivocal or to exclude other pathology in the undifferentiated patient with poorly localized abdominal and pelvic pain.[16] Multiplanar CT reconstructions of the fallopian tubes can depict the tubal anatomy to better visualize a tubo-ovarian abscess, but it has the disadvantages of ionizing radiation and increased cost compared with ultrasonography.[17] Multidetector CT detected 90% of adnexal masses in a study of cadavers.[18] Similarly, the multiplanar capability of MRI improved characterization of tissue and provided excellent detail and resolution.[19] However, despite the fact that the use of CT and MR multiplanar technology has increased substantially in recent years, ultrasonography continues to be recommended as the initial imaging modality of choice in the evaluation of most pelvic diseases.[12,17]

Therapy

For outpatient management, the first line of treatment for PID is ceftriaxone, 250 mg intramuscular in a single dose, plus doxycycline, 100 mg orally twice a day for 14 days.[2] Concurrent use of oral metronidazole may be considered. If parenteral cephalosporin therapy is not feasible, oral levofloxacin or ofloxacin, with or without metronidazole, can be used if the prevalence of *Neisseria gonorrhoeae* is low, and should be further guided by culture and sensitivity findings. Patients admitted for PID should receive doxycycline, 100 mg intravenously (IV) every 12 hours, plus cefotetan, 2 g (IV) every 12 hours, or cefoxitin, 2 g (IV) every 6 hours. Clindamycin or metronidazole should be added if tubo-ovarian abscess is suspected. Patients with penicillin allergy should receive clindamycin, 900 mg (IV) every 8 hours, plus gentamicin.

Disposition

Most patients with PID can be managed as outpatients. Criteria for hospitalization include pregnancy, tubo-ovarian abscess, severe illness, inability to tolerate oral regimen or lack of response to oral therapy, and inability to exclude surgical emergency.[20]

Screening and Prevention

Although some evidence suggests that screening for chlamydia reduces the rate of PID, the effectiveness of a single test has been disappointing. In one prospective European study treatment of chlamydia-positive patients reduced the incidence of progression to PID from 9.5% to 1.6%. However, most episodes of PID occurred in women who initially tested negative for chlamydia.[21] This suggests that screening may need to occur more frequently to detect those patients who subsequently develop STD but remain asymptomatic. Treatment of any symptomatic patient in the ED and counseling for frequent screening and follow-up is recommended.

OVARIAN CYSTS AND MASSES

The diagnosis and appropriate management of adnexal masses can be challenging because the differential diagnosis is broad (**Tables 1** and **2**), but they are most commonly functional cysts or benign tumors. Evaluation is important to identify patients who are at higher risk for torsion or ovarian cancer. The lifetime risk of a woman developing ovarian cancer is about 1 in 70.[22] Masses in premenopausal

Table 1
Imaging modalities for the evaluation of pelvic masses

Modality	Sensitivity (%)	Specificity (%)	Positive Likelihood Ratio
Doppler ultrasonography	86	91	9.6
Magnetic resonance imaging	91	88	7.6
Computed tomography	90	75	3.6

Data from Agency for Healthcare Research and Quality. Management of adnexal mass. Evidence based report/technology assessment no. 130. AHRQ publication no. 06–E004. Rockville (MD): AHRQ; 2006.

women are more likely to be gynecologic (ie, functional cysts), whereas adnexal masses in postmenopausal women are more likely to be benign neoplasms (ie, cystadenomas). Physical examination has limited ability to detect adnexal masses. Transvaginal ultrasound remains the recommended diagnostic imaging modality and is superior to other techniques in terms of overall accuracy.

Management of Pelvic Masses

Adnexal masses in premenopausal women are generally benign but require gynecologic follow-up if symptomatic once ovarian torsion has been excluded. In a prospective trial, premenopausal women diagnosed with benign ovarian cysts smaller than 6 cm in diameter were followed for a median of 42 months with conservative management. Most lesions, which included endometriomas, simple cysts, dermoid cysts, hemorrhagic cysts, and hydrosalpinx, remained unchanged in size during this period. All the cysts disappeared after 2 years and no patient developed signs or symptoms of ovarian cancer.[23]

Table 2
Differential diagnosis of pelvic mass

Type of Adnexal Mass	Benign	Malignant
Gynecologic	Ectopic pregnancy Endometrioma Functional cyst Hydrosalpinx Leiomyomata Mature teratoma Mucinous cystadenoma Serous cystadenoma Tubo-ovarian abscess	Epithelial carcinoma Germ cell tumor Stromal tumor Metastatic breast cancer
Nongynecologic	Appendiceal abscess Bladder diverticulum Nerve sheath tumor Paratubal cyst Pelvic kidney Ureteral diverticulum	Gastrointestinal cancer Metastasis Retroperitoneal sarcoma

Data from American College of Obstetricians and Gynecologists. Management of adnexal masses. ACOG practice bulletin no. 83. Obstet Gynecol 2007;110:202.

Polycystic ovary syndrome is another common condition that affects 5% to 10% of women of reproductive age and may be diagnosed incidentally in the ED. Changes in treatment strategies have been developed based on its complex pathogenesis and association with insulin resistance and increased risk of cardiovascular disease. Further follow-up with a primary care physician and gynecologist can aid management with diet changes, oral contraceptives, clomiphene citrate, gonadotropins, antiandrogens, and insulin-sensitizing agents.[24]

Ovarian masses in postmenopausal women have a greater chance of malignancy and most pelvic masses (excluding simple cysts) require further diagnostic evaluation by a gynecologist. The ovary is a common site for metastasis of uterine, breast, and colorectal cancer.

A prospective trial of more than 2500 postmenopausal women with unilocular cysts 10 cm or smaller in diameter who were evaluated with serial ultrasonography showed that more than two-thirds of patients had spontaneous resolution.[25] No cancers were found after a mean follow-up of 6.3 years. This suggests that the risk of malignancy is extremely low in this subset of patients and therefore, simple cysts 10 cm or less in diameter may be monitored without intervention.[22] Increases in cancer antigen 125 (CA-125) levels are helpful in discriminating benign from malignant lesions but are more specific in postmenopausal patients and are not routinely ordered in the ED.

Referral for a newly diagnosed pelvic mass is recommended if the examination or imaging reveals ascites, abdominal or distant metastases, first degree family history of breast or ovarian cancer, or increased levels of CA-125 (>200 units/mL in women <50 years and >35 units/mL in women >50 years of age).[26]

Complications

Most ovarian masses and disorders are benign and are frequently incidental findings. However, they may cause symptoms, such as hormonal overproduction, hemorrhage, rupture, mass effects, or torsion. Ovarian cyst rupture and hemorrhage is generally self-limiting but can present with a surgical abdomen, and may require laparoscopy if the diagnosis is questionable or the patient is hemodynamically compromised. Recurrent cyst rupture or hemorrhage may be prevented with oral contraceptives to suppress ovulation.

OVARIAN TORSION

Ovarian torsion is a gynecologic emergency. Twisting of the ovarian vascular pedicle causes obstruction to venous outflow and arterial inflow (**Fig. 1**). It is most often associated with a benign cyst or tumor, which causes partial or complete rotation. The incidence of torsion is 3% amongst acute gynecologic complaints and may result in the loss of ovarian function.[27]

History and physical examination may not reveal classic findings, with sudden onset of unilateral pelvic pain. In one study, the diagnosis was accurate at the first clinical examination in less than 60% of cases.[28]

Typical ultrasonographic findings include a unilateral enlarged ovary, uniform peripheral cystic structures, a mass within the affected ovary, free fluid in the pelvis, lack of arterial or venous blood flow, and a rotated vascular pedicle (**Fig. 2**). The presence of flow on color Doppler imaging suggests that the ovary may still be viable but does not exclude the diagnosis.[29] Because the ovary has dual blood supply from both the uterine and ovarian arteries, surgically proven cases of torsion often show documented blood flow on Doppler ultrasonographic examination.[30] Classic findings on ultrasonograms have high false-positive rates approaching 50%, and may be

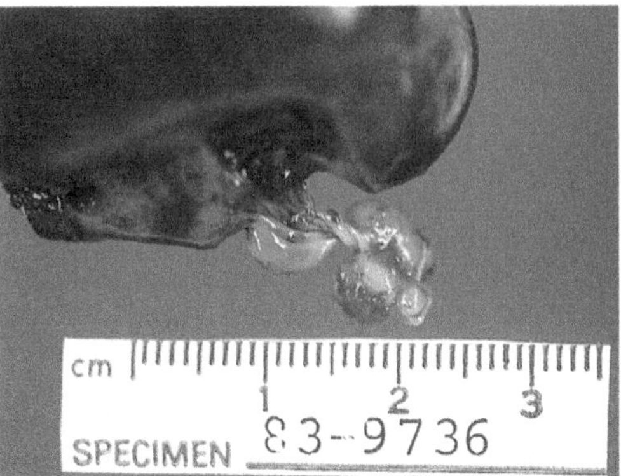

Fig. 1. Surgical pathology specimen following oophorectomy demonstrating torsed pedicle seen in ovarian torsion. (*From* Andreotti RF, Shadinger LL, Fleischer AC. The sonographic diagnosis of ovarian torsion: pearls and pitfalls. Ultrasound Clin 2007;2:11 (Figure 9B); with permission.)

improved with the additional finding of the sonographic whirlpool sign.[31] The whirlpool sign is direct sonographic visualization of the twist in the pedicle on standard gray-scale ultrasound. It has a reported accuracy of 88% for torsion when visualized.[32]

Common CT findings include an enlarged ovary, uterine deviation to the affected side, smooth wall thickening of the twisted adnexal cystic mass or fallopian tube, peripheral cystic structures, and ascites (**Fig. 3**). A CT scan with well-visualized, normal ovaries may assist in excluding ovarian torsion, whereas abnormal findings or the inability to visualize the adnexae necessitate further diagnostic evaluation.[33]

A retrospective study of 34 patients with pathologically proven ovarian torsion compared the accuracy of preoperative diagnosis by imaging modality.[34] Of these patients, 21 had ultrasonography and 13 had CT performed as the initial diagnostic study. The correct diagnosis of ovarian torsion was made in 15/21 (71%) of the patients initially evaluated with ultrasonography, compared with 5/13 (38%) of patients initially evaluated with CT. The sensitivity increased to 14/16 (88%) in patients who had ultrasonography performed with Doppler imaging as the initial study. However, 5/26

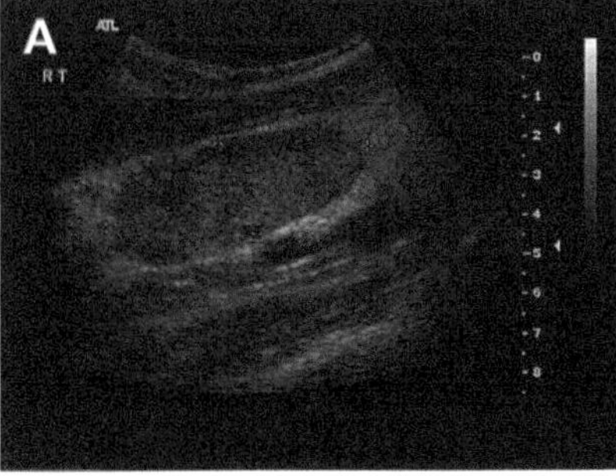

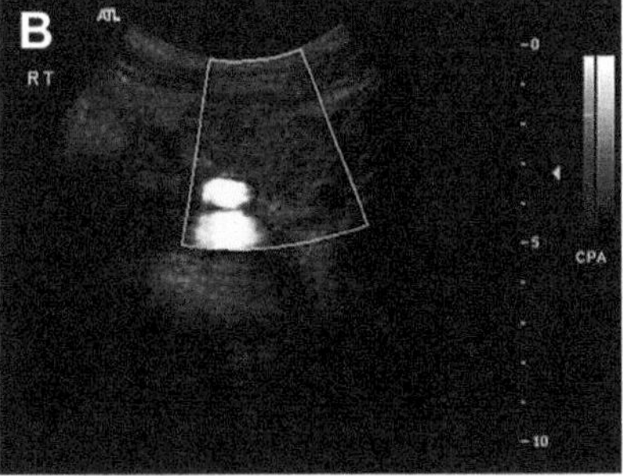

Fig. 2. Typical ultrasonographic findings in ovarian torsion. Enlarged ovary containing homogeneous echoes centrally (*plate A*); power Doppler evaluation fails to demonstrate color signal within the ovary (*plate B*). (*From* Andreotti RF, Shadinger LL, Fleischer AC. The sonographic diagnosis of ovarian torsion: pearls and pitfalls. Ultrasound Clin 2007;2:160 (Figure 8B, C); with permission.)

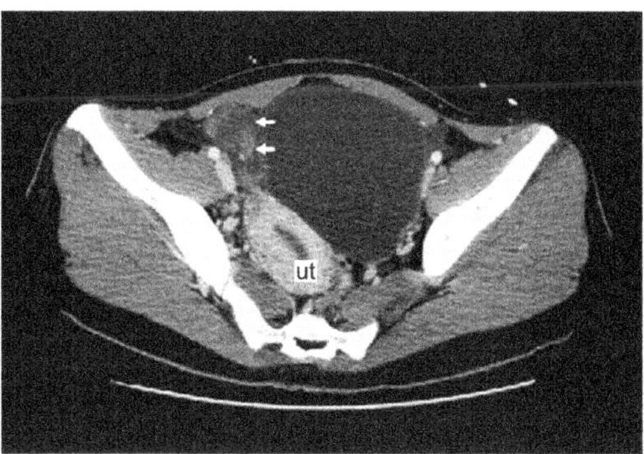

Fig. 3. CT of the pelvis in a patient with pathology proven ovarian torsion demonstrating a right-sided adnexal mass (*arrows*), thickened right fallopian tube, and deviation of the uterus (ut) toward the twisted adnexa. (*From* Andreotti RF, Shadinger LL, Fleischer AC. The sonographic diagnosis of ovarian torsion: pearls and pitfalls. Ultrasound Clin 2007;2:163 (Figure 12B); with permission.)

(19%) of all patients evaluated with Doppler ultrasonography demonstrated normal findings (false-negatives), thus failing to make the correct diagnosis.

The bottom line is that although imperfect, ultrasonography with Doppler is the best available initial diagnostic imaging technique if the clinical suspicion for ovarian torsion is high. The limitations include the fact that ultrasonography is less likely to rule out other diagnoses and may produce falsely reassuring results (false-negatives). CT may be useful initially if the localization of the pain is poor and alternate diagnoses are equally or more likely. The limitations of CT include exposure to ionizing radiation and possible delay in diagnosis if the patient requires further imaging after a nondiagnostic CT. Neither test has perfect sensitivity and further evaluation may be warranted even in the case of a normal study if sufficient clinical concern remains. Because the only definitive diagnosis of ovarian torsion involves surgical intervention, emergent specialty consultation may be necessary to aid in decision making in some cases.

Emergency management consists of rapid evaluation, diagnosis, and consultation with the gynecologist. The prolonged duration of symptoms may not preclude ovarian salvage and urgent management may improve the outcome.[35] Although intuitively postmenopausal women may not require emergent intervention for ovarian salvage, prudent management and disposition should be determined in consultation with gynecologic specialists. Definitive treatment depends on several factors and may be managed with either resection of the adnexa or with ovarian conservation using detorsion, and aspiration or resection of the cyst.

ABNORMAL VAGINAL BLEEDING

Background

Abnormal vaginal bleeding is frequently the chief complaint in patients presenting to the ED. Pregnancy-related bleeding, including ectopic pregnancy, needs to be considered in every patient of reproductive age. Causes of vaginal bleeding in the nonpregnant patient may range from benign anovulatory bleeding to sexual abuse to life-threatening hemorrhage.

History

Elements of the history that are important include menstrual history, onset and duration of symptoms, presence of clots, abuse, trauma, foreign bodies, use of hormone replacement therapy, and other associated symptoms. Past medical history is also essential because other medical conditions including thyroid, liver, and kidney disease as well as coagulation disorders are associated with abnormal vaginal bleeding. It is helpful to quantify the amount of bleeding with an estimation of pads and tampons used on an hourly or daily basis. Sexual history, presence of pain or bleeding with intercourse, and history of any abnormal Pap smears or cancer should be ascertained.

Physical Examination

Initial assessment includes evaluation of hemodynamic stability; the patient's vital signs should be assessed for hypotension or tachycardia. The abdomen should be palpated for any abnormal masses, distension, or tenderness. External examination of the genitalia, rectum, and perineum allows inspection for trauma or foreign bodies. Patients may attribute hematuria or rectal bleeding to vaginal bleeding but other potential bleeding sources should be considered. A speculum examination allows better visualization of the vaginal mucosa and cervix for lacerations, ulcers, friable mucosa, and ongoing bleeding. Bimanual examination may reveal cervical motion tenderness, adnexal tenderness, or the presence of a mass. A rectal examination may be performed to evaluate for other potential sources of bleeding.

Differential Diagnosis

The differential diagnosis for abnormal vaginal bleeding is broad and easiest to characterize by age group. Prepubertal bleeding includes trauma, sexual abuse, congenital abnormalities, vaginitis, foreign bodies, and malignancy. Women in their reproductive years are pregnant until proven otherwise and this diagnosis should always be considered and excluded. Other possible causes include fibroids, polyps, infection or inflammation, intrauterine device or foreign body, malignancy, vascular malformation, sexual intercourse or abuse, and other medical illnesses. Systemic disorders including thyroid disease, hepatic and renal disease, clotting disorders, certain types of cancer, and other causes of autoimmune disease and thrombocytopenia can lead to uterine bleeding.

Dysfunctional uterine bleeding is a diagnosis of exclusion and is a common cause of menorrhagia. It is caused by either failure of endometrial hemostasis (ovulatory dysfunctional uterine bleeding) or failure of the ovary to expel an ovum and decreased progesterone production (anovulatory, dysfunctional uterine bleeding). The latter results in overgrowth of the endometrium that eventually sloughs when it outgrows its vascular supply. Postmenopausal women are most likely to bleed from endometrial atrophy but malignancy should always be considered because the incidence of endometrial cancer increases with age. Some types of hormone replacement therapy contain progesterone, which results in withdrawal bleeding when given cyclically. Antithrombotic agents or hormone treatment may cause vaginal bleeding but further follow-up with gynecology is needed to exclude alternate causes.[36]

Laboratory and Imaging Studies

Laboratory studies may be helpful if the bleeding is thought to be significant or would change the management or disposition of the patient. A pregnancy test should be performed to rule out pregnancy-associated bleeding. A complete blood count provides information on hemoglobin, hematocrit, and platelet count. Coagulation studies may be helpful for patients who are anticoagulated, have liver disease, or clotting disorders. Blood typing is helpful if the patient is likely to require blood product transfusion. Pelvic ultrasound in the nonpregnant patient should be reserved for patients with significant bleeding or in other cases where it may affect acute management or disposition. Ultrasonography may reveal sources of bleeding including fibroids, polyps, endometrial thickening, masses, or a tubo-ovarian abscess. A potentially unstable patient should not be sent out of the ED for imaging; rather bedside evaluation and emergent specialty consultation are prudent. At the other end of the spectrum, a stable patient with a normal hemoglobin level or hematocrit may be referred for further outpatient evaluation including outpatient ultrasonographic imaging.

Treatment and Referral

Unstable patients require aggressive resuscitation and possible blood transfusion, admission, and surgical management. Stable patients should have follow-up gynecologic consultations for further evaluation because the underlying cause of bleeding is not always evident in the ED. Treatment of the nonpregnant patient may be medical or surgical and depends on the age of the patient, the cause of the bleeding, and the patient's desire to become pregnant or maintain fertility.

A trial or taper of oral contraceptives may be used or recommended in patients younger than 35 years, who do not smoke, because this population is at less risk for cancer and blood clots. One treatment option for outpatient management is estrogen, 10 mg/day in 4 divided doses.[37] Ten milligrams of medroxyprogesterone acetate is added for 7 to –10 days after bleeding has stopped to prompt withdrawal bleeding on completion and help establish a regular cycle.[30] Another option for patients with a history of anovulation is medroxyprogesterone alone or as a combined oral contraceptive to promote organized endometrial sloughing and withdrawal bleeding. Contraceptives containing ethinyl estradiol 35 μg and norethindrone 1 mg can be given 4 times daily until the bleeding stops, followed by a 10-day taper, which results in withdrawal bleeding. Several other hormonal and medical therapies may be used and can be initiated in consultation with the gynecologist.

Patients who do not respond to medical therapy may undergo dilation and curettage or other endometrial ablation procedures. Hysterectomy can be performed in severe cases or electively in patients who are postmenopausal and understand the risks, benefits, and fertility implications of surgery.

BARTHOLIN CYSTS AND ABSCESSES

Obstruction of the distal Bartholin duct may result in its dilation and formation of a cyst. The cyst may become infected and an abscess may develop in the Bartholin gland. However, a Bartholin duct cyst does not necessarily have to be present for a gland abscess to develop.

There are many different management options for Bartholin cysts and abscesses. Certain techniques should not be used when an abscess is present, whereas others are preferred in the setting of gland abscesses. Management options include sitz baths, antibiotic treatment, needle aspiration, simple drainage, incision and drainage followed by primary closure, the creation of a new duct opening through fistulization, marsupialization, gland excision, destruction with silver nitrate or alcohol, and laser cyst ablation. The most common fistulization technique involves insertion of a small inflatable catheter (Word catheter) into the cyst or abscess cavity. Novel fistulization techniques, such as using a small loop of secured plastic tubing in place of a Word catheter, have also been described in the EM literature.[38] A Jacobi ring catheter creates 2 drainage tracts rather than 1 and is thought to be as effective as a Word catheter.[39,40] Marsupialization involves surgical eversion of the cyst wall followed by its approximation to the surrounding vaginal mucosa. It should not be performed when an abscess is present. A prospective randomized study comparing marsupialization with silver nitrate application found similar recurrence rates for the two methods, but the group randomized to silver nitrate completed healing faster with less scar formation.[41]

A recent systematic review evaluated several methods of treatment and compared their recurrence rates and time to healing.[42] The recurrence rate after treatment was highest for needle aspiration. There were no reported recurrences after marsupialization, but this procedure was found to have significantly longer healing time compared with incision and drainage followed by primary closure, without any significant difference in recurrence. Premature loss of the Word catheter was the most frequent adverse event in patients who received catheter placement after fistulization. Recurrence of Bartholin cyst or abscess ranged from 4% to 17% after fistulization with either a Word catheter or a Jacobi ring. Comparative studies were too heterogeneous for meta-analysis, and recurrence and healing times varied between studies although healing generally occurred within 2 weeks. Thus, this literature review was unable to identify a best treatment approach, and optimal management for Bartholin duct cysts and abscesses remains unclear until larger, randomized, controlled trials comparing therapeutic strategies are performed. The existing literature supports the use of any of these methods and is dependent on the comfort of the provider and patient characteristics.

Bartholin Cyst and Abscess Drainage

Patients tend to present for emergency evaluation with progressive cyst pain or associated abscess formation. There is a lack of compelling evidence supporting any single management technique over others. The two methods most commonly used in the ED setting for cysts and abscesses are simple incision and drainage or incision followed by the placement of a Word catheter.[43]

For simple incision and drainage, the labia are spread open to allow adequate visualization and a 1-cm vertical incision is made on the mucosal surface of the labia minora. Care should be taken to avoid incision on the more lateral, nonmucosal (skin) side of the labia minora, because this may lead to fistula formation and other complications. The incision is extended through the abscess or cyst and the contents of the cavity are expressed manually. A wick is then placed within the cavity to prevent premature closing.

For incision and insertion of a Word catheter, a small 0.5-cm stab wound is made to the mucosal surface of the labia minora into the abscess cavity. The contents are again expressed manually and the tip of the Word catheter is guided into the wound cavity (**Fig. 4**). The balloon is inflated by injecting 2 to 4 mL of sterile saline into the free end of the catheter, which should remain in place if the inflated balloon is larger than the initial puncture made during incision. The free end of the catheter is placed inside the vaginal canal and left in place for up to 4 weeks before removal. Wound culture and the use of antibiotics are controversial and left to the discretion of the physician.[44] Recurrence is the most common complication with either technique. Patients with recurrent cysts and abscesses, the presence of deeper or more extensive infection, or patients at higher risk for carcinoma should be referred to gynecology for further evaluation and management.

EMERGENCY CONTRACEPTION

Emergency contraception is a common reason for ED visits for victims of sexual assault as well as patients who have not used adequate protection during sexual intercourse. In 2007, the US Food and Drug Administration (FDA) approved over-the-

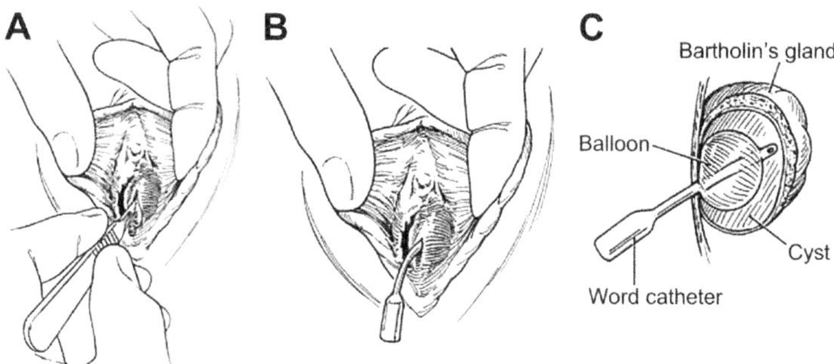

Fig. 4. Bartholin cyst and abscess drainage: (*A*) vaginal mucosal incision, (*B*) Word catheter placement into cyst cavity, (*C*) Word catheter balloon inflated within cyst cavity. (*From* Campbell CJ. Incision and drainage of Bartholin's abscess. In: Rosen P, Chan TC, Vilke GM, et al, editors. Atlas of emergency procedures. St Louis (MO): Mosby; 2001. p. 153; with permission.)

counter (OTC) availability of levonorgestrel, marketed as Plan B.[45] In 2009, the FDA lowered the required age for OTC availability of levonorgestrel to include patients aged 17 years and older. Levonorgestrel is available for patients younger than 17 years by prescription. Levonorgestrel 0.75 mg orally should be administered as soon as possible following intercourse, followed by a second dose 12 hours later. Although it is recommended that patients take the medication as soon as possible, it can be given up to 120 hours later. The most common side effect is nausea, experienced in about 18% of patients, which may be lessened with the use of antiemetics.[46] It is not associated with the contraindications of other forms of birth control because of its short course. Single dose levonorgestrel 1.5 mg orally, known as Plan B One-Step, is an alternative dosing regimen.

Despite the widespread availability of emergency contraception, it failed to reduce unplanned pregnancies in a randomized controlled trial.[47] Use of emergency contraception was lower in women with higher number of previous pregnancies, recent reported history of unprotected sex, and less aversion to pregnancy. Thus, increased access to emergency contraceptives may have a greater impact on those women who are less likely to become pregnant anyway and may explain the lack of benefit seen in clinical trials.[48] A survey of emergency care providers demonstrated that almost half of the respondents were not very familiar with emergency contraception and identified 5 barriers to prescribing them: lack of follow-up (72%), time constraints (40%), lack of clinical resources ([illegible]), discouraging regular contraceptive use (29%), and concern about birth defects (27%).[49] Despite such concerns, there has been no demonstrated association between the use of levonorgestrel and any pregnancy complication, congenital malformation, or adverse pregnancy outcome.[50] Another study found no association between the use of emergency contraception and future risk of pregnancy and sexually transmitted infection.[51] A 2007 survey of New York schools demonstrated that less than half the students had heard about emergency contraceptive pills, despite extensive publicity.[52] Even in the United Kingdom, where 91% of the women surveyed were familiar with the morning after pill, fewer than 7% of women had actually used it in the preceding year.[53] This was thought to be secondary to poor understanding of fertility, contraception, and pregnancy risk. Addressing educational gaps in both higher risk patients as well as health care providers may therefore be the most beneficial action to increase access to emergency contraceptive pills in the ED or OTC.

SUMMARY

Pelvic pain occurring in a female patient is a common ED presentation. In patients presenting with pelvic pain or vaginal bleeding, excluding pregnancy is the most important initial diagnostic undertaking. Once pregnancy has been ruled out, attention focuses on other potential life or fertility threats. Time-sensitive conditions, such as unstable pelvic hemorrhage, ovarian torsion, or tubo-ovarian abscess, should be aggressively managed in consultation with a gynecologist. Ultrasonography remains the most helpful initial diagnostic modality in evaluating acute pelvic pain, bleeding, or infection in most cases.

Because many patients may not have access to a primary care provider or gynecologist, emergency physicians should also be familiar with the treatment of common STDs, diagnosis and treatment of PID, drainage of Bartholin cyst abscesses, use of emergency contraception, and general education for patients regarding pelvic infection or other pathology. Large ovarian cysts or masses, abnormal vaginal bleeding (particularly in postmenopausal women), and recurrent or extensive Bartholin cyst infections should be referred for urgent gynecologic follow-up.

Most nonpregnant women with pelvic complaints can be safely managed in the outpatient setting after ED evaluation. However, emergency practitioners should be aware of possible emergencies and the latest recommendations for diagnosis and treatment.

REFERENCES

1. Abatangelo L, Okereke L, Parham-Foster C, et al. If pelvic inflammatory disease is suspected empiric treatment should be initiated. J Am Acad Nurse Pract 2010; 22:117–22.
2. Centers for Disease Control and Prevention. Sexually transmitted disease treatment guidelines, 2010. MMWR Recomm Rep 2010;59(No. RR-12):44–9, 63–7.
3. Stokes T. Screening for Chlamydia in general practice: a literature review and summary of the evidence. J Public Health Med 1997;19(2):222–32.
4. Rein DB, Kassler WJ, Irwin KL, et al. Direct medical cost of pelvic inflammatory disease and its sequelae: decreasing but still substantial. Obstet Gynecol 2000;95:39.
5. Behrman AJ, Shoff WH, Shepherd SM. Pelvic inflammatory disease. In: Tintinalli JE, Kelen G, Stapczynski JS, editors. Emergency medicine: a comprehensive study guide. 6th edition. New York: McGraw-Hill; 2004. p. 697.
6. Trent M, Chung SE, Forrest L. Subsequent sexually transmitted infection after outpatient treatment of pelvic inflammatory disease. Arch Pediatr Adolesc Med 2008;162:1022–5.
7. Marks C, Tideman RL, Estcourt CS, et al. Assessment of risk for pelvic inflammatory disease in urban sexual health population. Sex Transm Infect 2000;76:470.
8. Centers for Disease Control and Prevention. 2002 Guidelines for treatment of sexually transmitted diseases. MMWR Recomm Rep 2002;51(RR-6):1.
9. Simms I, Warburton F, Westrom L. Diagnosis of pelvic inflammatory disease: time to rethink. Sex Transm Infect 2003;7:491–4.
10. Close RJ, Sachs CJ, Dyne PL. Reliability of bimanual pelvic examinations performed in emergency departments. West J Med 2001;175:240–4.
11. Tayal VS, Crean CA, Noton HJ, et al. Prospective comparative trial of endovaginal sonographic bimanual examination versus traditional digital bimanual examination in nonpregnant women with lower abdominal pain with regard to body mass index classification. J Ultrasound Med 2008;27:1171–7.

12. Morishita K, Gushimiyagi M, Hashiguchi M, et al. Clinical prediction rule to distinguish pelvic inflammatory disease from acute appendicitis in women of childbearing age. Am J Emerg Med 2007;25:152–7.
13. Benacerraf BR. Why has computed tomography won and ultrasound lost the market share of imaging for acute pelvic conditions in the female patient? J Ultrasound Med 2010;29:327–8.
14. Adhikari S, Blaivas M, Lyon M. Role of bedside transvaginal ultrasonography in the diagnosis of tubo-ovarian abscess in the emergency department. J Emerg Med 2008;34:429–33.
15. Occhipinti KA, Frankel SD, Hricak H. The ovary. Computed tomography and magnetic resonance imaging. Radiol Clin North Am 1993;31:1115–32.
16. Alonso R, Nacenta S, Martinez P. Role of multidetector CT in the management of acute female pelvic disease. Emerg Radiol 2009;16:453–72.
17. Yitta S, Hecht EM, Slywotzky CM. Added value of multiplanar reformation in the multidetector CT evaluation of the female pelvis: a pictorial review. Radiographics 2009;29:1987–2003.
18. Tsili AC, Tsampoulas C, Charisiadi A. Adnexal masses: accuracy of detection and differentiation with multidetector computed tomography. Gynecol Oncol 2008; 110:22–31.
19. Levine CD, Patel UJ, Ghanekar D. Benign extraovarian mimics of ovarian cancer. Distinction with imaging studies. Clin Imaging 1997;21:350–8.
20. Balamuth F, Zhai H, Mollen C. Toward improving the diagnosis and the treatment of adolescent pelvic inflammatory disease in emergency departments: results of a brief, educational intervention. Pediatr Emerg Care 2010;26: 85–92.
21. Oakeshott P, Kerry S, Aghaizu A. Randomised controlled trial of screening for *Chlamydia trachomatis* to prevent pelvic inflammatory disease: the POPI (prevention of pelvic infection) trial. BMJ 2010;340:C1642.
22. Graham L. ACOG releases guidelines on management of masses. Am Fam Physician 2008;77:1320–3.
23. Alcazar JL, Castillo G, Jurado M, et al. Is expectant management of sonographically benign adnexal cysts an option in selected asymptomatic premenopausal women? Hum Reprod 2005;20:3231–4.
24. Krysiak R, Okopien B, Gdula Dymek A. Update on the management of polycystic ovary syndrome. Pharmacol Rep 2006;58:614–25.
25. Modesitt SC, Pavlik EJ, Ueland FR, et al. Risk of malignancy in unilocular cystic tumors less than 10 centimeters in diameter. Obstet Gynecol 2003;102: 594–9.
26. Im SS, Gordon AN, Buttin BM, et al. Validation of referral guidelines for women with pelvic masses. Obstet Gynecol 2005;105:36.
27. Oelsner G, Shashar D. Adnexal torsion. Clin Obstet Gynecol 2006;49:459.
28. Bouguizane S, Bibi H, Farhat Y. Adnexal torsion: a report of 135 cases. J Gynecol Obstet Biol Reprod 2003;32:535–40.
29. Chang HC, Bhatt S, Dogra VS. Pearls and pitfalls in diagnosis of ovarian torsion. Radiographics 2008;28:1355–68.
30. Tibbles C. Selected gynecologic disorders. In: Marx J, Hockberger R, Walls R, et al, editors. Rosen's emergency medicine concepts and clinical practice. Philadelphia: Mosby Elsevier; 2010. p. 1325–32.
31. Valsky DV, Esh-Broder E, Cohen SM, et al. Added value of the gray-scale whirlpool sign in the diagnosis of adnexal torsion. Ultrasound Obstet Gynecol 2010; 36(5):630–4.

32. Lee EJ, Kwon HC, Joo HJ, et al. Diagnosis of ovarian torsion with color Doppler sonography: depiction of twisted vascular pedicle. J Ultrasound Med 1998;17:83.
33. Moore C, Meyers AB, Capotasto J. Prevalence of abnormal CT findings in patients with proven ovarian torsion and a proposed triage schema. Emerg Radiol 2009;16:115–20.
34. Chiou SY, Lev-Toaff AS, Masuda E, et al. Adnexal torsion: new clinical and imaging observations by sonography, computed tomography, and magnetic resonance imaging. J Ultrasound Med 2007;26:1289–301.
35. Anders JF, Powell EC. Urgency of evaluation and outcome of acute ovarian torsion in pediatric patients. Arch Pediatr Adolesc Med 2005;159:532–5.
36. Daniels RV, McCuskey C. Abnormal vaginal bleeding in the nonpregnant patient. Emerg Med Clin North Am 2003;21(3):751–2.
37. Morrison L, Spence J. Vaginal bleeding and pelvic pain in the nonpregnant patient. Emergency medicine: a comprehensive study guide. St Louis (MO): McGraw-Hill; 2000. p. 669–80.
38. Kushnir VA, Mosquera C. Novel technique for management of Bartholin's gland cyst and abscesses. J Emerg Med 2009;36:388–90.
39. Patil S, Sultan AH, Thakar R. Bartholin's cysts and abscesses. J Obstet Gynaecol 2007;27:241–5.
40. Gennis P, Li SF, Provataris J, et al. Jacobi ring catheter treatment of Bartholin's abscesses. Am J Emerg Med 2005;23:414–5.
41. Ozdegirmenci O, Kayikcioglu F, Haberal A. Prospective randomized study of marsupialization versus silver nitrate application in the management of Bartholin's gland cyst and abscesses. J Minim Invasive Gynecol 2009;16:149–52.
42. Wechter ME, Wu J, Marzano D, et al. Management of Bartholin's duct cyst and abscesses: a systematic review. Obstet Gynecol Surv 2009;64:395–404.
43. Krystaleah L. Bartholin's gland and abscess or cyst incision and drainage. In: Reichman EF, Simon RR, editors. Emergency medicine procedures. 1st edition. New York: McGraw-Hill; 2004. p. 1084–90.
44. Bhide A, Nama V, Patel S, et al. Microbiology of cysts/abscesses of Bartholin's gland: review of empirical antibiotic therapy against microbial culture. J Obstet Gynaecol 2010;30(7):701–3.
45. U.S. Food and Drug Administration. Plan B (0.75 mg levonorgestrel) and Plan B One-Step (1.5 mg levonorgestrel) tablets information. FDA approves Plan B One-Step emergency contraceptive; lowers age for obtaining Two-Dose Plan B emergency contraceptive without a prescription. Available at: http://www.fda.gov/drugs/drugsafety/postmarketdrugsafetyinformationforpatientsandproviders/ucm109775.htm. Accessed February 2, 2011.
46. Raymond EG, Creinin MD, Barnhart KT, et al. Meclizine for prevention of nausea associated with use of emergency contraceptive pills: a randomized trial. Obstet Gynecol 2000;95:271.
47. Lo SS, Fan SY, Ho PC, et al. Effect of advanced provision of emergency contraception on women's contraceptive behavior: a randomized controlled trial. Hum Reprod 2004;19:2404–10.
48. Beacher L, Weaver MA, Raymond EG. Increased access to emergency contraception: why it may fail. Hum Reprod 2009;24:815–9.
49. Goyal M, Zhao H, Mollen C. Exploring emergency contraception knowledge, prescription practices, and barriers to prescription for adolescents in the emergency department. Pediatrics 2009;123:765–70.

50. Zhang Z, Chen J, Wang Y, et al. Pregnancy outcome after Levonorgestrel-only emergency contraception failure: a prospective cohort study. Hum Reprod 2009;24:1605–11.
51. Sander PM, Raymond EG, Weaver MA. Emergency contraceptive use as a marker of future risky sex, pregnancy, and sexually transmitted infection. Am J Obstet Gynecol 2009;201:146.e1–6.
52. Teen pregnancy in New York City, 1997–2007. New York: New York City Department of Health and Mental Hygiene; 2007. Available at: http://www.nyc.gov/html/doh/html/ms/ms-nyctp-97-07.shtml. Accessed February 24, 2011.
53. Westley E, Glasier A. Emergency contraception: dispelling the myths and misperceptions. Bull World Health Organ 2010;88:243.

Pediatric Urinary Tract Infections

Rahul G. Bhat, MD[a,b], Tamara A. Katy, MD[a,*], Frederick C. Place, MD[c]

KEYWORDS

- Urinary tract infections • Urine culture • Urinalysis
- *Escherichia coli* • Pediatric

Urinary tract infections (UTIs) in children are commonly seen in the emergency department (ED) and pose several challenges to establishing the proper diagnosis and determining management. The emergency medicine provider cannot ignore the possibility of UTI when evaluating a neonate (<1 month), infant (1 month to 1 year), or child (≥1 year) with fever without a significant, definite source. Accurate and timely diagnosis of pediatric UTI can prevent short-term complications, such as severe pyelonephritis or sepsis, and long-term sequelae including scarring of the kidneys, hypertension, and ultimately chronic renal insufficiency and need for transplant.[1,2] This article reviews pediatric UTI and addresses epidemiology, diagnosis, treatment, and imaging, and their importance to the practicing emergency medicine provider. The term "febrile UTI" is used to describe upper tract UTI, which typically refers to progression of infection beyond the confines of the bladder with associated systemic symptoms. The term "lower UTI" is used to describe UTI without fever or other systemic symptoms, which is typically diagnosed only in children who can specifically verbalize urinary or other associated complaints.

ETIOLOGY

Bacterial Pathogens

Escherichia coli are responsible for over 80% of pediatric UTIs.[3–8] Other common gram-negative organisms include *Klebsiella, Proteus, Enterobacter*, and occasionally *Pseudomonas*.[6] Gram-positive pathogens include group B *Streptococcus* and *Enterococcus* in neonates and infants, and *Staphylococcus saprophyticus* in adolescent girls.[2,9] Fungal infections are much less common and are usually seen in patients who

[a] Department of Emergency Medicine, Georgetown University Hospital, 3800 Reservoir Road, NW, Washington, DC 20007, USA
[b] Department of Emergency Medicine, Washington Hospital Center, 110 Irving Street, NW, Washington, DC 20010, USA
[c] Department of Emergency Medicine, INOVA Fairfax Hospital, Virginia Commonwealth University, 3300 Gallows Road, Falls Church, VA 22042, USA
* Corresponding author.
E-mail address: tamkaty76@gmail.com

Emerg Med Clin N Am 29 (2011) 637–653
doi:10.1016/j.emc.2011.04.004 emed.theclinics.com
0733-8627/11/$ – see front matter

are diabetic, immunocompromised, or have bladder catheters, particularly those also on long-term antibiotic therapy.[10] Common contaminants include *Lactobacillus* spp, *Corynebacterium* spp, coagulase-negative staphylococci, and α-hemolytic streptococci.[11]

Pathogenesis

As with all infectious processes, UTI represents a battle between host defenses and bacterial virulence factors.[3,12] Host defenses, such as frequent voiding and unidirectional urine flow, work to prevent bacteriuria and urinary stasis, whereas Tamm-Horsfall glycoprotein inhibits bacterial adherence to the urinary mucosa.[13]

Epidemiology

There have been hundreds of heterogeneous studies over the decades examining numerous cohorts that all differ in terms of age range, inclusion criteria, racial composition, circumcision status, and location of enrollment. One of the greatest limitations is that beyond the neonatal period, most studies are observational and inclusion rates (eg, for febrile infants) are at the discretion of the clinician and are well below 100%. However, consistently observed is an increased prevalence of febrile UTI in uncircumcised male neonates and girls under the age of 2 years.[14] A 2007 community-based, multicenter study demonstrated that the cumulative risk of UTI in children under the age of 6 years was 4.2%.[15] The highest prevalence of UTI is consistently found to be in uncircumcised boys less than 3 months of age, followed by girls under 12 months of age.[3,4,14,16] In the ED setting, UTIs are the most common serious bacterial illness encountered in febrile children between 0 and 24 months, with a prevalence ranging from 1.9% to 21%, depending on the population studied.[4,5,14–21]

HOST RISK FACTORS

Gender and Circumcision Status

Interestingly, girls are less likely than uncircumcised boys to present with a febrile UTI in the first few months of life based on the available data.[14] In a representative study by Zorc and coworkers,[4] uncircumcised, febrile boys less than 60 days of age had the greatest incidence of UTI, with a rate of 21% compared with 5% in female infants and only 2.3% in circumcised boys. Beyond the first 6 months of age, however, girls have a significantly greater risk of UTI than boys.[14,16,20] Most authorities recommend routine examination and culture of the urine in febrile girls 0 to 24 months of age.[16,20,22]

Uncircumcised males have a significantly higher rate of UTI than any other population, particularly in early infancy.[4,16,23,24] Most studies have consistently confirmed a 10- to 20-fold increase in the risk of UTI in uncircumcised males.[4,5,16,21,23,24] Uncircumcised males experience a higher rate of UTI through several mechanisms, including heavy periurethral colonization by uropathogens, and an inability to fully retract the foreskin.[24–26] When evaluating a febrile, uncircumcised infant in the ED, the best available evidence suggests that a significant risk of UTI persists up until 12 months of age, and work-up should include urinalysis and culture.[22] Febrile circumcised boys over 6 months of age have a statistically lower risk of UTI and generally do not require a work-up with urinalysis and culture.[22]

Race

White race, as compared with African American and Hispanic ethnicities, has consistently been found to be a significant risk factor for febrile UTIs.[14,16,19,27,28] A meta-analysis of four separate studies found that white children had about twice the rate of UTI compared with black children (8% vs 4.7%).[21] In particular, febrile white girls under the age of 2 years with a temperature greater than or equal to 39°C are at greatest risk, with reported rates as high as 16%.[16,19]

Behavioral

In older children, parents often ask why their child has developed a UTI and whether it has anything to do with hygienic habits. Bubble baths and direction of wiping after defecation have little support as independent risk factors for the development of UTI.[3,29] Urgency–frequency syndrome (excessively frequent voiding) and primary nocturnal enuresis (nighttime bedwetting) likewise have not been definitively linked to increased risk of UTI.[3] Dysfunctional elimination syndrome (incomplete or infrequent voiding, often caused by overly active urinary sphincter tone) may increase the risk of febrile UTI,[30–32] although this association has recently been questioned.[33] UTI has also been linked to the presence of severe constipation, and successful treatment of constipation has been shown to reduce the risk of recurrent UTI.[34,35]

Anatomic Issues

Any abnormality resulting in obstruction to flow of urine can lead to an increased risk of UTI by promoting urinary stasis. These obstructions can be anatomic (urethral stricture, posterior urethral valves) or neurogenic, generally from congenital or acquired abnormalities of the spinal cord.

Vesicoureteral reflux (VUR) is an abnormality of urine flow, with reflux of urine from the bladder proximally into the ureters. Normally, the distal ureter courses obliquely through the bladder wall and intramural pressure of the bladder wall compresses this segment, preventing retrograde flow.[36] Children with VUR typically have a shorter, less oblique intramural segment, resulting in an ineffectual vesicoureteral junction. As the grade of reflux increases (on a five-point scale), the risk of renal scarring increases.[36] It is unclear whether this scarring is the result of a higher rate of febrile UTI or caused by the hydrostatic pressures alone.[37]

DIAGNOSIS

History and Physical Examination

The evaluation of UTI is generally dependent on the age of the child. The presentation generally shifts from quite nonspecific to more focused complaints as the child grows older. However, signs and symptoms may continue to be subtle even in older children, and one should maintain a reasonable index of suspicion, particularly in highly febrile (>39°C) children. Young infants in particular may present with vague and nonspecific symptoms, such as poor feeding, decreased urinary output, lethargy, increased sleeping, vomiting, failure to thrive, and jaundice.[5,12,38–40] Fever is not necessary to raise the suspicion of UTI in neonates. Occult UTI has been significantly associated with the presence of jaundice, particularly if the onset of jaundice was after 8 days of age and an elevated conjugated bilirubin fraction is present.[39]

Beyond the neonatal period, fever is generally the primary symptom that leads to the diagnosis of UTI, and most ED-based studies explicitly identify fever as inclusion criteria for pediatric UTI.[4,5,16,19,41,42] The duration and height of the fever at presentation are clearly identified risk factors.[43] In a 2007 meta-analysis, more than 2 days of fever greater than or equal to 38°C without a source carried a positive likelihood ratio of 3.6 (95% confidence interval [CI], 1.4–8.8), whereas temperatures greater than or equal to 39°C had a positive likelihood ratio of 4 (95% CI, 1.2–13).[43] This association between higher fevers and occult UTI has been confirmed in other large studies.[4,5,16]

Other nonspecific features commonly reported in children with occult UTI include vomiting; loose stools (often mistaken for diarrhea); and abdominal discomfort.[40] However, other investigators have found that these associations lack statistical significance.[16,19]

It is important to note that in children under the age of 2 years, the presence of another possible source of fever, such as gastroenteritis, bronchiolitis, upper respiratory infection, or otitis media, does not entirely exclude UTI.[16,19] Positive viral antigen studies (eg, respiratory syncytial virus or influenza) have been associated with a significant decrease in UTI risk.[4,11,44,45] However, the risk is not insignificant in young infants; respiratory syncytial virus–positive infants less than 60 days of age have a 5.4% risk of UTI, compared with 10% in respiratory syncytial virus–negative infants.[45]

Likewise, presence of an unequivocal source for the fever (eg, varicella, pneumonia, croup, herpangina, or stomatitis) has been associated with only a modest decrease in the risk of UTI from 5.9% to 3.3%.[16] Hoberman and colleagues[19] found that children with a "possible" source still had an intermediate risk of occult UTI (3.5%) compared with children with an unequivocal source (1.6%) and no clear source (7.5%). Shaw and colleagues[16] studied 2411 febrile children 12 to 24 months of age and found that the prevalence of UTI in children without a source was 5.9%, compared with 2.7% in those with a potential source. Fully 64% of children with UTI were thought to have another source for their fever by the examining clinician.[16] In febrile infants, no single sign or symptom maintains a sufficiently low negative likelihood ratio to exclude UTI.[43]

In older, verbal children, the classic symptoms of dysuria, frequency, abdominal or flank pain, new-onset (often nocturnal) incontinence, and fever all carry significant and useful positive likelihood ratios.[40,43] However, these findings are not adequately specific to diagnose UTI and mandate laboratory evaluation. Adolescent girls with urethritis from an unrecognized sexually transmitted disease (often chlamydia or gonorrhea) are at high risk of misdiagnosis and inappropriate therapy.[46] Many young children experience a brief period in which any urge to void is manifested as urgency or frequency, yet do not have an infectious etiology. Additionally, dysuria is frequently the presenting complaint for nonspecific vaginitis in young girls and occasionally dysuria and hematuria may be the presenting symptoms of urethral prolapse.[47,48] This emphasizes the value of genitourinary examination in all ages, along with a detailed history in children with suspected UTI.

Children with a history of documented UTI are at significant risk of recurrence and should be evaluated aggressively. A recent, large, community-based study found that children with documented UTI under the age of 6 have a 12% risk of recurrence per year.[15]

Laboratory Assessment

The gold standard for the diagnosis of UTI is the urine culture. However, culture results are not typically available until 24 to 48 hours after the initial patient evaluation.[20,40,49,50] Rapid screening tests (ie, dipstick and urinalysis) have long been used to identify children likely to have a positive urine culture.[51] Early identification is particularly important in attempting to avoid renal involvement.[20,51] However, rapid screening tests suffer significant problems with sensitivity and specificity in young children. As such, although they can be used to select children for immediate treatment, they should never be a substitute for obtaining a urine culture.[20,40,50,52]

Urine dipstick

Rapid screening performed by a urine dipstick test primarily looks for the presence of leukocyte esterase (LE) or nitrites in the urine sample. LE is released when leukocytes are broken down with the subsequent release of esterases from lysed urine granulocytes. Nitrites are a byproduct of dietary nitrate metabolism by uropathogenic bacteria.[53] In a 2010 meta-analysis evaluating the accuracy of rapid urine tests in children, Williams and colleagues[54] examined the data from 95 studies with a total of 95,703 children. Summary estimates for the sensitivity and specificity for LE were 79% (95% CI, 73–84) and 87% (95% CI, 79–91), respectively. To emphasize the great variability within the published literature, they noted that across 30 different studies, the sensitivities of LE ranged from 47% to 95%. These results are quite consistent with other published estimates for LE.[14,20,52] Importantly, LE misses more than 20% of children with UTI and inappropriately suggests the presence of UTI in more than 10% of tested patients. Nitrites are far more specific than LE in identifying likely UTI; however, sensitivity is quite poor. The meta-analysis by Williams and colleagues[54] produced sensitivity and specificity estimates of 49% (95% CI, 41%–57%) and 98% (95% CI, 96%–99%), respectively. Again, the range of reported sensitivities across 46 different studies was extreme: 8.3%–95.2%. Nitrites have such a high false-negative rate because not all organisms produce nitrites (eg, gram-positive and *Acinetobacter* spp) or the urine is too dilute. More frequent voiding in non–toilet-trained infants reduces the time available for nitrite conversion.[52,53,55] Thus, although the absence of nitrites in the urine has little diagnostic meaning, their presence virtually guarantees that the child has bacteria in the urine.

Using an either/or strategy to define a positive dipstick has been shown to significantly improve the sensitivity of the urine dipstick without greatly reducing the specificity of the test.[20,52,54] Williams and colleagues[54] found that the presence of either nitrites or LE was more accurate than LE alone, with a sensitivity and specificity of 88% (95% CI, 82%–91%) and 79% (95% CI, 69%–87%), respectively.

Urine microscopy

The presence of pyuria (leukocytes in the urine) has been used for decades to identify patients likely to have a UTI.[56] The definition of pyuria, however, varies widely in the literature.[20] Researchers have traditionally determined a cutoff for pyuria of greater than or equal to five white blood cells per high power field (WBC/hpf) or 10 WBC/hpf, with each study arriving at a different area under the curve and each investigator choosing a different cutoff point for optimal sensitivity or specificity.[52,57] Other investigators have simply chosen one of these values before conducting the study.[18,52,57–60] This lack of standardization is further reflected in the different cutoffs used in nationally published practice guidelines. The most widely disseminated guideline for fever-without-a-source, published by Baraff and colleagues[61] in 1993, recommends using a cutoff of 10 WBC/hpf, whereas the 1999 American Academy of Pediatrics (AAP) UTI Practice Parameter considers a cutoff of 5 WBC/hpf.[20] The question of which cutoff should be used is not a trivial one because positive and negative likelihood ratios can vary significantly (**Table 1**).[40]

Two large meta-analyses in the past decade have tried to address the sensitivity and specificity of microscopic urinalysis, recognizing the extensive heterogeneity in the literature.[54,62] Gorelick and Shaw[52] evaluated five studies using 5 WBC/hpf as a cutoff and nine studies using 10 WBC/hpf. They produced a summary true-positive rate of 67% for 5 WBC/hpf (range, 55%–88%) and 77% using 10 WBC/hpf (range, 57%–92%). False-positive rates were 21% and 11%, respectively. Similarly, Williams and colleagues[54] evaluated 49 studies with 66,937 children and calculated a sensitivity for urine microscopy WBC of 74% (95% CI, 67%–80%) and specificity of 86% (95% CI, 82%–90%) using a cutoff of greater than 5 WBC/hpf in most of the included studies analyzed.

Table 1
Likelihood Ratios of Diagnosing UTI by Age Group

	Microscopy (>5 WBC/hpf for Pyuria and Few Bacteria for Bacteriuria)		Microscopy (>10 WBC/hpf for Byuria and Moderate Bacteria for Bacteriuria)		Dipstick Urine Testing (Both Leukocyte Esterase and Nitrite)	
Children	Younger than 2 years	2 years or older	Younger than 2 years	2 years or older	Younger than 2 years	2 years or older
LR+ (95% CI)	1.63 (1.24–2.13)	1.69 (1.52–1.87)	15.6 (4.16–58.44)	10.84 (5.95–19.75)	6.24 (1.14–34.22)	27.1 (11.44–64.21)
LR– (95% CI)	0.27 (0.07–0.99)	0.04 (0.00–0.59)	0.66 (0.44–0.97)	0.51 (0.35–0.73	0.31 (0.13–0.71)	0.17 (0.07–0.41)

Abbreviation: LR, likelihood ratio.

From National Collaborating Centre for Women's and Children's Health. Urinary tract infection in children: diagnosis, treatment and long-term management. Clinical Guideline. London (UK): RCOG Press; 2007; with the permission of the Royal College of Obstetricians and Gynaecologists.

Both Gorelick and Shaw[52] and Williams and colleagues[54] also examined the accuracy of bacteria noted on microscopic examination. Each investigator reported excellent sensitivity and specificity for the presence of bacteria noted on gram-stained and unstained samples, outperforming both dipstick analysis and microscopy for WBCs. Williams and colleagues[54] reported sensitivities of 91% (95% CI, 80%–96%) in gram-stained samples and 88% (95% CI, 75%–94%) in unstained samples. Specificities were also quite high at 96% and 92%, respectively.

Urine dipstick versus microscopic urinalysis

When the accuracy of dipstick analysis is compared with that of urine microscopy, it is not clear that microscopy, at least for WBCs, provides significant added value.[14,52,54] Gorelick and Shaw[52] and Williams and colleagues[54] both concluded that urine microscopy for white cells should not be used in the diagnostic work-up of UTI, noting comparable sensitivity and specificity to dipstick, along with delay in diagnosis and added cost.[52,54] However, this issue remains unsettled because other investigators have concluded that microscopy outperforms urine dipstick results, particularly in younger children, using higher cutoffs (ie, 10 WBC/hpf) when combined with presence of bacteria.[40,63,64] The real question that remains to be answered is the added value of urine microscopy after dipstick results have already been reported.[40] To date, there has not been a well-designed study that addresses this question.

Urine culture: defining UTI

A positive urine culture is necessary for the diagnosis of a UTI, although actually defining what constitutes a "positive" culture has proved to be difficult and somewhat imprecise.[50,65] It has been known for almost a century that because of the ubiquitous problem of contamination, the mere presence of microorganisms in a urine culture is not enough to prove infection.[50,66] A positive urine culture may be the result of pathogenic bacteriuria (UTI), collection contamination, or asymptomatic bacteriuria.[62] Since the 1950s, a positive urine culture has generally been defined as greater than 10^5 (100,000 or 100K) colony forming units per milliliter (CFU/mL) of urine.[66] This cutoff was initially established by Kass[66] with adults, and later confirmed by Pryles[50] in children, and was based on the bimodal distribution between true bacteriuria and contamination. However, even Kass recognized that some UTIs probably resulted in colony counts less than 10^5, and since then variable cutoffs (often 10K, 50K, or 100K) have been used in various studies to define a positive urine culture, depending on the investigator and the method of collection.[11,19,67] The traditional cutoff for urine obtained by noninvasive collection methods (clean-catch or clean bag) has remained 10^5 (100K) CFU/mL for decades.[5,11,14,15,40,42,67,68] Most investigators use a cutoff of 10^4 (10K) CFU/mL to define infection with specimens obtained by catheterization.[11,16,18,19,69] Because it was recognized very early on that urine obtained by suprapubic aspiration (SPA) in noninfected children is almost invariably sterile, most authorities use 10^2 (0.1K) CFU/mL as the cutoff for defining a positive culture in an SPA sample.[5,18,27] Other published thresholds include 50,000 CFU/mL from a catheterized specimen,[4,44,70,71] 10,000 CFU/mL from a catheterized specimen with a positive urinalysis,[4,44] or any growth from SPA.[64]

A high suspicion for contamination should be maintained for cultures with low colony counts, heavy mixed growth of bacteria, or growth of a pure organism not known to cause infection.[72] Examples of nonpathogenic organisms include *Lactobacillus*, *Corynebacterium*, α-hemolytic streptococci, *Micrococcus*, *Candida*, and coagulase-negative staphylococci.[11,14,67] Investigators often consider the presence of more than one organism to signify contamination; however, mixed growth may represent primary bacteriuria with secondary contamination and clinical judgment should be applied in this scenario.[14,40,45,67] The bottom line is that decisions in the ED setting are often made well before availability of urine culture results. With this said, in evaluating recent urine culture results available at the time of the ED visit, or when interpreting culture results after the ED visit, the important things to remember include the following: more than 100K of a single organism is essentially diagnostic of UTI, more than 50K is suggestive, more than 10K is highly suspicious in a catheterized specimen, and any bacterial growth after SPA should be considered a UTI.

Asymptomatic bacteriuria

A small but defined number of normal, healthy, asymptomatic children have bacteriuria if cultured.[73,74] It is unclear whether these patients will go on to have symptomatic UTIs in the future or would benefit from immediate treatment. Because there is no way to differentiate symptomatic UTI from asymptomatic bacteriuria in the ED setting, patients with positive urine cultures, as defined in the prior section, must be assumed to have symptomatic UTI and treated as such.

Methods of Collection

It has long been recognized that the reliability of urine culture for the diagnosis of UTI depends on the method of collection.[69,75–78] Although urethral catheterization largely eliminated problems with contamination, concerns about invasiveness and the introduction of infection by the procedure itself led to the development of SPA as an alternative, initially considered no more invasive than “an intramuscular injection, and the required skill is no greater.”[78,79] In practice, however, convincing a parent to allow this invasive procedure to be performed on their child may not be so straightforward.

Bagged specimens

Medical personnel and parents alike often prefer the use of noninvasive clean bag urine collection, and a negative urine culture collected by this method can effectively exclude UTI.[20] However, even with meticulous cleaning, bagged specimens produce an unacceptably high rate of contaminated cultures, generally around 63%.[20,56,73,75,78] In one representative study, of the 3440 contaminated cultures evaluated in the study, 132 (1.7%) resulted in one or more adverse clinical outcomes, including unnecessary treatment, admission, or radiologic investigation.[75]

Other investigators have tried to suggest that clean-bag specimens may be more reliable than once believed.[42,80] A large Pediatric Research in Office Setting study of 1646 febrile infants published in 2005 suggested that bagged specimens may have a role in the office setting.[42] Bagged specimens produced more ambiguous cultures compared with catheterization (7.4% vs 2.7%). However, one would need to catheterize 21 children to avoid one ambiguous culture by bag method. Catheterized specimens were more accurate in this study, although the magnitude of the difference was small. In the acute care setting, published guidelines by the AAP, the National Institute for Health and Clinical Excellence, and the World Health Organization clearly discourage the use of bagged specimens, because most studies suggest an unacceptably high culture contamination rate.[20,64,81] A positive culture obtained by bag specimen cannot be used to reliably diagnose UTI.[20] Additionally, because urine dipstick and microscopy (using any method of collection) are not sufficiently sensitive to rule out a UTI, a urine culture is essential. As a result, the urine must be obtained by catheter or SPA in non–toilet-trained children.

Suprapubic aspiration

To distinguish true bacteriuria from contamination, Pryles and several subsequent investigators successfully demonstrated that with proper technique, SPA consistently provides an uncontaminated specimen (**Fig. 1**).[76–79] However, the perception and demonstration of increased discomfort and procedural failure rate has led to a precipitous decline in its use, particularly outside of the neonatal intensive care unit.[82–84] Nevertheless, SPA continues to be considered the gold standard method of urine collection.[12,20,77] Despite the lack of experience by most currently practicing clinicians, the procedure may still be necessary in girls with labial adhesions and boys with phimosis. The relatively recent introduction of ultrasound technology has led to a significant improvement in success rates, and likely in the comfort of the clinician performing the procedure.[82,85–87]

Transurethral bladder catheterization

Despite initial concerns regarding the potential to introduce infection, urinary catheterization has become the standard of practice for febrile children under the age of 2 years.[12,20,40,50,61,78] Early studies demonstrated dramatically reduced contamination

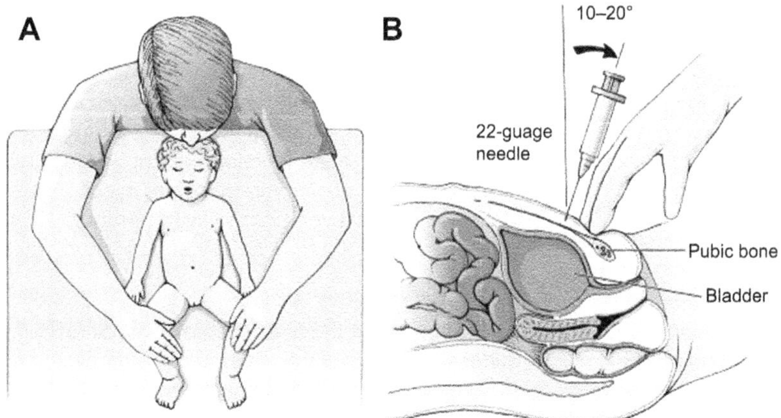

Fig. 1. (*A, B*) SPA procedure. (*From* Silverman MA, Schneider RE. Urologic Procedures. In: Roberts JR, Hedges JR, editors. Clinical procedures in emergency medicine. 5th edition. Philadelphia; Saunders; 2009. Figure 55-24; with permission.)

rates over previous methods, without the discomfort of SPA.[69,79,84] Nevertheless, compared with SPA, catheterized specimens still demonstrate a higher rate of contamination, particularly in the ambiguous range between 1000 and 10,000 colony counts.[69,79] If antibiotics have not been given, a repeat urine culture usually clarifies the issue of contamination.[68,79] To reduce discomfort with bladder catheterization, intraurethral or topical lidocaine have been shown to be effective in several studies.[88–90] Ultrasound may be strategically useful just before transurethral bladder catheterization in determining the likelihood of a successful catheterization based on bladder volume (**Fig. 2**).[91,92]

Clean-catch urine collection

Midstream clean-catch urine collection has been shown to obviate the need for catheterization in older, toilet-trained children.[69,78] With proper technique, contamination rates are within acceptable limits.[67,69,93–95] Even clean-catch midstream urine culture from infants has been shown to be accurate when collected properly.[96] The importance of proper cleaning and the limitations of clean-catch urine collection are both emphasized by Vaillancourt and coworkers[67] in a study of 350 randomized, toilet-trained children presenting to a pediatric ED. The rate of contamination for the noncleaning group far exceeded that of the group that received cleansing instructions (24% vs 8%).

Additional Testing

Both procalcitonin and C-reactive protein, along with the peripheral WBC count, have been studied for their ability to accurately differentiate upper from lower UTI.[97] Although C-reactive protein and procalcitonin have demonstrated reasonable sensitivity, the specificity of C-reactive protein for upper tract infection is low, limiting its usefulness.[98–100] Similarly, peripheral WBC count does not reliably differentiate upper from lower UTI.[99,100] The use of procalcitonin testing seems promising but more investigation is necessary before moving beyond the research stage.[101,102]

Blood cultures are frequently drawn as part of the standard evaluation for fever-without-a-source for infants, or in the older febrile child who looks moderately or severely ill. Positive blood cultures associated with UTI may occur at all ages but rates tend to be significantly higher in younger infants (>10%), particularly those under 6 months of age.[5,18,41,103,104] Most children with bacteremia are clinically indistinguishable from those without bacteremia, and bacteremia is cleared within 24 hours with

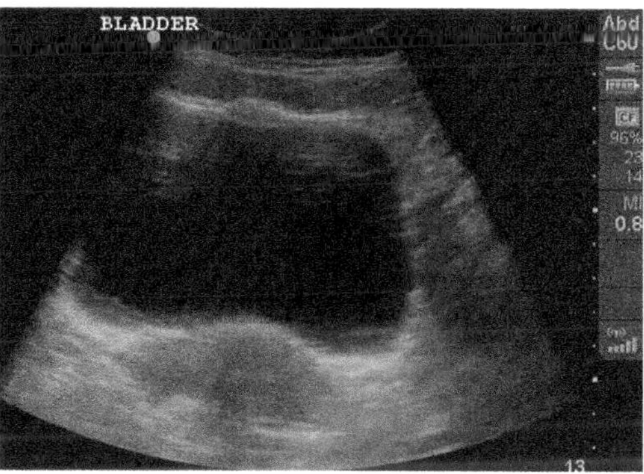

Fig. 2. Full bladder as visualized with transabdominal (suprapubic) ultrasound. (*Courtesy of* Medstar Health, Washington, DC.)

appropriate therapy, regardless of the route of antibiotic delivery.[6,38] Regardless of age, the presence of bacteremia rarely impacts management because the organism is invariably the same as the urine culture, and antibiotic treatment is also the same.[5,6,38,103,104] The usefulness of obtaining blood cultures in the context of febrile UTI is likely to be minimal.[6,38]

Frequently, the question arises whether one still needs to perform a lumbar puncture on young infants (<60 days) who have been diagnosed with a febrile UTI. Many authorities recommend a lumbar puncture to exclude meningitis caused by hematogenous dissemination before initiation of antibiotic therapy. Meningitis concomitant with UTI in young infants does not seem to be common; however, sterile cerebrospinal fluid pleocytosis may be noted.[105] However, the authors recommend sending cerebrospinal fluid for culture before starting intravenous antibiotics in infants younger than 8 weeks of age because of a lack of definitive evidence that it is safe to omit this procedure.[103]

DISPOSITION AND INITIAL MANAGEMENT

Most children, including young infants, with febrile UTI can be managed as outpatients.[3,6,41] The availability of highly effective oral third-generation cephalosporins has also allowed the shift toward increased outpatient management. As resistance patterns evolve, however, the wisdom of this approach may change.[6]

Children younger than 2 to 3 months of age, or children of any age who are toxic, dehydrated, unable to tolerate oral fluids or medications, or those who are at high risk for missed follow-up, are generally best managed with admission for parenteral antimicrobial therapy.[20,40] Admitted children should be treated with an intravenous third-generation cephalosporin or an aminoglycoside.[20]

For children discharged with febrile UTIs, choice of antimicrobial is largely driven by local resistance patterns and previous antimicrobial exposure, which currently favor third-generation cephalosporins.[6,8,20,106] Nitrofurantoin should never be used for febrile UTI because it does not achieve therapeutic serum or renal concentrations, and quinolones should be reserved for resistant organisms in the pediatric patient.[12,20] An initial parenteral dose of ceftriaxone has not been proved to improve outcome, but this may be advisable in younger infants because of their increased risk of sepsis.[41,107]

Significant improvement should not be expected for 24 to 48 hours; in one study, the mean time to defervescence was 24 hours for both the intravenous and oral therapy arms.[6,108] The AAP recommends prompt ultrasonography (to exclude abscess, obstruction, pyonephrosis, and so forth) in children who fail to respond within 48 hours, although a recent study suggests that the likelihood of finding significant abnormalities is extremely small.[20,108] Antimicrobial treatment should be for 7 to 14 days depending on the appearance of the child.[20,109] Shorter courses of therapy may be associated with treatment failure in the pediatric population, even for lower tract infection.[109]

FOLLOW-UP IMAGING

The diagnosis of UTI in a young child often triggers further diagnostic evaluation for genitourinary tract abnormalities that is time-consuming, uncomfortable, and expensive.[110,111] Even though follow-up imaging studies are outside the scope of routine ED practice, it is important to understand the patient's subsequent evaluation and cascade of testing that may follow. The traditional approach, currently advocated by the AAP and many other experts, is to obtain a renal ultrasound followed by voiding cystourethrography or radionuclide cystography in all infants under 2 years of age diagnosed with UTI.[3,20] This approach has been questioned and is not as aggressively recommended in the recent United Kingdom National Institute for Health and Clinical Excellence guidelines, with imaging only recommended for infants under 6 months of age or children with an "atypical" presentation, including severely ill, poor urine flow, elevated creatinine, abdominal mass, sepsis, failure to respond to antibiotic therapy in 48 hours, or infection with organisms other than *E coli*.[40]

Renal ultrasound can describe static anatomic abnormalities, such as abnormal kidney size, hydroureter, duplicated collecting system, or bladder diverticuli.[36,63,101] It is not accurate in identifying renal scarring from prior UTIs or parenchymal involvement with current UTI, and in the modern era of prenatal ultrasound, the yield for this test is quite low.[71,112] The primary purpose of the voiding cystourethrography is to identify the presence of VUR or posterior urethral valves. VUR is graded on a 1 to 5 scale, with grades 4 and 5 representing moderate to severe dilation of the ureters and renal pelvis.[36,101] For a long time, VUR has been considered to be a risk factor for recurrent UTI and renal scarring. This time-honored assumption is based on flawed studies and more recent studies question this association.[111,112] Radionuclide studies (eg, technetium-99 dimercaptosuccinic acid) are useful for the detection of renal scarring.[112,113]

The goal of radiographic evaluation is to identify patients with functional or anatomic abnormalities that might place them at risk for recurrent UTI and subsequent renal scarring and possibly chronic renal failure.[81] This approach (and these underlying assumptions) has recently received great scrutiny and has been questioned.[67,114] These radiographic studies are only useful if subsequent intervention can be shown to change a patient's risk and outcome (ie, if surgical intervention or prophylactic antimicrobials reduces further risk of infection and subsequent renal damage).[71,81] However, prophylaxis has not been shown to effectively prevent recurrent infection, even in children with documented VUR.[15,40,115,116] Surgical intervention also has not been proven to improve outcome compared with watchful waiting and early identification and treatment of recurrent UTIs.[111]

SUMMARY

The general approach to pediatric UTI is relatively straightforward: a child presents with fever (typically without a definite source), the clinician decides to obtain a urinalysis and urine culture, evaluates the urinalysis results, initiates antibiotics if indicated, and follows-up on the urine culture result in 24 to 48 hours. However, the decision on who to obtain a urine sample from can be particularly difficult in febrile infants and toddlers who look well and present in the context of a likely viral process. This is particularly true in younger children who typically require urinary catheterization to obtain an appropriate specimen for culture. Statistically speaking, most febrile children do not have a UTI, and the process of urine collection can be invasive and unpleasant. However, children without fever may have certain nonspecific complaints that should also trigger the clinician to think about the possibility of UTI. Significant limitations in the sensitivity and specificity of rapid urine screening tests make interpretation of the urinalysis results challenging. Therefore, concomitant sterile acquisition of urine for culture is critical. Finally, evaluation of ambiguous urine culture results must be approached with caution. The implications of initial decision-making are significant for the patient and family, and can drive a potentially uncomfortable and costly follow-up process. This, in turn, potentially labels a child as at risk for recurrent UTI, lowering the threshold for future invasive tests, thereby reinitiating a viscous cycle. Although there is the potential for treachery and diagnostic dilemma when approaching pediatric UTI, most patients can be safely and effectively managed in the ED and referred for close outpatient follow-up by a primary care provider.

REFERENCES

1. Jacobson SH, Eriksson CG, Lins L, et al. Development of hypertension and uraemia after pyelonephritis in childhood: 27 year follow up. BMJ 1989;299:703–6.
2. Zorc JJ, Kiddoo DA, Shaw KN. Diagnosis and management of pediatric urinary tract infections. Clin Microbiol Rev 2005;18:417–22.
3. Sedberry-Ross S, Pohl HG. Urinary tract infections in children. Curr Urol Rep 2008;9:165–71.
4. Zorc JJ, Levine DA, Platt SL, et al. Clinical and demographic factors associated with urinary tract infection in young febrile infants. Pediatrics 2005;116:644–8.
5. Newman TB, Bernzweig JA, Takayama JI, et al. Urine testing and urinary tract infections in febrile infants seen in office settings. Arch Pediatr Adolesc Med 2002;156:44–54.
6. Hoberman A, Wald ER, Hickey RW, et al. Oral versus initial intravenous therapy for urinary tract infections in young febrile children. Pediatrics 1999;104:79–86.
7. Doganis D, Siafas K, Mavrikou M, et al. Does early treatment of urinary tract infection prevent renal damage. Pediatrics 2007;120:e922.
8. Paschke AA, Zaoutis T, Conway PH, et al. Previous antimicrobial exposure is associated with drug-resistant urinary tract infections in children. Pediatrics 2010;125:664–72.
9. Ronald A. The etiology of urinary tract infection: traditional and emerging pathogens. Am J Med 2002;113(Suppl 1A):14S.
10. Sobel JD, Vazquez JA. Fungal Infections of the urinary tract. World J Urol 1999;17:410.
11. Smitherman HF, Caviness C, Macias CG. Retrospective review of serious bacterial infections in infants who are 0 to 36 months of age and have influenza A infection. Pediatrics 2005;115:710–8.
12. Chang SL, Shortliffe LD. Pediatric urinary tract infections. Pediatr Clin North Am 2006;53:379–400.
13. Kuo H, Mak RH. Pathogenesis of urinary tract infection: an update. Curr Opin Pediatr 2006;18:148–252.
14. Bachur R, Harper MB. Reliability of the urinalysis for predicting urinary tract infections in young febrile children. Arch Pediatr Adolesc Med 2001;155:60–5.
15. Conway PH, Cnaan A, Zaoutis T, et al. Recurrent urinary tract infections in children: risk factors and association with prophylactic antimicrobials. JAMA 2007;298:179–86.
16. Shaw KN, Gorelick M, McGowan KL, et al. Prevalence of urinary tract infection in febrile young children in the emergency department. Pediatrics 1998;102:e16–21.
17. Sahsi RS, Carpenter CR. Does this child have a urinary tract infection? Ann Emerg Med 2009;53:680–4.
18. Crain EF, Gershel JC. Urinary tract infections in febrile infants younger than 8 weeks of age. Pediatrics 1990;86:363–7.
19. Hoberman A, Chao H, Keller DM, et al. Prevalence of urinary tract infection in febrile infants. J Pediatr 1993;123:17–23.
20. Practice parameter: the diagnosis, treatment, and evaluation of the initial urinary tract infection in febrile infants and young children American Academy of Pediatrics; Committee on Quality Improvement, Subcommittee on Urinary Tract Infection. Pediatrics 1999;103:843–52.
21. Shaikh N, Morone NE, Bost JE, et al. Prevalence of urinary tract infection in childhood: a meta-analysis. Pediatr Infect Dis J 2008;27:302.

22. Baraff LJ. Management of fever without source in infants and children. Ann Emerg Med 2000;36:602–14.
23. Wiswell TE, Smith FR, Bass JW. Decreased incidence of urinary tract infections in circumcised male infants. Pediatrics 1985;75:901–3.
24. Schoen EJ, Colby CJ, Ray GT. Newborn circumcision decreases incidence and costs of urinary tract infections during the first year of life. Pediatrics 2000;105: 789–93.
25. Fusell EN, Kaack MB, Cherry R, et al. Adherence of bacteria to human foreskins. J Urol 1988;140:997–1001.
26. Hiraoka M, Tsukahara H, Ohshima Y, et al. Meatus tightly covered by the prepuce is associated with urinary infection. Pediatr Int 2002;44:658.
27. Gorelick MH, Shaw KN. Clinical decision rule to identify febrile young girls at risk for urinary tract infection. Arch Pediatr Adolesc Med 2000;154:386–90.
28. Chen L, Baker MD. Racial and ethnic differences in the rates of urinary tract infections in febrile infants in the emergency department. Pediatr Emerg Care 2006; 22:485.
29. Persad S, Watermeyer S, Griffiths A, et al. Association between urinary tract infection and postmicturition wiping habit. Acta Obstet Gynecol Scand 2006;85(11): 1395–6.
30. Wan J, Kaplinsky R, Greenfield S. Toilet habits of children evaluated for urinary tract infection. J Urol 1995;154:797.
31. Naseer SR, Steinhardt GF. New renal scars in children with urinary tract infections, vesicoureteral reflux and voiding dysfunction: a prospective evaluation. J Urol 1997;158:566.
32. Snodgrass W. Relationship of voiding dysfunction to urinary tract infection and vesicoureteral reflux in children. Urology 1991;38:341.
33. Shaikh N, Hoberman A, Wise B, et al. Dysfunctional elimination syndrome: is it related to urinary tract infection or vesicoureteral reflux diagnosed early in life? Pediatrics 2003;112:1134–7.
34. Blethyn A, Jones K, Newcombe R, et al. Radiological assessment of constipation. Arch Dis Child 1995;73:532–3.
35. Loening-Baucke V. Urinary incontinence and urinary tract infection and their resolution with treatment of chronic constipation of childhood. Pediatrics 1997; 100:228–32.
36. Lim R. Vesicoureteral reflux and urinary tract infection: evolving practices and current controversies in pediatric imaging. AJR Am J Roentgenol 2009;109:1197–208.
37. Garin EH, Campos A, Homsy Y. Primary vesicoureteral reflux: review of current concepts. Pediatr Nephrol 1998;12:249.
38. Honkinen O, Jahnukainen T, Mertsola J, et al. Bacteremic urinary tract infection in children. Pediatr Infect Dis J 2000;19(7):630–4.
39. Garcia FJ, Nager AL. Jaundice as an early diagnostic sign of urinary tract infection in infancy. Pediatrics 2002;109(5):845–51.
40. National Institute for Health and Clinical Excellence. Urinary tract infection in children: diagnosis, treatment and long-term management. London: National Institute of health and Clinical Excellence; 2007. p. 1–136.
41. Dore-Bergeron M, Gauthier M, Chevalier I, et al. Urinary tract infections in 1- to 3-month-old infects: ambulatory treatment with intravenous antibiotics. Pediatrics 2009;124:16–22.
42. Schroeder AR, Newman TB, Wasserman RC, et al. Choice of urine collection methods for the diagnosis of urinary tract infection in young, febrile infants. Arch Pediatr Adolesc Med 2005;159:915–22.

43. Shaikh N, Morone NE, Lopez J, et al. Does this child have a urinary tract infection? JAMA 2007;298:2895–904.
44. Krief WI, Levine DA, Platt SL, et al. Influenza virus infection and the risk of serious bacterial infections in young febrile infants. Pediatrics 2009;124:30–9.
45. Levine DA, Platt SL, Dayan PS, et al. Risk of serious bacterial infection in young febrile infants with respiratory syncytial virus infections. Pediatrics 2004;113: 1728–34.
46. Huppert JS, Biro FM, Mehrabi J, et al. Urinary tract infection and *Chlamydia* infection in adolescent females. J Pediatr Adolesc Gynecol 2003;16:133–7.
47. Pierce AM, Hart CA. Vulvovaginitis: causes and management. Arch Dis Child 1992;67:509–12.
48. Fernandes ET, Dekermacher S, Sabadin MA, et al. Urethral prolapse in children. Urology 1993;41:240–2.
49. Pyrles CV, Steg NL. Specimens of urine obtained from young girls by catheter versus voiding: a comparative study of bacterial cultures, gram stains, and bacterial counts in paired specimens. Pediatrics 1959;23:441–52.
50. Pryles CV. The diagnosis of urinary tract infection. Pediatrics 1960;26:441–51.
51. Fernandez-Menendez JM, Malaga S, Matesanz JL, et al. Risk factors in the development of early technetium-99m- dimercaptosuccinic acid renal scintigraphy lesions during first urinary tract infection in children. Acta Paediatr 2003;92:21–6.
52. Gorelick MH, Shaw KN. Screening tests for urinary tract infection in children: a meta-analysis. Pediatrics 1999;104:e54.
53. Israni AK, Kasiske BL. Laboratory assessment of kidney disease: clearance, urinalysis and kidney biopsy. In: Brenner BM, editor. Brenner & Rector's the kidney. 8th edition. Philadelphia: Saunders Elsevier; 2007. p. 736–7.
54. Williams GJ, Macaskill P, Chan SF, et al. Absolute and relative accuracy of rapid urine tests for urinary tract infection in children: a meta-analysis. Lancet Infect Dis 2010;10:240–50.
55. American College of Emergency Medicine. Clinical policy for children younger than 3 years presenting to the ED with fever. Ann Emerg Med 2003;42:530–45.
56. Lam CN, Bremner AD, Maxwell JD, et al. Pyuria and bacteriuria. Arch Dis Child 1967;42:275–80.
57. Hoberman A, Wald ER, Reynolds EA, et al. Pyuria and bacteriuria in urine specimens obtained by catheter from young children with fever. J Pediatr 1994;124: 513–9.
58. Jaskiewicz JA, McCarthy CA, Richardson AC, et al. Febrile infants at low risk for serious bacterial infection: an appraisal of the Rochester criteria and implications for management. Pediatrics 1994;94:390–6.
59. Baker MD, Bell LM, Avner JR. Outpatient management without antibiotics of fever in selected infants. N Engl J Med 1993;329:1437–41.
60. Baskin MN, O'Rourke EJ, Fleisher GR. Outpatient treatment of febrile infants 28-89 days of age with intramuscular administration of ceftriaxone. J Pediatr 1992; 120:22–7.
61. Baraff LJ, Schriger DL, Bass JW, et al. Practice guideline for the management of infants and children 0 to 36 months of age with fever without source. Pediatrics 1993;92:1–12.
62. Hoberman A, WAld ER. Urinary tract infections in young febrile children. Pediatr Infect Dis J 1997;16:11–7.
63. Huicho L, Campos-Sanchez M, Alamo C. Meta-analysis of urine screening tests for determining the risk of urinary tract infection in children. Pediatr Infect Dis J 2002;21:1–11.

64. Price E, Pallett A, Gilbert RD, et al. Microbiological aspects of the UK National Institute for Health and Clinical Excellence (NICE) guidance on urinary tract infection in children. J Antimicrob Chemother 2010;65:836–41.
65. Helmholz HF, Milleken F. The bacteriology of normal infants' urine. Am J Dis Child 1922;23:309.
66. Kass EH. Bacteriuria and the diagnosis of infections of the urinary tract. Arch Intern Med 1957;100:709–13.
67. Vaillancourt S, McGillivray D, Zhang X, et al. To clean or not to clean: effect on contamination rates in midstream urine collections in toilet-trained children. Pediatrics 2007;119:e1288–91.
68. Coulthard MG, Kalra M, Lambert HJ, et al. Redefining urinary tract infections by bacterial colony counts. Pediatrics 2010;125:335–41.
69. Wald ER, DeMuri GP. Imaging and antimicrobial prophylaxis following the diagnosis of urinary tract infection in children. Pediatr Infect Dis J 2008;27: 553–4.
70. Hoberman A, Wald ER, Penchansky L, et al. Enhanced urinalysis as a screening test for urinary tract infection. Pediatrics 1993;125:1196–9.
71. Hoberman A, Charron M, Hickey RW, et al. Imaging studies after a first febrile urinary tract infection in young children. N Engl J Med 2003;348:195–202.
72. Sobel JD, Kaye D. Urinary tract infections. In: Mandell GL, Douglas RG, editors. Bennett's principles and practice of infectious diseases. 7th edition. Philadelphia: Churchill Livingstone Elsevier; 2009. p. 957–85.
73. Wettergren B, Jodal U, Jonasson G. Epidemiology of bacteriuria during the first year of life. Acta Paediatr Scand 1985;74:925–33.
74. Abbott GD. Neonatal bacteriuria: a prospective study in 1,460 infants. Br Med J 1972;1:267–9.
75. Al-Orifi F, McGillivray D, Tange S, et al. Urine culture from bag specimens in young children: are the risks too high? J Pediatr 2000;137:221–6.
76. Pyrles CV. Percutaneous bladder aspiration and other methods of urine collection for bacteriologic study. Pediatrics 1965;36:128–31.
77. Nelson JD, Peters PC. Suprapubic aspiration of urine in premature and term infants. Pediatrics 1965;36:132–4.
78. Newman CG, O'Neill P, Parker A. Pyruria in infancy, and the role of suprapubic aspiration of urine in diagnosis of infection of urinary tract. Br Med J 1967; 2(5547):277–9.
79. Pryles CV, Atkin MD, Morse TS, et al. Comparative bacteriologic study of urine obtained from children by percutaneous suprapubic aspiration of the bladder and by catheter. Pediatrics 1959;24:983–91.
80. Schlager TA, Dunn ML, Dudley SM, et al. Bacterial contamination rate of urine collected in a urine bag from healthy non-toilet-trained male infants. J Pediatr 1990;116:738–9.
81. Quigley R. Diagnosis or urinary tract infections in children. Curr Opin Pediatr 2009; 21:194–8.
82. Pollack CV, Pollack ES, Andrew ME. Suprapubic bladder aspiration versus uretheral catheterization in ill infants: success, efficiency, and complications rates. Ann Emerg Med 1994;23:225–30.
83. Kozer E, Rosenbloom E, Goldman D, et al. Pain in infants who are younger than 2 months during suprapubic aspiration and transurethral bladder catheterization: a randomized, controlled study. Pediatrics 2006;118:e51.
84. El-Naggar W, Yiu A, Mohamed A, et al. Comparison of pain during two methods of urine collection in preterm infants. Pediatrics 2010;125:1224–9.

85. Buys H, Pead L, Hallett R, et al. Suprapubic aspiration under ultrasound guidance in children with fever of undiagnosed cause. BMJ 1994;308:690.
86. Munir V, Barnett P, South M. Does the use of volumetric bladder ultrasound improve the success rate of suprapubic aspiration of urine? Pediatr Emerg Care 2002;18:346–9.
87. Chu RW, Wong YC, Luk SH, et al. Comparing suprapubic urine aspiration under real-time ultrasound guidance with conventional blind aspiration. Acta Paediatr 2002;91(5):512–6.
88. Gerard LL, Cooper CS, Duethman KS, et al. Effectiveness of lidocaine lubricant for discomfort during pediatric urethral catheterization. J Urol 2003;170:564–7.
89. Vaughan M, Paton EA, Bush A, et al. Does lidocaine gel alleviate the pain of bladder catheterization in young children? A randomized, controlled trial. Pediatrics 2005;116(4):917–20.
90. Mularoni PP, Cohen LL, DeGuzman M. A randomized clinical trial of lidocaine gel for reducing infant distress during urethral catheterization. Pediatr Emerg Care 2009;25(7):439–43.
91. Milling TJ Jr, Van Amerongen R, Melville L, et al. Use of ultrasonography to identify infants for whom urinary catheterization will be unsuccessful because of insufficient urine volume: validation of the urinary bladder index. Ann Emerg Med 2005;45(5): 510–3.
92. Chen L, Hsiao AL, Moore CL, et al. Utility of bedside bladder ultrasound before urethral catheterization in young children. Pediatrics 2005;115(1):108–11.
93. Lohr JA, Donowitz LG, Dudley SM. Bacterial contamination rates in voided urine collections in girls. J Pediatr 1989;114:91–3.
94. Lohr JA, Donowitz LG, Dudley SM. Bacterial contamination rates for non-clean-catch and clean-catch midstream urine collections in boys. J Pediatr 1986;109: 659–60.
95. Saez-Llorens X, Umana MA, Odio CM, et al. Bacterial contamination rates for non-clean catch and clean catch midstream urine collections in uncircumcised boys. J Pediatr 1989;114:93–4.
96. Ramage I, Chapman JP, Hollman AS, et al. Accuracy of clean-catch urine collection in infancy. J Pediatr 1999;135:765–7.
97. Benador N, Siegrist C, Gendrel D, et al. Procalcitonin is a marker of severity of renal lesion in pyelonephritis. Pediatrics 1998;102:1422–5.
98. Pecile P, Miorin E, Romanello C, et al. Procalcitonin: a marker of severità of acute pyelonephritis among children. Pediatrics 2004;114:e249–54.
99. Garin EH, Olavarria F, Araya C, et al. Diagnostic significance of clinical and laboratory findings to localize site of urinary infection. Pediatr Nephrol 2007;22:1002–6.
100. Biggi A, Dardanelli L, Pomero G, et al. Acute renal cortical scintigraphy in children with a first urinary tract infection. Pediatr Nephrol 2001;16:733–8.
101. Bauer R, Kogan BA. New developments in the diagnosis and management of pediatric UTIs. Urol Clin North Am 2008;35:47–58.
102. Hellerstein S. Acute urinary tract infection: evaluation and treatment. Curr Opin Pediatr 2006;18:132–8.
103. Bacchur R, Caputo GL. Bacteremia and meningitis among infants with urinary tract infections. Pediatr Emerg Care 1995;11:280–4.
104. Pitetti RD, Choi S. Utility of blood cultures in febrile children with UTI. Am J Emerg Med 2002;20:271–4.
105. Goldman RN, Matlow A, Linett L. What is the risk of bacterial meningitis in infants who present to the emergency department with fever and pyuria? CJEM 2003; 5(6):393–9.

106. Matoo TK. Are prophylactic antibiotics indicated after a urinary tract infection? Curr Opin Pediatr 2009;21:203–6.
107. Baker PC, Nelson DS, Schunk JE. The addition of ceftriaxone to oral therapy does not improve outcome in febrile children with urinary tract infections. Arch Pediatr Adolesc Med 2001;155:135–9.
108. Bachur R. Nonresponders: prolonged fever among infants with urinary tract infections. Pediatrics 2000;105:e59.
109. Keren R, Chan E. A meta-analysis of randomized, controlled trials comparing short- and long-course antibiotic therapy for urinary tract infections in children. Pediatrics 2002;109:e70.
110. Jones KV. Time to review the value of imaging after urinary tract infection in infants. Arch Dis Child 2005;90:663–5.
111. Marks SD, Gordon I, Tullus K. Imaging in childhood urinary tract infections: time to reduce investigation. Pediatr Nephrol 2008;23:9–17.
112. Montini G, Zucchetaa P, Tomasi L, et al. Value of imaging studies after a first febrile urinary tract infection in young children: data from Italian Renal Infection Study 1. Pediatrics 2009;123:e239–46.
113. Siomou E, Giapros V, Fotopoulos A, et al. Implications of 99mTc-DMSA scintigraphy performed during urinary tract infection in neonates. Pediatrics 2009;124:881–7.
114. Sreenarasimhaiah S, Hellerstein S. Urinary tract infections per se do not cause end-stage kidney disease. Pediatr Nephrol 1998;12:210–3.
115. Garin EH, Olavarria F, Nieto VG, et al. Clinical significance of primary vesicoureteral reflux and urinary antibiotic prophylaxis after acute pyelonephritis: a multicenter, randomized, controlled study. Pediatrics 2005;117:626.
116. Williams G, Craig JC. Prevention of recurrent urinary tract infection in children. Curr Opin Infect Dis 2009;22:72–6.

Pediatric Genitourinary Emergencies

Norine A. McGrath, MD[a,*], John M. Howell, MD[b],
Jonathan E. Davis, MD[a]

KEYWORDS

- Genitourinary • Pediatric • Traumatic injury • Torsion
- Infection • Paraphimosis • Priapism

Children in the emergency department (ED) require a unique behavioral skill set and a specialized knowledge base. Pediatric medical complaints and differential diagnoses often vary from adults. Taking a history and conducting a physical examination often involves a frightened and nonverbal patient. Discussions of diagnosis and care involve both patients and their caregivers. Into this complex milieu, subspecialty clinical concerns constitute an additional level of complexity, and sometimes anxiety, for emergency physicians (EPs). In this clinical setting, the EP must consider the unique aspects of a child's urologic system.

The female urethra is a relatively short tract traversing muscle sphincters at the opening of the vaginal vault. In part because of this anatomy, female neonates and infants are prone to urinary tract infections (UTI). In the male patient the urethra follows the length of the penis and the corpus cavernosum and corpus spongiosum, exiting the glans penis at the urethral meatus (**Fig. 1**). The coronal sulcus distinguishes the glans penis from the penile shaft. With more complex external genitalia that both follow and intertwine with the urinary tract, male children are prone to a variety of unique medical complaints. The infant penis is proportionately smaller than the adult penis. This makes male children more prone to structural, and in some cases infectious, problems compared with female children.

This article addresses a variety of congenital and acquired pediatric genitourinary (GU) disorders. In some instances the EP is required to identify and treat common disorders. At other times the EP must be vigilant for serious or lethal problems. At all times, the EP must remember that treating the child in a kind and empathetic manner

The authors report no financial disclosures.

[a] Department of Emergency Medicine, Georgetown University Hospital, Washington Hospital Center, 3800 Reservoir Road, Washington, DC 20007, USA
[b] Department of Emergency Medicine, Inova Fairfax Hospital/Inova Fairfax Hospital for Children, 3300 Gallows Road, Falls Church, VA 22042, USA
* Corresponding author.
E-mail address: norinemcgrath@gmail.com

Emerg Med Clin N Am 29 (2011) 655–666
doi:10.1016/j.emc.2011.04.003 emed.theclinics.com
0733-8627/11/$ – see front matter

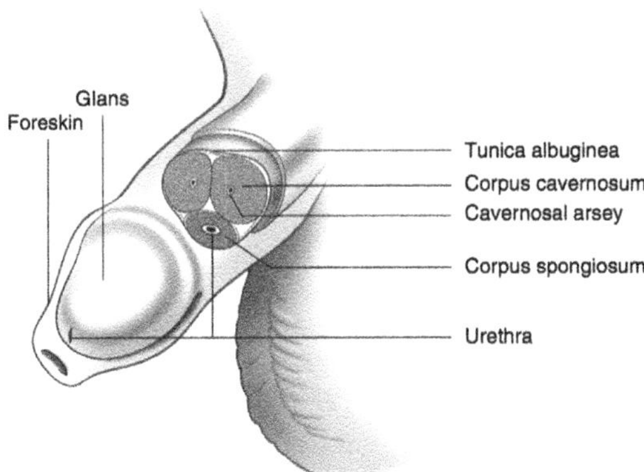

Fig. 1. Anatomy of the penis. (*From* Davis JE. Penile complaints. In: Amieva-Wang NE, editor. A practical guide to pediatric emergency medicine: caring for children in the emergency department. Cambridge (United Kingdom): Cambridge University Press; 2011; with permission.)

is at least as important as the first two considerations. GU emergencies include paraphimosis, priapism, serious infection, significant traumatic injury, and gonadal torsion.

CIRCUMCISION COMPLICATIONS

In neonates, circumcision is performed under local anesthesia and without sutures. Serious complications occur infrequently in neonates or infants.[1] Minor complications may include local infection, adhesions, and bleeding. Bleeding is usually venous oozing that can be controlled with local pressure. Rarely, a proclotting agent may be required. Obtain a thorough birth history, because neonates who are born at home may not receive vitamin K. Later in the healing process patients may develop urethral meatal stenosis from adhesions of the healing glans. If the baby is able to void, these adhesions generally are lysed in a urologist's office (ie, meatotomy). If the baby is unable to void, obtain urgent urologic consultation. Infection, although rare, can progress to neonatal sepsis. Clinically significant erythema, induration, or drainage is treated with antibiotics, especially if associated with fever. In general, febrile babies under 1 month of age are admitted for a short course of intravenous (IV) antibiotics until blood cultures are negative. Treat older babies with outpatient oral antibiotics if the child is well-appearing, not fussy, and feeds normally. There is a significant prevalence of methicillin-resistant *Staphylococcus aureus* (MRSA) in nurseries.[2] Consequently, cover both MRSA and methicillin-sensitive *S aureus* based on local sensitivity patterns.

BALANITIS AND BALANOPOSTHITIS

Balanitis, in the circumcised, or balanoposthitis, in the uncircumcised, is inflammation of the glans (balanitis) and foreskin (posthitis). Balanoposthitis occurs in approximately 6% of uncircumcised children.[3] Symptoms include redness and swelling of the glans and foreskin, usually without penile shaft involvement. There may be visible discharge from the urethral meatus.

In children, these disorders are caused by poor hygiene; chemical irritation from detergent or creams; local trauma; contact dermatitis (eg, diaper dermatitis); candidal infection; bacterial infection (eg, streptococcus, staphylococcus, and gram negatives); and less commonly drug eruptions. Attempt to identify recent exposures that could cause symptoms. Culture meatal discharge if clinically warranted. Consider sexual abuse, especially if the symptoms are recurrent.

Treatment involves improved hygiene, frequent bathing, and parental involvement in small children to ensure washing and flushing under the foreskin. Discourage forced retraction of the foreskin. Irritation and inflammation may be relieved with Sitz baths. Children may be reluctant to urinate because of dysuria from skin contact. Encourage such children to urinate into warm bath water. A topical antifungal is frequently effective. Prescribe a low-potency hydrocortisone cream or ointment if chemical irritation is suspected. Bacterial infections are generally treated with a first-generation cephalosporin, unless clinical suspicion or risk factors for MRSA infection are present. Rarely, patients may require admission for cellulitis or urinary obstruction. Importantly, necrotizing fasciitis of the perineum (Fournier's gangrene) has been rarely reported in children, primarily in the setting of diabetes or immune compromise.[4]

PHIMOSIS

Phimosis is constriction of the foreskin that limits retraction of the foreskin (or prepuce) over the glans. Infants have a physiologic phimosis caused by adhesions between the prepuce and glans. A physiologic phimosis consists of a pliant, unscarred preputial orifice on physical examination. The foreskin gradually becomes retractile over time as a result of intermittent erections and keratinization of the inner epithelium. By 3 years of age, 90% of glans can easily be retracted, with nearly all becoming retractile by late adolescence.[5,6]

A pathologic phimosis exists when the failure to retract results from distal scarring of the prepuce. This is typically a subacute condition that may present acutely to the ED when a patient is unable to void spontaneously as a result of distal urethral obstruction. Pathologic phimosis is caused by local trauma; infection; chemical irritation; complications of circumcision (insufficient tissue removal); and poor hygiene. Patients with acute phimosis are either fussy or complain of penile pain over hours to days. Children also may develop hematuria or urinary retention because of obstruction or dysuria. On physical examination, the physician discovers a tender foreskin that is not easily retracted. Although the prepuce may be gently manipulated to allow a better examination, do not attempt forced retraction. Forceful retraction causes future adhesions and strictures. There are no diagnostic tests required.

The mainstay of treatment is improved hygiene. First-line topical treatment is a 2-week course of corticosteroid cream (eg, 0.1% triamcinolone or 0.6% betamethasone). Several studies have shown that topical treatment leads to a reduction in instrumentation and surgical procedures, and in some cases may be curative.[7,8] Obtain urgent urologic consultation for acute urinary retention. All patients require urology follow-up and some may go on to require meatal dilatation or circumcision.

PARAPHIMOSIS

Paraphimosis is the inability to reduce proximal foreskin over the coronal sulcus at the glans (**Fig. 2**). Prolonged retraction of the foreskin leads to venous congestion and swelling. The foreskin may be retracted because of infection, trauma, masturbation, a hair tourniquet, a urethral foreign body, or iatrogenically after failure to reduce the foreskin during an examination. Symptoms can develop within hours. Diagnosis is made by history and physical examination, although a radiograph may be useful if a constricting foreign body is suspected.

Paraphimosis can frequently be managed in the ED without the need for emergent specialty consultation. There are many reported methods of successful paraphimosis

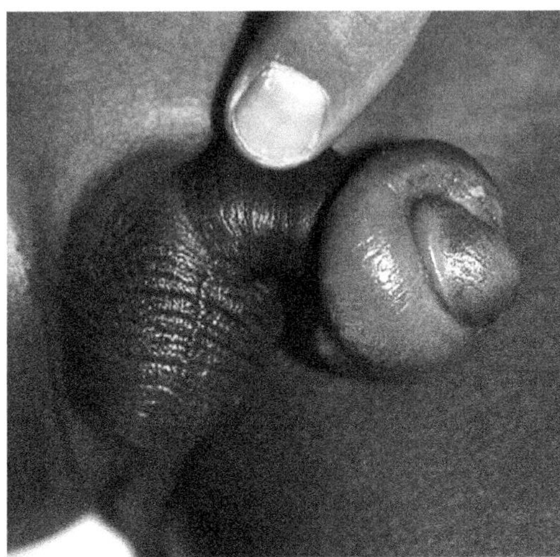

Fig. 2. Paraphimosis. (*From* Kliegman RM, Behrman RE, Henson HB, et al, editors. Nelson textbook of pediatrics. 17th edition. Philadelphia: Saunders; 2007. p. 2256; with permission.)

reduction. Regardless of method, the underlying strategy typically involves decreasing edema (glans or foreskin), followed by reduction of the glans penis back through the proximal constricting band of foreskin.[9]

Gentle, circumferential pressure on the glans penis may allow reduction. Alternatively, the foreskin may be punctured with a 21-gauge needle multiple times to allow drainage of edematous fluid, followed by reduction of the glans penis (**Fig. 3**). Reduction of the foreskin is urgent. Prolonged retraction and swelling can lead to arterial compression, necrosis, and gangrene. If reduction cannot be made through conservative efforts, obtain urologic consultation for a dorsal slit procedure or urgent circumcision.[10]

TRAUMATIC INJURY

Tourniquet injuries have different causes depending on age. In neonates and infants, a tourniquet may occur accidently from maternal hair or thread.[11] Clitoral hair tourniquets occur infrequently and cause unexplained fussiness in infants. An occult hair tourniquet should be considered in the evaluation of an infant with inconsolable crying.

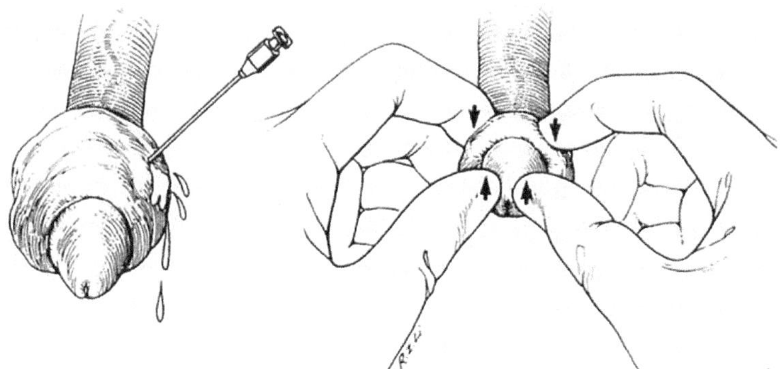

Fig. 3. Paraphimosis reduction. (*From* Barone JG, Fleisher MH. Treatment of paraphimosis using the "puncture" technique. Ped Emerg Care 1993;9:299; with permission.)

In adolescents, tourniquet injuries occur from prolonged intentional application of a foreign body or penile ring. History may be limited depending on the patient's age. Venous or arterial occlusion causes swelling distal to the tourniquet. An accidental tourniquet may require a thorough physical examination because swelling may obscure landmarks and the offending item.

Hair tourniquets may require local anesthesia or procedural sedation to remove. Over-the-counter hair removal products have been used successfully for the removal of digital (finger or toe) hair tourniquets,[12] leading some to suggest its use for simple penile hair tourniquets. These products, however, are very caustic and should not be used near mucous membranes, such as the urethral meatus or inner preputial tissue. Topical antibiotics may be indicated for skin breakdown or ulceration. Depending on the severity of swelling and duration of injury, a retrograde urethrogram and ultrasound may be performed to confirm urethral patency and vascular integrity, respectively.

Among the most potentially severe forms of accidental genital injury is domestic animal attack.[13] Perform local wound cleansing, irrigation, and closure. Although the scrotum is quite vascular, prescribe oral antimicrobials in selected cases. Provide rabies immunoprophylaxis if indicated. Consult urologic or plastic surgery in the setting of partial penile detachment or degloving injury. Toddlers are prone to blunt penile trauma from a falling toilet seat while potty training.[14] Penile or scrotal injury also may be caused by zipper entrapment. This injury occurs more commonly in smaller children. Do not retract the zipper manually because tissue may be further torn. Release the zipper by cutting the median bar of the zipper mechanism (**Fig. 4**).

Blunt scrotal trauma frequently results from organized athletic activities, straddle injuries, falls, or major trauma. Assess blood flow and anatomic integrity with Doppler ultrasound. Blunt testicular trauma may be associated with testicular torsion.[15] Indications for urgent surgical repair include rupture of the tunica albuginea (testicular rupture) or large hematocele.[16]

Delay in the diagnosis and treatment of a significant testicular injury can lead to a three to four times increased risk of testicular loss.[17] Penetrating scrotal or vulvar injuries mandate thorough examination, frequently under local anesthesia. In girls

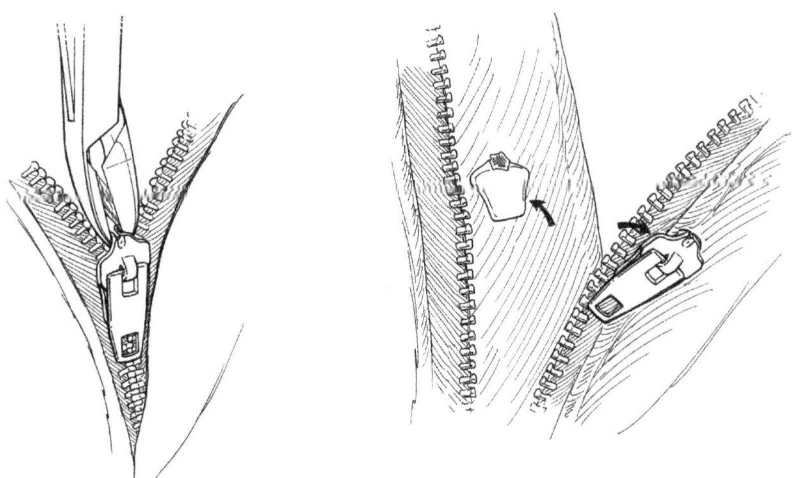

Fig. 4. Zipper removal. (*From* Vilke GM. Zipper removal. In: Rosen P, Chan TC, Vilke GM, et al, editors. Atlas of emergency procedures. St Louis (MO): Mosby; 2001. p. 137; with permission.)

this includes a vaginal examination for possible intravaginal penetrating injuries that extend to the rectum or peritoneal cavity.

PRIAPISM

Priapism is prolonged penile erection without sexual stimulation. Patients complain of swelling and pain (caused by tissue ischemia) after 4 hours of erection. Among children, priapism is nearly always caused by sickle cell disease or leukemia. Twenty-nine percent to 42% of patients with sickle cell disease develop priapism.[18] Less commonly in children, priapism occurs with hypercoagulable states, acute brain or spinal injuries, or medication side effects. Question adolescents about the use of sildenafil and tadalafil, because priapism has been rarely associated.[19] Priapism may also occur in younger children resulting from accidental ingestion of these drugs.[20] Priapism also is linked to heavy alcohol and nasal cocaine use.

Priapism is divided into two categories because these distinctions are important therapeutically. Ischemic or low-flow priapism indicates little or no intracorporal blood flow. This type of priapism is worrisome and warrants urgent intervention. Nonischemic or high-flow priapism is less worrisome acutely. Ischemic priapism is a true compartment syndrome of the penis. A blood sample from the corpus cavernosum demonstrates hypoxia, hypercarbia, and low pH. The penis is usually tender and fully rigid following spontaneous onset. Nonischemic priapism typically results from injury, although atraumatic etiologies exist. The penis is not completely rigid and blood sample results usually are normal. Neurogenic priapism (eg, brain or spinal cord injury) is not related to blood flow occlusion.

Therapeutic evaluation is focused. During the history, identify timing of the episode, previous episodes, comorbidities, and any ingestion. Prolonged or recurrent priapism is associated with both the inability to maintain an erection during sexual excitement and cosmetic abnormalities from chronic fibrosis. If indicated, order a complete blood count and reticulocyte count to exclude leukemia, undiagnosed sickle cell disease, and aplastic crisis.

Blood gas analysis of penile blood is helpful in some cases. Draw a few milliliters of blood from the corpus cavernosa into a heparinized syringe. In ischemic priapism, the Po_2 is typically less than 30 mm Hg, the Pco_2 is greater than 60 mm Hg, and the pH is below 7.25. In nonischemic etiologies, the Po_2 is typically above 90 mm Hg, the Pco_2 is less than 40 mm Hg, and the pH is above 7.40.[21] In selected cases, ultrasound helps identify fistulas that cause high-flow states; however, this testing should not delay treatment.

The treatment of priapism most frequently is managed by a urologist. However, in certain circumstances, it may be necessary for the EP to initiate treatment for low-flow priapism in the ED. The goals of first-line treatment are pain relief, withdrawal of cavernous blood, irrigation with normal saline, and if needed instillation of an alpha sympathomimetic agent that induces cavernous smooth muscle contraction and facilitates blood exiting the penis. Pain relief is achieved with a dorsal penile nerve block or a field block at the base of the penile shaft. Patients may also require parenteral pain management during the initial evaluation. Once the penis is anesthetized, insert a 19- or 21-gauge needle or angiocatheter into the corpus cavernosum and withdraw up to 5 mL of blood. Approximately 30% of patients are treated successfully with aspiration (with or without irrigation) alone; corporal sympathomimetic agent infusion is the next step in treatment.[21]

After aspiration, the cavernosum is infused with the α_1-selective adrenergic agonist phenylephrine. This method is successful in 43% to 81% of patients.[21] As a pure alpha agent, phenylephrine may cause hypertension, which may be associated with reflex bradycardia. These patients, therefore, should be monitored for several hours. Children carry a lower cardiovascular risk profile than adults and are less prone to cardiovascular side effects. One approach is to instill 1 mL of dilute phenylephrine (100–500 μg phenylephrine per milliliter of normal saline) into the corpus cavernosum every 3 to 5 minutes for up to 1 hour.[21] Smaller volumes are indicated for children and adults with cardiovascular disease. Observe these patients for several hours because repeat evacuation and irrigation may be required.

If these measures fail, obtain emergent urologic consultation because a surgical shunt may be required. Patients with underlying predisposing disorders may benefit from systemic treatment. For example, sickle cell patients frequently improve with oxygenation, hydration, blood transfusion, or plasmapharesis, although evidence-based guidelines are lacking.[22,23] Nonischemic priapism generally resolves spontaneously without significant intervention and rarely leads to tissue or flow damage, even when prolonged.

GONADAL TORSION

Gonadal torsion is a surgical emergency. Torsion of the testicular or ovarian vascular pedicle leads to ischemia and infarction of the affected gonad, with clear implications for future fertility. Testicular torsion and ovarian torsion are covered more extensively elsewhere in this issue. However, there are several key considerations specific to the pediatric population.

Children with testicular torsion typically present as an "acute scrotum," which is an acute painful swelling of the scrotum or its contents, accompanied by local signs or general symptoms.[24] Although the differential diagnosis is extensive, the three principle causes of an acute scrotum are (1) testicular torsion; (2) acute epididymitis; and (3) testicular (or epididymal) appendage torsion.[25] Incarcerated inguinal hernia is a surgical emergency that may also present as an acute scrotum, particularly in the first year of life.[26] Significant overlap exists in the clinical signs and symptoms for all of these conditions.[27] The incidence of testicular torsion peaks in the newborn and peripubertal periods.[28,29] Historical and examination features that may be helpful in distinguishing testicular torsion are listed in **Table 1**.

The presence of an ipsilateral cremasteric reflex makes testicular torsion less likely.[28] However, the presence of an intact cremasteric reflex lacks sufficient power to thoroughly exclude the diagnosis.[27] The clinical use of an absent cremasteric reflex is very limited. Healthy boys may lack the reflex altogether, particularly in their first few years of life.[30] Further, inflammation or swelling from any cause may blunt the reflex. Doppler ultrasound is the initial diagnostic study of choice. Sonography is used not only to assess for testicular torsion, but also to search for an alternative cause of acute scrotal pain.[31] One large series reported a negative predictive value of ultrasound approaching 97%.[32] However, several case reports, and at least two series, have reported false-negative rates of around 25% for pathologically confirmed testicular torsion.[33,34] The bottom line is that if the ultrasound is nondiagnostic for testicular torsion, and the clinical story is concerning, emergent surgical consultation is prudent.

Ovarian torsion may be encountered in adolescents or young girls. It is associated with a benign cyst or tumor in some, but not all, cases.[35] Patients with ovarian torsion may present with vague symptoms, and initial misdiagnosis is common.[36] Remaining vigilant to this potential diagnosis is the key. Ultrasound is the initial diagnostic study of choice. The presence of flow on color Doppler imaging suggests the ovary may still be viable, but does not exclude the diagnosis of pedicle torsion.[37,38] Importantly, the ovary has dual blood supply from both the uterine and ovarian arteries. Adnexal

Table 1
Historical and examination features of testicular torsion

	Feature	OR Favoring Diagnosis of TT[a] (95% confidence interval)	NPV for Excluding TT[b]
History	Nausea and vomiting	8.9 (2.6–30.1)	—
	<24 hours symptoms	6.7 (1.5–33.3)	—
Physical examination	High-riding	58.8 (19.2–166.6)	95%
	Transverse lie	—	95%
	Anterior rotation of epididymis	—	92%

Abbreviations: NPV, negative predictive value for excluding the diagnosis of TT from other conditions; OR, odds ratio favoring the diagnosis of TT over other causes of an acute scrotum; TT, testicular torsion.

[a] *Data from* Beni-Israel T, Goldman M, Bar Chaim S. Clinical predictors of testicular torsion as seen in the pediatric ED. Am J Emerg Med 2010;28:786–9.

[b] *Data from* Ciftci AO, Senocak ME, Tanyel FC, et al. Clinical predictors for differential diagnosis of acute scrotum. Eur J Pediatr Surg 2004;14(5):333–8.

abnormalities on computed tomography (CT) may suggest the diagnosis. More importantly, CT may be helpful in excluding alternative diagnoses. Risks of CT imaging include radiation exposure, which is of particular concern for young patients. The only definitive diagnosis of ovarian torsion involves surgical intervention. As such, emergent gynecology consultation may be necessary to aid in decision-making if clinical suspicion is high.

INFECTIONS OF THE URINARY TRACT AND KIDNEY

UTI occurs at any age and in either gender. Prevalence is highest in girls under the age of 2 years and boys under the age of 1 year. Several organisms cause UTI in children, with *Escherichia coli* the most common offender. A novel form of *E coli* produces an extended-spectrum β-lactamase (ESBL). *Klebsiella* species may also produce ESBL. ESBL *E coli* are multidrug resistant and frequently require inpatient management with a carbapenem antibiotic.[39]

Symptoms in children vary by age. Patients under the age of 2 years present with fussiness, poor feeding, fever, and vomiting. Children over the age of 2 years have more specific symptoms: dysuria, hematuria, abdominal pain, and enuresis. Pursue a history of prior UTI, urinary reflux, and recent catheterization because these are risk factors for UTI. Physical examination is nonspecific, although the perineum of young girls should be examined to exclude other causes of GU complaints.

The differential diagnosis includes poor hygiene; chemical irritants (eg, detergent, bubble bath, or lotions); vaginal or urethral foreign bodies; pinworms; traumatic injury; and sexual abuse. Infants and toddlers, especially girls, should be examined externally by placing them supine with the hips externally rotated and abducted (ie, frog-leg position). Performing this examination while distracting the child helps identify poor hygiene, vaginitis, inflammation, injuries, and foreign bodies. Young girls may accidentally or intentionally place objects or toilet paper within the introits or vagina causing dysuria, discharge, and bleeding that is mistaken for hematuria. Female toddlers and older children may unintentionally scratch themselves while exploring.

Consider sexual abuse if discharge, vaginitis, or an unexplained injury or foreign body is identified. Studies have suggested that each year 1% of children experience some form of sexual abuse, resulting in the abuse of 12–25% of girls and 8–10% of boys by 18 years of age.[40] Patients with symptoms of UTI or vaginal or penile discharge with suspected sexual abuse should be tested for sexually transmitted infections and referred to specialists with experience in evaluating pediatric sexual abuse and child protective services, when appropriate.[40]

The first step in diagnosing UTI is urinalysis. In the setting of unexplained fever, consider urinalysis in girls less than 2 years of age, uncircumcised boys less than 1 year of age, and circumcised boys less than 6 months of age. In young children who are not continent, obtain the urine sample using either bladder cauterization or (uncommonly) suprabupic aspiration. Labial adhesions make urethral catheterization difficult or impossible. Even with meticulous cleaning, bagged specimens produce an unacceptably high rate of contaminated specimens. In older children who are toilet trained, a clean catch specimen is adequate. A parent may assist the child. Send a urine culture for smaller children because urinalysis is false-negative in up to 10% of this population.[41]

Analysis of urine reports several results. The diagnostic performances of these outcomes were recently evaluated in a thorough meta-analysis reported in *Lancet* in 2010 (**Table 2**).[41] Interestingly, this study supports the idea that the urinary white blood cell count on microscopy does not add to the diagnostic performance of the dipstick, and that Gram stain for bacteria is the most accurate diagnostic method.

Treatment varies depending on age. Babies less than 1 month of age are admitted for a full sepsis work-up and IV antibiotics (eg, ampicillin and either cefotaxime or gentamicin). Although experts do not provide consistent recommendations, strongly consider admitting young infants, especially if febrile or vomiting, for IV antibiotics (eg, ceftriaxone, or ampicillin plus either cefotaxime or gentamicin) because of the risk of renal scarring. Children 3 months to 2 years of age should be given either IV or oral antibiotics with close follow-up if they are nontoxic, able to feed, and have responsible caregivers. Patients older than 2 years with uncomplicated UTI are treated with oral antimicrobials.

The duration of therapy also varies by age. Treat adolescents in a similar fashion to adults (eg, 3- to 5-day course may be acceptable). Younger children, especially infants, toddlers, and preschool children are treated for 10 days. Use local susceptibility patterns to guide antimicrobial selection. An acceptable first choice for younger children is a third-generation cephalosporin, such as cefdinir (14 mg/kg/d in one or two divided doses) or cefixime (8 mg/kg/d in two divided doses). Cephalexin (25–50 mg/kg/d divided every 6–12 hours), amoxicillin clavulanate (50 mg/kg/d in two divided

Table 2
Diagnostic performance of urine microscopy and dipstick parameters for the diagnosis of urinary tract infection in children

	Sensitivity (95% CI)	Specificity (95% CI)
Urine microscopy		
WBC count	74% (67–80)	86% (82–90)
Gram stain	91% (80–96)	96% (92–98)
Unstained bacteria	88% (75–94)	92% (83–96)
Urine dipstick		
LE alone	79% (73–84)	87% (80–92)
Nitrite alone	49% (41–57)	98% (96–99)
Either LE or nitrite	88% (82–91)	79% (69–87)
Both LE and nitrite	45% (30–61)	98% (96–99)

Abbreviations: CI, confidence interval; LE, leukocyte esterase; WBC, white blood cell.

Data from Williams GJ, Macaskill P, Chan SF, et al. Absolute and relative accuracy of rapid urine tests for urinary tract infection: a meta-analysis. Lancet 2010;10:240–50.

doses), and trimethoprim–sulfamethoxazole (8–10 mg/kg/d based on trimethoprim component) may be useful based on local susceptibility patterns for afebrile children without vomiting. Close follow-up should be arranged for all patients, and guardians should be informed to seek medical care more urgently if the patient is unable to urinate, tolerate oral intake, or remains febrile for more than 48 hours.

If the urinalysis is negative, set the expectation with the caregiver that the culture may be positive, requiring antimicrobial therapy. It is important to have systems in place to ensure identification of positive cultures and follow-up with the child's pediatrician or caregiver.

Pyelonephritis, a bacterial infection of the kidney, can lead to scaring of the renal calyx with diminished renal function and obstruction later in life. Infants may present with nonspecific symptoms including fever, vomiting, and fussiness. As such, distinguishing kidney infection from lower UTI in younger children is especially challenging. Older children may complain of fever and flank or abdominal pain. Urinalysis reflects the presence of UTI, but also may demonstrate bacterial casts, indicating that infection is present in the tubules of the kidneys.

Treat these patients with a longer course of antibiotics. Neonates are hospitalized as described previously. Older patients may be treated as outpatients for 14 days with close follow-up. Patients should have resolution of fever and flank pain within 72 hours. Failure to improve may require further diagnostic imaging to rule out perinephric abscess or ureteral calculus. These children should have a repeat urinalysis to confirm clearance of infection. Some patients require a second course of appropriate antibiotics based on sensitivity pattern results. Pregnant adolescents virtually always require hospitalization and IV antibiotics. During pregnancy, decreased ureteral peristalsis caused by increased levels of progesterone makes the clearance of bacteria more difficult. This requires greater supervision of both mother and fetus during initial treatment.

SUMMARY

Serious complications following circumcision occur infrequently in young children. Minor complications may include local infection, adhesions, and bleeding. Balanitis and balanoposthitis are treated with improved hygiene, topical antifungal agents, and in some cases antibiotics.

Phimosis is constriction of the foreskin so that it cannot be retracted back over the glans penis. It is an emergency only when a child is unable to void spontaneously. Paraphimosis is the inability to reduce the proximal foreskin over the coronal sulcus of the glans. The prepuce can generally be returned to anatomic position once foreskin or glans swelling has been sufficiently alleviated. Inability to reduce a paraphimosis in the ED is an indication for urologic consultation.

Priapism in children is typically related to sickle cell disease or leukemia. It must be treated aggressively to reduce tissue ischemia, long-term tissue damage, and diminished future function. Treatment may involve aspiration of blood, irrigation with normal saline, and instillation of dilute phenylephrine.

Gonadal torsion is a surgical emergency. Presenting symptoms may be nonspecific, so maintain vigilance for this condition in male or female patients of any age. Ultrasound is the initial diagnostic study of choice in all patients with suspected torsion. Beware of the potential for false-negative ultrasound findings, and have a low threshold for engaging specialty consultants to aid in decision-making in compelling or unclear cases.

UTIs in pediatric patients must be treated aggressively with appropriate antibiotics and close follow-up to avoid progression to sepsis, pyelonephritis, or renal injury.

REFERENCES

1. Weiss HA, Larke N, Halperin D, et al. Complications of circumcision in male neonates, infants and children: a systematic review. BMC Urol 2010;10:2.
2. Nguyen DM, Bancroft E, Mascola L, et al. Risk factors for neonatal methicillin-resistant *Staphylococcus aureus* infection in a well-infant nursery. Infect Control Hosp Epidemiol 2007;28(4):406–11.
3. Herzog LW, Alvarez SR. The frequency of foreskin problems in uncircumcised children. Am J Dis Child 1986;140(3):254–6.
4. Adams JR, Mata JA, Venable DD, et al. Fournier's gangrene in children. Urology 1990;35(5):439–41.
5. McGregor TB, Pike JG, Leonard MP. Pathologic and physiologic phimosis: approach to the phimotic foreskin. Can Fam Physician 2007;53:445–8.
6. Oster J. Further fate of the foreskin: incidence of preputial adhesions, phimosis, and smegma among Danish schoolboys. Arch Dis Child 1968;43(228):200–3.
7. Ashfield JE, Nickel KR, Siemens DR, et al. Treatment of phimosis with topical steroids in 194 children. J Urol 2003;169(3):1106–8.
8. Sookpotarom P, Porncharoenpong S, Vejchapipat P. Topical steroid is effective for the treatment of phimosis in young children. J Med Assoc Thai 2010;93(1):77–83.
9. Choe JM. Paraphimosis: current treatment options. Am Fam Physician 2000; 16(12):2623–6.
10. Mackway-Jones K, Teece S. Ice, pins, or sugar to reduce paraphimosis. Emerg Med J 2004;21:77–8.
11. Barton DJ, Sloan GM, Nichter LS, et al. Hair-thread tourniquet syndrome. Pediatrics 1998;82(6):925–8.
12. Douglas DD. Dissolving hair wrapped around an infant's digit. J Pediatr 1977; 91:162.
13. Gomes CM, Ribiero-Filho L, Giron AM, et al. Genital trauma due to animal bites. J Urol 2000;165:80–3.
14. McAleer IM, Kaplan GW. Pediatric genitourinary trauma. Urol Clin North Am 1995; 22:177–88.
15. Seng YJ, Moissinac K. Trauma induced testicular torsion: a reminder for the unwary. J Accid Emerg Med 2000;17:381–2.
16. Morey AF, Metro MJ, Carney KJ, et al. Consensus on genitourinary trauma: external genitalia. BJU Int 2004;94:507–15.
17. Mulhall JP, Gabram SG, Jacobs LM. Emergency management of blunt testicular trauma. Acad Emerg Med 1995;2:639–43.
18. Burnett AL. Therapy insight: priapism associated with hematologic dyscrasias. Nat Clin Pract Urol 2005;2(9):449–56.
19. Goldmeier D, Lamba H. Prolonged erections produced by dihydrocodeine and sildenafil. BMJ 2002;324:1555.
20. Wills BK, Albinson C, Wahl M, et al. Sildenafil citrate ingestion and prolonged priapism and tachycardia in a pediatric patient. Clin Toxicol (Phila) 2007;45(7): 798–800.
21. Montague DK, Jarow J, Broderick GA, et al. American Urological Association guideline on the management of priapism. J Urol 2003;170:1318–24.
22. Maples BL, Hagemann TM. Treatment of priapism in pediatric patients with sickle cell disease. Am J Health Syst Pharm 2004;61:355–63.
23. Adeyoju AB, Olujohungbe ABK, Morris J, et al. Priapism in sickle-cell disease; incidence, risk factors and complications. An international multicentre study. BJU Int 2002;90:898–902.

24. Cavusoglu YH, Karaman A, Karaman I, et al. Acute scrotum: etiology and management. Indian J Pediatr 2005;72(3):201–3.
25. Ben-Chaim J, Leibovitch I, Ramon J, et al. Etiology of acute scrotum at surgical exploration in children, adolescents and adults. Eur Urol 1992;21(1):45–7.
26. Primatesta P, Goldacre J. Inguinal hernia repair: incidence of elective and emergency surgery, readmission and mortality. Int J Epidemiol 1996;25(4):835–9.
27. Beni-Israel T, Goldman M, Bar Chaim S. Clinical predictors of testicular torsion as seen in the pediatric ED. Am J Emerg Med 2010;28:786–9.
28. Melekos MD, Asbach HW, Markou SA. Etiology of acute scrotum in 100 boys with regard to age distribution. J Urol 1988;139:1023–5.
29. Makela E, Lahdes-Vasama T, Rajakorpi H, et al. A 19-year review of paediatric patients with acute scrotum. Scand J Surg 2007;96(1):62–6.
30. Caesar RE, Kaplan GW. The incidence of the cremasteric reflex in normal boys. J Urol 1994;152:779–80.
31. Sidhu PS. Clinical and imaging features of testicular torsion: role of ultrasound. Clin Radiol 1999;54:343–52.
32. Lam WW, Yap T, Jacobsen AS, et al. Colour Doppler ultrasonography replacing surgical exploration for acute scrotum: myth or reality? Pediatr Radiol 2005; 35(6):597–600.
33. Baud C, Veyrac C, Couture A, et al. Spiral twist of the spermatic cord: a reliable sign of testicular torsion. Pediatr Radiol 1998;28:950–4.
34. Kalfa N, Veyrac C, Lopez M, et al. Multicenter assessment of ultrasound of the spermatic cord in children with acute scrotum. J Urol 2007;177(1):297–301.
35. Anders JF, Powell EC. Urgency of evaluation and outcome of acute ovarian torsion in pediatric patients. Arch Pediatr Adolesc Med 2005;159(6):532–5.
36. Kokoska ER, Keller MS, Weber TR. Acute ovarian torsion in children. Am J Surg 2000;180:462–5.
37. Chang HC, Bhatt S, Dogra VS. Pearls and pitfalls in diagnosis of ovarian torsion. Radiographics 2008;28:1355–68.
38. Breech LL, Hillard PJ. Adnexal torsion in pediatric and adolescent girls. Curr Opin Obstet Gynecol 2005;17(5):483–9.
39. Jacoby G, Han P, Tran SO. Comparative in vitro activities of carbapenem L-749,345 and other antimicrobials against multiresistant gram-negative clinical pathogens. Antimicrob Agents Chemother 1997;41(8):1830–1.
40. Kellogg N. American Academy of Pediatrics Committee on Child Abuse and Neglect. The evaluation of sexual abuse in children. Pediatrics 2005;116(2): 506–12.
41. Williams GJ, Macaskill P, Chan SF, et al. Absolute and relative accuracy of rapid urine tests for urinary tract infection: a meta-analysis. Lancet 2010;10:240–50.

Index

Note: Page numbers of article titles are in **boldface** type.

A

Acetylcysteine, to prevent contrast-induced nephropathy, 582
Appendage torsion, 478–479
  testicular torsion, and epididymitis, differentiating characteristics of, 472
    relative incidence of, 472, 473
Appendages, position of, 471, 473
Azotemia, prerenal, 575

B

Bacteriuria, in pediatric urinary tract infections, 643
Balanitis, 493–494, 656–657
Balanoposthitis, 493–494, 656–657
Bartholin cysts and abscesses, abscess drainage in, 630, 631
  treatment of, 630
Bladder, contusions of, 502
  imaging of, 502
  injuries of, 502
    clinical indicators of, 503
    immediate repair of, indications for, 504
Bladder catheterization, transurethral, in pediatric urinary tract infections, 644–645

C

Candidiasis, vulvovaginal, 594
Cephalosporins, in gonorrhea, 592
Cervicitis, and urethritis, sexually transmitted infections presenting with, 588–593
Chancroid, 494, 598
Children, genitourinary emergencies in, **655–666**
  infections of urinary tract and kidney in, 662–664
  ultrasonography in, 564
  urinary tract infections in. See *Urinary tract infection(s), pediatric.*
Chlamydia, 589
Circumcision, complications of, 656, 664
Contraception, emergency, 630–631
Contrast-induced nephropathy, 580–582
Corticosteroids, in urolithiasis, 529
Creatinine, serum, 570
Creatinine clearance, 570
CT scan, in ovarian torsion, 626–627
  noncontrast helical, in urolithiasis, 525–526
  of genitourinary tract, 557, 558

Emerg Med Clin N Am 29 (2011) 667–674
doi:10.1016/S0733-8627(11)00058-7

Cystitis, uncomplicated, treatment of, 543–545
Cystography, retrograde, 555

D

Desmopression, intranasal, in urolithiasis, 529
Diuretics, in urolithiasis, 528
Dopamine, in acute tubular necrosis, 580

E

End-stage renal disease, management of, 578–579
Epididymitis, testicular torsion, and appendage torsion, differentiaing characteristics of, 472
    relative incidence of, 472, 473
  treatment of, 478

F

Fenoldopam, in acute tubular necrosis, 580
Fournier's gangrene, 479

G

Genital herpes, 595–596
Genital injury, accidental, 659
Genital trauma, female, 513–514
Genital ulcers, sexually transmitted infections causing, 595–600
Genital warts, 599–600
Genitalia, external, trauma to, 512–514
Genitourinary emergencies, in nonpregnant woman, **621–635**
  pediatric, **655–666**
Genitourinary system, anatomy of, 501–502
  imaging of, in emergency department, 553–567
Genitourinary trauma, 479–480, **501–518**
Glomerular disease, acute, 577
Glomerular filtration rate, 570
Gonadal torsion, 661–662, 664
Gonorrhea, 589–592

H

Herpes, genital, 595–596
Herpes simplex virus infections, 494
HIV nPEP, for sexual assault victim, 613, 614
Hyperkalemia, 576

I

Inguinal hernia, incarcerated, 479
Intravenous pyelogram, 556

K

Kidney, anatomy of, 570
and urinary tract, infections of, in children, 662–664
injuries of, acute, 571, 572–580
biomarkers for, 571
classification of, 573–574
treatment of, 578, 579
types of, 571
flow chart for, 508, 509
in blunt and penetrating trauma, 507–510
severity scale of, 508
ultrasonography of, 559–561, 562
Kidney stones. See *Urolithiasis*.
Kidney-ureter-bladder radiography, 554–559

L

Levonorgestral, 631
Lymphogranuloma venereum, 598

M

Mannitol, in acute tubular necrosis, 580
MRI, of genitourinary tract, 557–558

N

Nephropathy, contrast-induced, 580–582
Nephrotic syndrome, 577
Nitromidazoles, in trichomonal infections, 592–593
Nuclear medicine, use in genitourinary tract, 558–559

O

Ovarian cysts and masses, complications of, 625
differential diagnosis of, 623–624
Ovarian torsion, CT in, 626–627
ultrasonography in, 625–626
Ovaries, ultrasonography of, 563–564

P

Pain, in renal colic, 520, 523
management of, in urolithiasis, 527–528
Paraphimosis, 657–658
causes of, 490
iatrogenic, 489
symptoms of, 489
treatment of, 490–491

Pelvic inflammatory disease, background of, 621–622
  diagnosis of, 622
  disposition in, 623
  imaging in, 622–623
  screening and prevention of, 623
  therapy for, 623
Pelvic masses, differential diagnosis of, 624
  imaging for evaluation of, 624
  management of, 624–625
Penile calciphylaxis, 495
Penile emergencies, **485–499**
Penile trauma, 491–493
  due to foreign body, 492–493
Penis, anatomy of, 485, 486, 655, 656
  emergent conditions of, 485–493
  entrapment of, 491–492
  fracture of, 494–495
  in sexually transmitted disease, 494
  trauma to, 512–513
Peyronie's disease, 495
Phimosis, 493, 657, 664
Posthitis, 493–494
Pregnancy, prevention of, for sexual assault victim, 612–613
  urolithiasis in, 532
Prehn's sign, 475
Priapism, 485–489, 660
  causes of, 486–487
  evaluation in, 488
  ischemic, 486, 487–488
  nonischemic, 486
    treatment of, 489
  stuttering, 487
    treatment of, 489
  treatment of, 488–489, 660–661, 664
Pyelogram, intravenous, 556
Pyelonephritis, acute, complications of, 547–548
    treatment of, 546–547
  and urinary tract infections, diagnosis and management of, **539–552**
  in children, 664

R

Radiation exposure, cumulative, 553–554
Radiography, kidney-ureter-bladder, 554–559
Renal colic, mechanisms of pain in, 520, 523
  mimics of, 524
Renal disease, chronic, 571–572
    management of, 578–579
  end-stage, management of, 578–579
  obstructive, 576
Renal failure, emergency evaluation and management of, **569–585**

pathophysiology of, 569–571
postrenal or obstructive, 575–576
Renal function, steps in, 569
Renal replacement therapy, 572
in acute kidney injury, 579
Renal stents, in urolithiasis, 531–532

S

Scrotal emergencies, **469–484**
differential diagnosis of, 469–473
evaluation in emergency department, 473–476
management in emergency department, 476–478
Scrotal pain, differential diagnosis of, 470–471
examination in, 474–476
history taking in, 474
Scrotal trauma, 480, 513
Scrotum, ultrasonography of, 561–562
Sexual assault, **605–620**
after-assault prophylactic medications in, 615
drug-facilitated, 617
-specific diagnostic testing in, 612
Sexual assault nurse examiner, 605–606
Sexual assault victim, clinical presentation of, 606
disposition of, 614–616
evaluation of, 606–612
anorectal examination in, 611
consent for, 607
genital examination in, 609–611
history taking in, 607
oropharyngeal examination in, 609
physical examination in, 608–609
intimate partner violence and, 616
male, management of, 616
management of, 612–614
medical treatment for, 612
pediatric, examination of, 616
pregnancy prevention for, 612–613
psychosocial support for, 612
sexually transmitted infection treatment for, 613–614, 615
suspect examination and, 616–617
Sexually transmitted disease, penis in, 494
Sexually transmitted infections, causing genital ulcers, 595–600
characterized by vaginal discharge, 593–594
emergency department disposition in, 600
emergency department management of, **587–603**
epidemiology of, 588
possible, emergency department approach in, 588
presenting with urethritis and cervicitis, 588–593
treatment for, for sexual assault victim, 613–614, 615
treatment recommendations for, 587–588, 590–591

Sickle cell disease, priapism in, 660
Suprapubic aspiration, in pediatric urinary tract infections, 644
Syphilis, 596–598

T

Testicular injuries, pediatric, 659
Testicular torsion, 661–662
  diagnostic imaging in, 477–478
  epididymitis, and appendage torsion, differentiating characteristics of, 472
    relative incidence of, 472, 473
  manual detorsion in, 478
  testicular salvage and atrophy rates in, 476
Tourniquet injuries, pediatric, 658–659
Trichomonal infections, 592–593
Tubular necrosis, acute, 577, 578
    pharmacologic therapies in, 579–580
Tunica vaginalis, testis position within, 474, 475

U

Ultrasonography, future directions in, 564–565
  general principles of, 559
  in ovarian torsion, 626–627
  in urolithiasis, 526
  ovarian, 563–564
  pediatric, 563–564
  renal, 559–561, 562
  scrotal, 561–562
Ureter, avulsion of, 506
  contusions of, 506
  injuries of, 504–506
    diagnosis of, 505, 506
    severity scale for, 505
    treatment of, 506
Urethra, anatomy of, 655
  injuries of, 510–512
    hematuria in, 511
    management of, 511–512
  male, anatomy of, 510
Urethritis, 494
  and cervicitis, sexually transmitted infections presenting with, 588–593
Urethrography, retrograde, 555, 556
Urinalysis, in urinary tract infection, 542
  in urolithiasis, 524–525
Urinary retention, from obstruction, 576
Urinary tract, and kidney, infections of, in children, 662–664
Urinary tract infection(s), and pyelonephritis, diagnosis and management of, **539–552**
  clinical presentation of, 541
  complicated, treatment of, 545–546
  definitions of, 539–540
  diagnosis of, 542–543

epidemiology and risk factors for, 540–541
in pregnancy, treatment of, 548
microbiology of, 541
pediatric, anatomic issues and, 639
behavioral habits and, 639
circumcision status and, 638
diagnosis of, 639–646
disposition and initial management in, 646
epidemiology of, 638
etiology of, 637–638
follow-up imaging in, 646–547
history and physical examination in, 639–640
host risk factors in, 638–639
laboratory assessment in, 640–643
race and, 638–639
urine collection in, methods of, 643–646
treatment of, 543–548
Urine collection, clean-catch, in pediatric urinary tract infections, 645
in urinary tract infection, 542
Urine culture, in pediatric urinary tract infections, 642–643
in urinary tract infection, 542–543
Urine dipstick, in pediatric urinary tract infections, 640–641
versus microscopic urinalysis, in pediatric urinary tract infections, 642
Urine microscopy, in pediatric urinary tract infections, 641–642
Urolithiasis, abdominal plain film in, 526
acute emergency department management of, 527–529
clinical presentation of, 521
corticosteroids in, 529
discharge instructions in, 530
during pregnancy, 532
emergency department evaluation of, 521–524
epidemiology of, 519
etiology of, 520–521
hydration and diuretics in, 528
in emergency department, **519–538**
infected, 531
intranasal desmopression in, 529
intravenous pyelogram in, 526–527
magnetic resonance imaging in, 527
medical expulsion therapy in, 528–529
noncontrast helical computed tomography in, 525–526
pain management in, 527–528
prognosis in, 529–530
renal stents in, 531–532
risk factors for, 522–523
special populations and complications in, 531–532
spontaneous stone passage in, 529, 530
terminology associated with, 520
ultrasonography in, 526
urinalysis in, 524–525
urology consultation in, 530–531

V

Vaginal bleeding, abnormal, background of, 627
    differential diagnosis of, 628
    history of, 627–628
    laboratory and imaging studies in, 628–629
    physical examination in, 628
    treatment and referral in, 629
Vaginal discharge, sexually transmitted infections characterized by, 593–594
Vaginosis, bacterial, 593–594

W

Warts, genital, 599–600

Z

Zipper entrapment, penile, management of, 659

Moving?

Make sure your subscription moves with you!

To notify us of your new address, find your **Clinics Account Number** (located on your mailing label above your name), and contact customer service at:

Email: journalscustomerservice-usa@elsevier.com

800-654-2452 (subscribers in the U.S. & Canada)
314-447-8871 (subscribers outside of the U.S. & Canada)

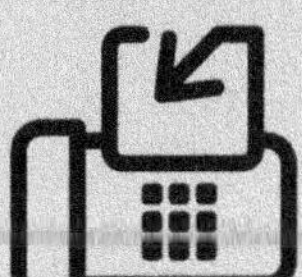

Fax number: 314-447-8029

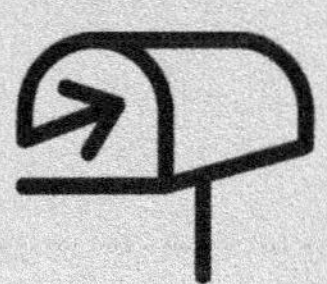

Elsevier Health Sciences Division
Subscription Customer Service
3251 Riverport Lane
Maryland Heights, MO 63043

*To ensure uninterrupted delivery of your subscription, please notify us at least 4 weeks in advance of move.

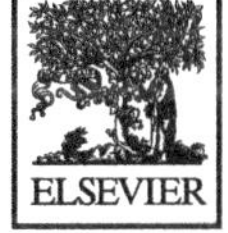

Printed and bound by CPI Group (UK) Ltd, Croydon, CR0 4YY
03/10/2024
01040457-0003